Event-Related Potentials

Event-Related Potentials

A Methods Handbook

edited by Todd C. Handy

A Bradford Book
The MIT Press
Cambridge, Massachusetts
London, England

MIT Press books may be purchased at special quantity discounts for business or sales promotional use. For information, please email special_sales@mitpress.mit.edu or write to Special Sales Department, The MIT Press, 5 Cambridge Center, Cambridge, MA 02142.

This book was set in Stone serif and Stone sans on 3B2 by Asco Typesetters, Hong Kong. Printed and bound in the United States of America.

Library of Congress Cataloging-in-Publication Data

Event-related potentials : a methods handbook / edited by Todd C. Handy.
    p. ; cm.
"A Bradford book."
Includes bibliographical references and index.
ISBN-13: 978-0-262-08333-1 (hc. : alk. paper)
ISBN-10: 0-262-08333-7 (hc. : alk. paper)
1. Evoked potentials (Electrophysiology)—Handbooks, manuals, etc. I. Handy, Todd C.
[DNLM: 1. Evoked Potentials. 2. Data Collection—methods. 3. Electrophysiology—methods.
4. Research Design. WL 102 E926 2004]
RC386.6.E86E945   2004
616.8′047547—dc22   2004040172

10 9 8 7 6 5 4 3 2

For ErinRose

Contents

Preface

Research using event-related potentials (ERPs) has expanded dramatically in the last decade. As a result, there has been a corresponding increase in the number of investigators who—with little formal training in the method—are applying ERP measures to questions of cortical function. Fueling this trend has been the growing availability of commercial ERP recording systems and their relatively inexpensive cost when compared to big-ticket neuroimaging items such as fMRI. Yet unlike the variety of methods books now available for fMRI, and despite the boom in ERP-driven research, a comparable tome presenting the fundamentals of ERP methodology has been noticeably absent. This book aims to meet this need for practical and concise information on the methods of ERPs—a book that should be intelligible to the novice ERP investigator, but sufficiently rigorous so as to be informative to the most seasoned of electrophysiology experts.

The book is divided into three parts. The first section, Experimental Design, comprises four chapters, all centering on issues germane to the initial planning of an ERP experiment. The section begins with a chapter by Otten and Rugg that introduces the basic ideas and assumptions underlying the interpretation of ERP data as it pertains to questions of perceptual, cognitive, and motor function. Luck then provides a practical compendium of ten essential points to consider when designing an ERP experiment, issues integral to understanding the effective application of ERP methods. Following that, Handy details the canonical ways in which ERP data are quantified, with a focus on how planned analyses constrain experimental design. Dien and Santuzzi conclude the section by reviewing the theoretical and practical aspects of ANOVAs as applied to ERP datasets. Taken together, these chapters provide a solid and practical foundation for understanding the design of ERP experiments and how to interpret ERP data.

The middle section of the book, Data Analysis, comprises seven chapters, presenting a variety of approaches to ERP data analysis. The first two chapters cover issues associated with the "preprocessing" of ERP data. Edgar, Stewart, and Miller detail the essential elements of digital filtering in ERP research, including a survey of fundamental terms and concepts tied to digital signal processing. Talsma and Woldorff review the different kinds of artifacts that can arise in ERP data, and the different types of procedures for removing such artifacts from ERP waveforms. The next five chapters then address specific analytic methods in depth. Slotnick discusses the nuances underlying the localization of ERP source generators in cortex, procedures derived from the topographic mapping of voltage over the surface of the scalp. In a chapter on high-resolution ERP recordings, Srinivasan proposes that the localization of cortical EEG sources can be improved by considering the surface Laplacian—or second spatial derivative—of skull current density. Moving from source localization to ERP componetry, Dien and Frishkoff provide an introductory treatment of principal components analysis (or PCA), a means of linearly decomposing ERP waveforms into more basic elements. Spencer considers how to interrogate single-trial ERP data, including the use of discriminant analysis, analytic approaches that—unlike standard signal averaging—can account for the intertrial variability in ERP data. Herrmann, Grigutsch, and Busch conclude the section with a discussion of wavelet analysis, procedures that isolate specific frequency bands in ERP data and that are a particularly powerful approach for examining event-related oscillatory behavior in EEG. Collectively, these chapters provide an important introduction to the different ways that ERP data can be analyzed, and the kinds of questions that these different techniques can address.

The final section of the book, Special Applications, covers the use of ERPs as they pertain to specific participant populations and other methodologies. To begin, DeBoer, Scott, and Nelson review the use of ERPs in the developmental domain, including the practical aspects of how to design experiments and record data when using infants and young children as participants. In the following chapter, Swick considers the use and interpretation of ERPs in neuropsychological populations, emphasizing how data from these patients has helped to elucidate the cortical systems underlying different ERP components. Switching gears, Soltani, Edwards, Knight, and Berger then explain the practical details of intracranial ERP recordings, and further, how intracranial ERPs relate to—and differ from—ERPs recorded from the scalp surface. In the final chapter, Hopfinger, Khoe, and Song detail how hemodynamic neuroimaging has helped inform traditional questions in ERP methodology, concluding with an eye toward recent developments in neuroimaging techniques that may help to solve long-standing problems in ERP research. In sum, the section gives insight into the broader context of ERP methodology, in terms of both the participants used in ERP research and how researchers can combine ERPs with related methodologies.

This book would not have been possible without the assistance of a number of key individuals. First and foremost are the contributors themselves, busy leaders in their fields who nevertheless committed their valuable time to the project; all cheerfully provided outstanding chapters, and I thank them warmly. Second, without a publisher the book would have gone nowhere. The MIT Press—and Barbara Murphy and Katherine Almeida, in particular—have provided stellar support throughout the lifespan of the project, and I greatly appreciate their professional efforts. Third, Michael Gazzaniga generously provided shelter and funding while I was planning and editing the book, even though it often took me away from duties more directly productive to his laboratory. Again, a warm thanks. Finally, I am deeply indebted to ErinRose Handy for gracefully—and all too frequently—allowing me to step away from my role as a husband in order to pursue my selfish academic whims. My career continues to depend on her faith and encouragement.

I Experimental Design

1 Interpreting Event-Related Brain Potentials

Leun J. Otten and Michael D. Rugg

Our ability to feel, think, and act can in some way be attributed to the workings of the brain. For over a century, scientists have used measures of brain activity to gain insights into perceptual, cognitive, and motor functions. As a result, researchers have developed a variety of methods to measure brain activity noninvasively (e.g., Rugg, 1999). These methods roughly fall into two classes: "electromagnetic" approaches that directly measure brain activity by recording the electromagnetic fields generated by certain neuronal populations, and "hemodynamic" approaches that indirectly measure brain activity by recording changes in vascular variables that are linked to changes in neural activity. Importantly, these methods differ in a number of aspects, including the preconditions for detecting a signal, the homogeneity with which neural activity is sampled from different parts of the brain, and the relative strengths in determining *when* versus *where* neural activity takes place. They therefore provide complementary views on neural activity.

This chapter focuses on electromagnetic measures of neural activity. Within this class of methods, there are several ways to examine electrical and magnetic activity, in both the temporal and spatial domains (e.g., Näätänen, Ilmoniemi, & Alho, 1994; Tallon-Baudry & Bertrand, 1999). Here we restrict discussion to event-related brain potentials (ERPs), which are small changes in the electrical activity of the brain that are recorded from the scalp and that are brought about by some external or internal event (see Coles & Rugg, 1995; Kutas & Dale, 1997). This electrical activity changes rapidly over time and has a spatially extended field. It is therefore usually recorded with a temporal resolution in the order of a few milliseconds from multiple scalp locations. The goal of this chapter is to explain how one can make functional interpretations from ERP data. After a brief introduction to the issues that ERP analysis aims to address, we outline the type of inferences that one can and cannot make from ERP data. The final two sections then examine the assumptions that underlie functional inferences, and how functional interpretations of ERP data may develop in future. The material considered here is similar to that covered by Kutas and Dale (1997) and Rugg and Coles (1995).

What Issues Can ERP Analysis Address?

A first step toward making functional interpretations from ERP data is to consider what purpose ERPs serve. One can study ERPs in their own right, that is, to gain a better understanding of aspects of ERPs themselves. For example, there has been substantial work to characterize individual features of ERP waveforms, and to identify the intracerebral origins of ERPs. More often, however, researchers use ERPs as a tool to resolve questions in disciplines such as psychology, psychiatry, and neuroscience. For example, ERPs have helped to delineate psychiatric and neurological conditions such as schizophrenia and ADHD (e.g., Ford et al., 1999; van der Stelt et al., 2001), why people take longer to respond in situations of conflicting information (e.g., Duncan-Johnson & Kopell, 1981), how attention normally works (e.g., Mangun & Hillyard, 1995), and why memory declines as we grow older (e.g., Rugg & Morcom, in press). Attempts have even been made to use ERPs as a lie-detection tool (Farwell & Donchin, 1991)!

In this chapter, we confine our discussion of functional interpretations from ERPs to their use in the field of cognitive neuroscience, although the logic and assumptions laid out here also apply to most other applications. Cognitive neuroscience "aims to understand how cognitive functions, and their manifestations in behavior and subjective experience, arise from the activity of the brain" (Rugg, 1997, 1). We focus on what ERPs can reveal about cognitive functions in healthy individuals, using within-group comparisons. Comparisons between groups of individuals, especially when special populations such as clinical or younger/older people are involved, require additional considerations (see Picton et al., 2000; or Rugg & Morcom, in press, for introductions to this topic).

Explanations in cognitive neuroscience can be articulated at many different levels, ranging from functional to cellular and even subcellular accounts (e.g., Marr, 1982). One can use ERPs to address questions at several of these levels. For example, at a functional level, some use ERPs to address whether the brain honors the distinction between syntax and semantics (e.g., Friederici, 1995). At a lower level, researchers use ERPs to investigate the speed of interhemispheric transmission (e.g., Lines, Rugg, & Milner, 1984), or the effects of pharmacological manipulations (e.g., Hsu et al., 2003). Often, interest spans across levels, and explanations at one level may constrain explanations at another level. In the next section, we discuss how one can use ERP data to make functional inferences.

Making Inferences from ERPs

We can classify inferences from ERP data in several ways. It is possible to order inferences on the basis of their complexity and underlying assumptions (Rugg & Coles,

1995), or on the emphasis placed on the temporal versus the spatial information that ERPs provide. Here, we draw a distinction between inferences that one can make with and without adopting a functional interpretation of some feature of an ERP waveform. ERPs have been in use since the 1960s, and many studies have attempted to associate particular features of ERP waveforms with specific cognitive processes. On the basis of the findings of such studies, it is sometimes possible to use specific ERP features (or "components"—see below) as markers for the engagement of the cognitive process with which they are correlated. One can also draw meaningful interpretations of ERP data without making assumptions about the functional significance of any particular waveform feature. In the following sections, we therefore distinguish between inferences made with and without such theoretical commitments. We discuss the latter class of interpretation first.

Inferences Not Based on Prior Knowledge

ERPs can be employed to study cognitive processes even when there is little or no prior useful information to bring to bear on the functional significance of any feature of the elicited ERP waveforms. In practice, this is a common situation. There are generally three kinds of inferences made in these circumstances: about the timing, degree of engagement, and functional equivalence of the underlying cognitive processes. These inferences rely on three aspects of ERP differences observed between conditions: their time course, amplitude, and distribution across the scalp, respectively. We will illustrate these inferences with a concrete example.

Consider an experiment in which ERPs are elicited at three electrode sites in two conditions (1 and 2), and in two situations (A and B; see figure 1.1). The simplest type of inference from these data is based on the observation that the ERP waveforms elicited in the two conditions differ. (For this and all subsequent types of inference, this observation can be substantiated by an appropriate quantification of the waveforms; see chapter 3 of this volume). On the assumption that specific cognitive processes are manifested in specific and invariant patterns of neural activity (see below), a reliable ERP difference between conditions implies that the cognitive processes associated with the two conditions differ in some respect. Understanding how the cognitive processes differ depends on a conceptual analysis of the differences between conditions.

Even this simple inference can lead to useful insights. For example, a longstanding question in cognitive psychology is the level to which unattended information is processed. One can address this question by recording ERPs for unattended information, and establishing whether the content of the unattended information influences the ERP waveforms. Using this logic, researchers have found that ERP waveforms for unattended information differ when an unattended, visually presented word is presented twice in succession (Otten, Rugg, & Doyle, 1993). This suggests that unattended visual information can be processed to the level of its identity.

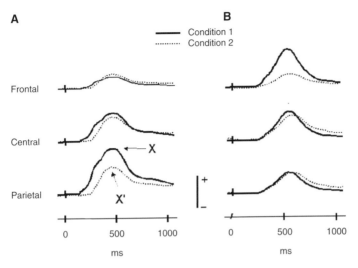

Figure 1.1
Hypothetical ERP waveforms elicited at three electrode sites in two experimental conditions in two experimental situations (*A* and *B*). The differences between the waveforms allow a number of functional interpretations. See text for details.

Expanding on the first type of inference, the second type of inference takes advantage of the high temporal resolution of ERP waveforms, which makes them especially valuable for drawing inferences about the timing of cognitive processes. In situation A of figure 1.1, the ERP waveforms in the two conditions start to differ at about 250 ms after the onset of the event of interest. This implies that the cognitive processes that differentiate the two conditions began to differ by 250 ms. Using this logic, researchers have demonstrated that the ERP waveforms elicited by attended and unattended stimuli can differ as early as 50 ms after stimulus onset (Woldorff & Hillyard, 1991). Accordingly, attentional processes must have been engaged within 50 ms, providing important information about the functional characteristics of selective attention.

The final two classes of inference discussed in this section are based on interpretation of the scalp distribution and amplitude of an ERP effect, respectively. Information about the scalp distribution of an ERP effect forms the basis of efforts to estimate the nature of the intracerebral sources that underlie the effect (e.g., Scherg, 1990). More importantly in the present context, however, this information contributes to the determination of whether functionally nonequivalent processes are engaged across conditions. Crucially, one can make such inferences even in the absence of knowledge about the intracerebral sources of the ERP effects in question.

In situation A of figure 1.1, the difference between the two conditions is largest at the parietal electrode site. By contrast, in situation B, the difference between conditions is largest at the frontal electrode site. As we discuss later, there are several reasons why scalp distributions may change. Regardless of the cause, however, different scalp distributions imply that different patterns of neural activity are associated with the two situations. So far as one is willing to accept the assumption that experimental conditions that are neurophysiologically dissociable are most likely functionally dissociable as well (see below), one can use ERPs to assess whether the cognitive processes engaged in different experimental conditions are functionally distinct.

We can apply the same logic to differences in scalp distribution that emerge over time. ERP effects can be compared not only across experimental conditions as exemplified above, but also across time points within a condition, or across time points across conditions. In any case, a difference in scalp distribution implies a difference in underlying neural pattern. In turn, different neural patterns imply that distinct functional processes were engaged across conditions, times, or both.

For example, when people are asked to decide whether or not they remember having experienced an item before, new and old items elicit different ERP waveforms. This difference is largest over left parietal scalp sites in an early time region of the waveforms, before becoming largest over right frontal scalp sites later on (see Rugg & Wilding, 2000, for review). These scalp distribution differences suggest that different patterns of neural activity are engaged over time. Accordingly, memory retrieval may rely on multiple, qualitatively different functional processes, operating at different points in time. Without evidence that the two effects are dissociable, however, the possibility that they act in concert to support a common process cannot be ruled out. As it happens, the left parietal and right frontal ERP effects are sensitive to distinct experimental manipulations (Rugg & Wilding, 2000).

If scalp distributions do not differ across conditions or time, does this have any functional implications? If experimental manipulations do not result in scalp distribution differences, but the associated ERP effects nonetheless differ in amplitude, this is usually taken to suggest a quantitative, as opposed to a qualitative, difference in the cognitive processing engaged in the two conditions. That is, the experimental manipulations are thought to have engaged the same cognitive process(es), but to differing degrees. Later on, we discuss caveats surrounding interpretations from such amplitude differences and null results.

Inferences Based on Prior Knowledge: ERP "Components"

As discussed in the previous section, we can make useful inferences about cognitive processes from ERP data without knowing what any particular waveform feature represents. However, we can gain additional information with knowledge about the functional significance of some aspect of an ERP waveform. ERPs can be thought of as time-varying scalp fields that result from the summation of electromagnetic activity generated by neuronal populations in different parts of the brain. Clearly, it would be informative to understand these fields both in terms of the neuronal populations responsible for them and the different cognitive processes with which they are associated. In essence, this is what the decomposition of ERP waveforms in terms of their underlying "components" attempts to achieve.

There is no universally accepted definition of what constitutes an ERP component. Because neural and cognitive processes overlap in both space and time, features of the waveform such as peaks or troughs can result from the summation of several contributing sources, and thus may not reflect functionally homogeneous neural or cognitive processes. Component definitions range between two extremes, sometimes referred to as the "physiological" and "functional" approaches to component identification. According to the physiological approach (e.g., Näätänen & Picton, 1987), an ERP component should be defined in terms of its anatomical source within the brain. To measure a component, it is therefore necessary to isolate the intracerebral sources underlying an ERP waveform. By contrast, according to the functional approach (e.g., Donchin, 1981), an ERP component should be defined predominantly in terms of the functional process with which it is associated. On this account, it is irrelevant whether one or several anatomical sources contribute to the component, as long as they constitute a functionally homogeneous system.

In practice, ERP components are usually defined with respect to both their functional significance and their underlying neural source(s). Along these lines, Donchin, Ritter, and McCallum (1978) give an operational definition of an ERP component. According to this view, a component is a part of the waveform with a circumscribed scalp distribution (alluding to the underlying neural configuration) and a circumscribed relationship to experimental variables (alluding to the cognitive function served by the activity of this configuration). Several procedures, based on the analysis of scalp distribution and sensitivity to experimental manipulations, have been proposed as methods to dissociate and measure overlapping components (see Picton et al., 2000).

What can we gain from the concept of an ERP component? Despite the difficulties surrounding their definition and measurement, components serve at least three purposes. First, they provide a language that allows communication across experiments, paradigms, and scientific fields. Second, they can provide a basis for integrating ERP data with other measures of brain activity. Third, components can serve as physiological markers for specific cognitive processes. In the case of some components, sufficient information has accumulated to indicate, in broad terms at least, their functional significance. Below, we illustrate how one can make functional interpretations from ERP data using the notion of a component (see also chapter 2 of this volume).

Again, consider the waveforms illustrated in figure 1.1. Assume that in situation A, the positive deflection in the waveforms (labeled X and X') is a known ERP component, associated with some specific cognitive process. (This assumption is for the purposes of exposition only. In reality, it is highly unlikely that such a large, temporally extended ERP deflection would reflect the activity of a single generator system, or a single cognitive process.) On this assumption, the first inference one can make from these data makes use of the time course of the component across conditions. The time course can be quantified with one of several temporal measures of the component, for example its onset, peak latency, rise time, or duration (see chapter 3 of this volume). In figure 1.1, the component onsets later in condition 2 than 1. This implies that the cognitive process presumed to be associated with the component is engaged at a later time in condition 2 than 1.

Next, figure 1.1 shows that the amplitude of the component in situation A differs between conditions. As with the time course of a component, we can define its amplitude in several ways. The observed amplitude difference in figure 1.1 implies that the cognitive process is engaged to a different degree across conditions. This inference relies crucially on previous work associating variance in the amplitude of the component with variance in the degree to which the associated cognitive process is engaged. To illustrate this type of inference, based on its scalp distribution and approximate time of occurrence, the positive peak seen in situation A of figure 1.1 may reflect the P300 or P3b component (Donchin, 1981; Donchin & Coles, 1988). Donchin and Coles (1988) proposed that P300 amplitude variations reflect variations in the degree to which an internal representation of the experimental context is updated. On this account, the differences between conditions shown in situation A of figure 1.1 support the inference that updating processes are greater in condition 1 than 2. Such inferences based on amplitude measures only apply when comparing the same component across conditions.

The reader may have noticed that all the inferences discussed in this and the previous sections were framed in terms of comparisons between experimental conditions. That is, they are based on an analysis of differential ERP effects. Functional interpretations of any measure of neural activity rely crucially on a carefully designed experiment. The processes of interest must be isolated with judiciously selected experimental conditions. Virtually without exception, this requires the researcher to manipulate the process across two or more experimental conditions. Accordingly, functional interpretations are usually made from differences in neural activity, computed between the conditions that are presumed to isolate the process(es) of interest.

What Cannot Be Inferred from ERPs?

ERP data can provide valuable information about cognitive functions in many situations. When using ERP data to make functional interpretations, it is important to keep these strengths in mind. Equally important, however, is to recognize the limitations of ERP data. For example, ERPs can provide no information about neural activity giving rise to "closed" electromagnetic fields (see below). In addition, many of the inferences discussed in the previous sections rely on assumptions that may be violated in any given case. In this section, we outline some of these issues. Note that most of these issues are equally relevant to noninvasive measures of brain activity other than ERPs.

Null Results

The first issue concerns null results. Several of the inferences discussed above follow from the finding that a comparison of interest failed to result in a statistically reliable difference in amplitude, scalp distribution, or latency. That is, the inference is based on the lack of an effect. For example, we described how the lack of a reliable scalp distribution difference across experimental manipulations may suggest that the same cognitive process is associated with each manipulation. However, for at least three reasons, interpretations based on the absence of an effect should be treated with caution. First, the experiment may not have had enough statistical power to bring out a difference, even when one exists. Second, the ERP waveforms may not have been quantified or analyzed in the optimal way. And perhaps most importantly, third, ERPs sample only a subset of the total activity that is going on in the brain at any one time. For its activity to be detectable at the scalp, the elements of a neuronal population must activate (or de-activate) synchronously, and their geometric configuration must be such that their activity summates (that is, they must have an "open field" configuration; see Wood, 1987). Accordingly, the neural activity differentiating the experimental conditions may not have the right dynamic or geometric properties to be detectable on the scalp. For these reasons, when two scalp distributions differ, it is possible to be confident that conditions engaged neurally nonequivalent processes. The converse, however, does not apply.

Scalp Distribution

Even when one finds a statistically reliable effect, its interpretation may not be straightforward. Effects on scalp distribution are a good example. As mentioned earlier, reliable differences in scalp distribution allow several possible conclusions. One is that functionally nonequivalent cognitive processes are engaged across conditions or time. Scalp distribution differences can only come about when the patterns of neural activity generating the distributions differ across conditions or time. However, it is unclear from ERP data alone what the exact nature of this difference is.

An ERP effect may be generated by a single, anatomically circumscribed neuronal population, or it may reflect the contribution of multiple, anatomically distributed populations. This means that there is more than one reason why the scalp distributions of two ERP effects may differ. In the simplest case, different distributions may signify the engagement of anatomically distinct generators. Alternatively, scalp distribution effects could reflect differences in the relative contributions of the different components of a common set of generators, in terms either of their strengths or time courses. In the first case, one would conclude that the two effects are truly distinct anatomically. In the second case, the effects might both reflect activity within a common functional network; whether such a finding constitutes evidence of a strong functional dissociation is arguably less obvious (e.g., Urbach & Kutas, 2002).

Polarity

A defining feature of an ERP effect is its polarity. It is important to note, however, that whether an effect is observed to be positive-going or negative-going depends on a variety of nonneurophysiological factors, such as the location of the reference electrode, the baseline against which the effect is compared, and the location and orientation of its intracerebral sources. The polarity of an ERP effect may also vary because of neurophysiological reasons. For example, the orientation of the electromagnetic field generated by the same neuronal population depends both on whether input is inhibitory or excitatory, and whether input is received via synapses distal or proximal to the cell bodies (Wood, 1987). For all of these reasons, in the absence of detailed information about the neural activity underlying it, the polarity of an ERP effect is of no particular neurophysiological or functional significance.

Intracerebral Sources

It should be obvious from the foregoing discussions that ERP data recorded from the scalp do not allow direct inferences about either the identity or the spatial location within the brain of the neural activity that gives rise to it. In other words, there is not a transparent relationship between an electrical field observed on the scalp and the brain regions giving rise to that field. For example, if an ERP effect is maximal over frontal scalp sites, this does not necessarily mean that the activity that gives rise to this effect is in frontal cortex. Clearly, it would be of considerable value to be able to discern the intracerebral sources of ERP data. Such knowledge would enhance the functional and neural interpretations of the data, and greatly facilitate its integration with findings from studies using other methods (e.g., fMRI). For detailed discussion of these issues, see chapters 7, 9, and 15 of this volume.

Amplitude

In addition to inferences based on scalp distribution, those based on the amplitude of an ERP effect also need qualification. Crucially, amplitude differences can occur in the absence of a change in the strength of the underlying neural activity. ERP waveforms are almost always formed by averaging across multiple EEG epochs, time-locked to a common class of events. Quantification of the waveforms therefore relies on the assumptions underlying the employment of signal averaging. One of these assumptions is that the signal is invariant across epochs. If there is variability in the time of occurrence of the signal ("latency jitter"), and the degree of variability differs between conditions, amplitude differences may occur in the averaged ERP waveforms even though the signal in the constituent epochs does not differ in amplitude. Methods do exist to estimate the signal in single trials rather than the averaged waveform (e.g.,

Childers et al., 1987; chapter 10 of this volume). However, because of the low signal-to-noise ratio, single-trial analyses are only successful when the signal of interest is large. Furthermore, such analyses are inappropriate when the effect of interest is inherent to the difference between different classes of trials (as is the case, for example, for ERP "repetition effects"; e.g., Bentin & Peled, 1990).

Arguably more important is a second way in which the assumption of across-trial invariance can be violated. According to this assumption, differences in amplitude between two ERP effects reflect differences in the degree to which their underlying generators are active, and hence the degree of engagement of the associated cognitive processes (see above). It is possible, however, that such differences merely reflect differences in the proportion of trials carrying an effect of constant amplitude. Under these circumstances, amplitude differences provide information not about the degree to which a process was engaged on any given trial, but about the probability of its engagement. Despite the markedly different theoretical interpretations that follow from these two scenarios, distinguishing between them can be formidably difficult, if not impossible.

Time Course

As already discussed, the time at which ERP waveforms diverge provides a measure of the time by which the neural activity, and hence the associated cognitive process, differs between experimental conditions. There are two considerations here. First, the onset of an effect does not necessarily reflect the actual point in time when the brain first distinguishes the conditions. It is possible that neural activity differed before this time, but that the ERPs were not sensitive to this difference (for example, because the activity was not detectable at the scalp). Thus, the onset latency of an ERP effect should be viewed as an upper bound on the time by which cognitive processing started to differ. Second, it is important to note that although we have focused above on onset latency, the full characterization of the time course of an ERP effect may require the estimation of several other parameters as well, for example, latency to peak, rise time, and duration. For some questions, such as when one wants to know not only about when a hypothetical process begins but also how long it lasts, these other parameters may be of equal importance.

Correlation versus Causation

All inferences from ERP data, and neuroimaging data in general, are correlational in nature. That is, they allow one to make statements about neural activity that is correlated with some cognitive process, but not whether this activity is necessary for that process to occur. Even when a tight correlation is found between some experimental manipulation and some neural measure, one cannot conclude that the measured activity is a direct manifestation of the cognitive process thought to be associated with the manipulation. Instead, it may reflect cognitive processes that occur downstream from the process of interest, or be incidental to it.

To determine whether a specific neural correlate is necessary for some cognitive process, one must investigate the consequences of interfering with the correlate. This might be achieved by studying patients with brain lesions, or by temporarily disrupting neural activity with techniques such as Transcranial Magnetic Stimulation (Cowey & Walsh, 2001), or pharmacological manipulations. Although a positive finding does not necessarily mean that the neural activity in question *is* necessary for the cognitive process of interest (Rugg, 1999), if the process is unaffected by interventions that abolish a neural correlate, one can confidently conclude that the activity in question plays no causal role in the process.

Interdomain Mapping

Using any measure of brain activity to understand functional processes requires a conceptualization of how functional states map onto physical brain activity. For example, several of the functional interpretations from ERP data discussed in this chapter are based on the assumption that different patterns of neural activity (as manifested in scalp distribution differences) imply qualitative differences in cognitive processes. Such interpretations are sustainable only when one assumes that there exists a one-to-one mapping between neural activity and cognitive processes. That is, that there is one, and only one, pattern of neural activity that underlies a distinct functional state. If, instead, one assumes that the same functional state can be caused by more than one physical state (as proposed by, for example, Mehler, Morton, & Jusczyk, 1984), it is difficult, if not impossible, to use measures of differential brain activity to infer functional processes (for a related discussion see Price and Friston, 2002; and Friston and Price, 2003).

Even when one assumes one-to-one mapping, different patterns of neural activity may not necessarily reveal distinct cognitive processes. To illustrate this point, Rugg and Coles (1995) described an example from the literature on ERPs and attention. The early deflections in ERP waveforms elicited by visual stimuli are modulated depending on whether the stimuli are attended or ignored. Importantly, the scalp distributions of these modulations differ depending on the visual field in which the stimuli are presented. When a stimulus occurs in the left visual field, the attention-related changes are largest at scalp sites over the right hemisphere, and vice versa (e.g., Mangun & Hillyard, 1995). These qualitative differences in scalp distribution have not, however, led to the conclusion that there exist distinct attentional processes for paying attention to the left versus right visual fields. Instead, the same attentional processes are supported by distinct neuroanatomical pathways (in this case, in homotopic regions of each cerebral hemisphere). Thus, there are at least some circumstances in which distinct patterns of neural activity do not reflect distinct cognitive processes. As a consequence, the demonstration that experimental conditions are associated with distinct scalp distributions (and therefore distinct patterns of neural activity) is a necessary, but not a sufficient, condition for concluding that distinct cognitive processes are engaged across conditions.

Finally, the question arises as to what constitutes evidence of distinct patterns of neural activity. It is presently unclear just how different two patterns need to be before they should be considered functionally distinct. Given a sufficiently sensitive measure, for example, one could in principle differentiate activity at the level of single neurons. This does not necessarily mean that it would be meaningful to apply a functional interpretation to differences at this level. As things stand at the moment, the trend in the ERP literature is for any statistically significant difference in scalp distribution to be considered of potential functional interest. The spatial resolution with which ERP scalp fields are sampled is continuously increasing, however, and along with it the power to detect subtle differences in scalp distribution. It will be of interest to see whether any limit emerges on the size of an effect that carries functional significance.

Conclusion

ERPs have provided important insights into perceptual, cognitive, and motor functions since the 1960s. In this chapter, we have highlighted the ways in which one can make functional interpretations from ERP data, the assumptions upon which they are based, and some of the difficulties surrounding functional interpretations. Because of their high temporal resolution and low cost, ERPs will likely remain an essential tool in cognitive neuroscience. An important development in future will be the integration of ERP data with neuroimaging tools that allow the specification of where neural activity originates inside the brain.

References

Bentin, S., & Peled, B. S. (1990). The contribution of task-related factors to ERP repetition effects at short and long lags. *Memory and Cognition, 18*, 359–366.

Childers, D. G., Perry, N. W., Fischler, I. A., Boaz, T., & Arroyo, A. A. (1987). Event-related potentials: A critical review of methods for single-trial detection. *Critical Reviews in Biomedical Engineering, 14*, 185–200.

Coles, M. G. H., & Rugg, M. D. (1995). Event-related brain potentials: An introduction. In M. D. Rugg & M. G. H. Coles (Eds.), *Electrophysiology of mind: Event-related brain potentials and cognition* (pp. 1–26). New York: Oxford University Press.

Cowey, A., & Walsh, V. (2001). Tickling the brain: studying visual sensation, perception and cognition by transcranial magnetic stimulation. *Progress in Brain Research, 134*, 411–425.

Donchin, E. (1981). Surprise!... surprise? *Psychophysiology, 18*, 493–513.

Donchin, E., & Coles, M. G. H. (1988). Is the P300 component a manifestation of context updating? *Behavioral and Brain Sciences, 11*, 355–372.

Donchin, E., Ritter, W., & McCallum, C. (1978). Cognitive psychophysiology: The endogenous components of the ERP. In E. Callaway, P. Tueting, & S. H. Koslow (Eds.), *Brain event-related potentials in man* (pp. 349–411). New York: Academic Press.

Duncan-Johnson, C. C., & Kopell, B. S. (1981). The Stroop effect: Brain potentials localize the source of interference. *Science, 214*, 938–940.

Farwell, L. A., & Donchin, E. (1991). The truth will out: Interrogative polygraphy ("lie detection") with event-related brain potentials. *Psychophysiology, 28*, 531–547.

Ford, J. M., Mathalon, D. H., Marsh, L., Faustman, W. O., Harris, D., Hoff, A. L., Beal, M., & Pfefferbaum, A. (1999). P300 amplitude is related to clinical state in severely and moderately ill patients with schizophrenia. *Biological Psychiatry, 46*, 94–101.

Friederici, A. D. (1995). The time course of syntactic activation during language processing: A model based on neuropsychological and neurophysiological data. *Brain and Language, 50*, 259–281.

Friston, K. J., & Price, C. J. (2003). Degeneracy and redundancy in cognitive anatomy. *Trends in Cognitive Sciences, 7*, 151–152.

Hsu, F. C., Garside, M. J., Massey, A. E., & McAllister-Williams, R. H. (2003). Effects of a single dose of cortisol on the neural correlates of episodic memory and error processing in healthy volunteers. *Psychopharmacology, 167*, 431–442.

Kutas, M., & Dale, A. (1997). Electrical and magnetic readings of mental functions. In M. D. Rugg (Ed.), *Cognitive neuroscience* (pp. 197–242). Hove, East Sussex: Psychology Press.

Lines, C. R., Rugg, M. D., & Milner, A. D. (1984). The effect of stimulus intensity on visual evoked potential estimates of interhemispheric transmission time. *Experimental Brain Research, 57*, 89–98.

Mangun, G. R., & Hillyard, S. A. (1995). Mechanisms and models of selective attention. In M. D. Rugg & M. G. H. Coles (Eds.), *Electrophysiology of mind: Event-related brain potentials and cognition* (pp. 40–85). New York: Oxford University Press.

Marr, D. (1982). *Vision*. San Francisco: Freeman.

Mehler, J., Morton, J., & Jusczyk, P. W. (1984). On reducing language to biology. *Cognitive Neuropsychology, 1*, 83–116.

Näätänen, R., Ilmoniemi, R. J., & Alho, K. (1994). Magnetoencephalography in studies of human cognitive brain function. *Trends in Neurosciences, 17*, 389–395.

Näätänen, R., & Picton, T. W. (1987). The N1 wave of the human electric and magnetic response to sound: A review and an analysis of the component structure. *Psychophysiology, 24*, 375–425.

Otten, L. J., Rugg, M. D., & Doyle, M. C. (1993). Modulation of event-related potentials by word repetition: The role of visual selective attention. *Psychophysiology, 30*, 559–571.

Picton, T. W., Bentin, S., Berg, P., Donchin, E., Hillyard, S. A., Johnson, R. Jr., Miller, G. A., Ritter, W., Ruchkin, D. S., Rugg, M. D., & Taylor, M. J. (2000). Guidelines for using human event-related potentials to study cognition: Recording standards and publication criteria. *Psychophysiology, 37*, 127–152.

Price, C. J., & Friston, K. J. (2002). Degeneracy and cognitive anatomy. *Trends in Cognitive Sciences, 6*, 416–421.

Rugg, M. D. (1997). *Cognitive neuroscience.* Hove, East Sussex: Psychology Press.

Rugg, M. D. (1999). Functional neuroimaging in cognitive neuroscience. In C. M. Brown & P. Hagoort (Eds.), *The neurocognition of language* (pp. 15–36). New York: Oxford University Press.

Rugg, M. D., & Coles, M. G. H. (1995). The ERP and cognitive psychology: Conceptual issues. In M. D. Rugg & M. G. H. Coles (Eds.), *Electrophysiology of mind: Event-related brain potentials and cognition* (pp. 27–39). New York: Oxford University Press.

Rugg, M. D., & Morcom, A. M. (in press). The relationship between brain activity, cognitive performance and aging: The case of memory. In R. Cabeza, L. Nyberg, & D. C. Park (Eds.), *The cognitive neuroscience of aging.* New York: Oxford University Press.

Rugg, M. D., & Wilding, E. L. (2000). Retrieval processing and episodic memory. *Trends in Cognitive Sciences, 4*, 108–115.

Scherg, M. (1990). Fundamentals of dipole source potential analysis. In F. Grandori, M. Hoke, & G. L. Romani (Eds.), *Auditory evoked magnetic fields and electric potentials. Advances in audiology, Vol. 5* (pp. 40–69). Basel, Switzerland: Karger.

Tallon-Baudry, C., & Bertrand, O. (1999). Oscillatory gamma activity in humans and its role in object representation. *Trends in Cognitive Sciences, 3*, 151–161.

Urbach, T. P., & Kutas, M. (2002). The intractability of scaling scalp distributions to infer neuroelectric sources. *Psychophysiology, 39*, 791–808.

van der Stelt, O., van der Molen, M., Boudewijn Gunning, W., & Kok, A. (2001). Neuroelectrical signs of selective attention to color in boys with attention-deficit hyperactivity disorder. *Cognitive Brain Research, 12*, 245–264.

Woldorff, M. G., & Hillyard, S. A. (1991). Modulation of early auditory processing during selective listening to rapidly presented tones. *Electroencephalography and Clinical Neurophysiology, 79*, 170–191.

Wood, C. C. (1987). Generators of event-related potentials. In A. M. Halliday, S. R. Butler, & R. Paul (Eds.), *A textbook of clinical neurophysiology* (pp. 535–567). New York: Wiley.

2 Ten Simple Rules for Designing ERP Experiments

Steven J. Luck

Peaks and Components

The term *ERP component* refers to one of the most important but most nebulous concepts in ERP research. An ERP waveform unambiguously consists of a series of peaks and troughs, but these voltage deflections reflect the sum of several relatively independent underlying or *latent* components. It is extremely difficult to isolate the latent components so as to measure them independently, which is the single biggest roadblock to designing and interpreting ERP experiments. Consequently, one of the keys to successful ERP research is to distinguish between the observable peaks of the waveform and the unobservable latent components. This chapter describes several of the factors that make it difficult to assess the latent components, along with a set of "rules" for avoiding misinterpreting the relationship between the observable peaks and the underlying components.

Panels A–C of figure 2.1 illustrate the relationship between the visible ERP peaks and the latent ERP components. Panel A shows an ERP waveform; panel B shows a set of three latent ERP components that when summed together equal the ERP waveform in panel A. When several voltages are simultaneously present in a conductor such as the brain, the combined effect of the individual voltages is exactly equal to their sum, so it is quite reasonable to think about ERP waveforms as an expression of several summed latent components. In most ERP experiments, the researchers want to know how an experimental manipulation influences a specific latent component, but we don't have direct access to the latent components and must therefore make inferences about them from the observed ERP waveforms. This is usually more difficult than it might seem, and the first step is to realize that the maximum and minimum voltages (i.e., the peak amplitudes) in an observed ERP waveform are not usually a good reflection of the latent components. For example, the latency of peak 1 in the ERP waveform in panel A is much earlier than the peak latency of component C1 in panel B. This leads to our first rule of ERP experimental design and interpretation:

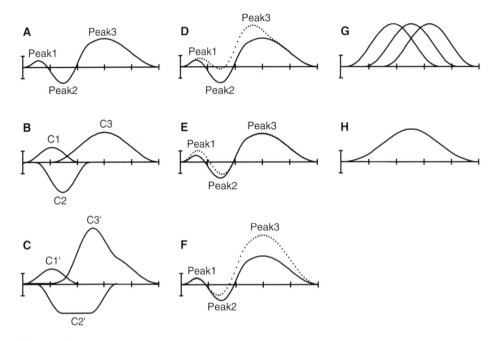

Figure 2.1
Examples of the latent components that may sum together to form an observed ERP waveform. Panels (*B*) and (*C*) show two different sets of latent components that could underlie the waveform shown in panel (*A*). Panel (*D*) shows the effect of decreasing the amplitude of component C2′ by 50% (broken line) compared to the original waveform (solid line). Panel (*E*) shows how an increase in the amplitude of component C1 (broken line) relative to the original waveform (solid line) can create an apparent shift in the latencies of both peak 1 and peak 2. Panel (*F*) shows how an increase in the amplitude of component C3 (broken line) relative to the original waveform (solid line) can influence both the amplitude and the latency of peak 2. Panel (*G*) shows a component at three different latencies, representing trial-by-trial variations in latency; panel (*H*) shows the average of these three waveforms, which is broader and has a smaller peak latency (but the same area amplitude) compared to each of the single-trial waveforms.

Rule #1   Peaks and components are not the same thing. There is nothing special about the point at which the voltage reaches a local maximum or minimum.

Researchers often quantify ERP waveforms by measuring the amplitude and latency of the voltage peaks, either implicitly or explicitly assuming that these measures provide a good means of assessing the magnitude and timing of a particular latent component. This is not usually a good assumption, and it leads to many errors in interpretation. We will discuss strategies for avoiding this problem later in this chapter.

Panel C of figure 2.1 shows another set of latent components that also sum together to equal the ERP waveform in panel A. In this case, the relatively short duration and rounded shape of peak 2 in panel A bears little resemblance to the long duration component C2' in panel C. This leads to our second rule:

Rule #2   It is impossible to estimate the time course or peak latency of a latent ERP component by looking at a single ERP waveform—there may be no obvious relationship between the shape of a local part of the waveform and the underlying latent components.

Violation of this rule is especially problematic when comparing two or more ERP waveforms. For example, consider the ERP waveforms in panel D of figure 2.1. The solid waveform represents the sum of the three latent components in panel C (and is the same ERP waveform as in panel A). The dashed waveform shows the effect of decreasing component C2' by 50 percent. To make this a bit more concrete, you can think of these waveforms as the response to an attended stimulus and an unattended stimulus, respectively, such that ignoring the stimulus leads to a 50 percent decline in the amplitude of component C2'. Without knowing the underlying component structure, it would be tempting to conclude from the ERP waveforms in panel D that the attentional manipulation does not merely cause a decrease in the amplitude of component C2' but also causes: (1) a decrease in the amplitude of component C1'; (2) an increase in the amplitude of component C3'; and (3) a decrease in the latency of component C3'. In other words, the finding of an effect that overlaps with multiple peaks in the ERP waveform tends to be interpreted as reflecting changes in multiple underlying components, but this is often not the case. Alternatively, you might conclude from the waveforms in panel D that the attentional manipulation adds an additional, long-duration component that would not otherwise be present at all. This would also be an incorrect conclusion, which leads us to:

Rule #3   It is extremely dangerous to compare an experimental effect (i.e., the difference between two ERP waveforms) with the raw ERP waveforms.

This example raises an important point about the relationship between amplitude and latency. Although the amplitude and latency of a latent component are conceptually independent, amplitude and latency often become confounded when ERP waveforms are measured. Consider, for example, the relatively straightforward correspondence between the peaks in panel A of figure 2.1 and the latent components in panel B. Panel E shows the effects of increasing the amplitude of the first latent component on the summed ERP activity. When the amplitude of component A is increased by 50 percent, this creates an increase in the latency of both peak 1 and peak 2 in the summed waveform; it also causes a decrease in the peak amplitude of peak 2. Panel F illustrates the effect of doubling the amplitude of the component C3, which causes a decrease in the amplitude and the latency of the second peak. Once again, this shows how the peak voltage in a given time range is a poor measure of the underlying ERP components in that latency range. This leads to our next rule:

Rule #4 Differences in peak amplitude do not necessarily correspond to differences in component size, and differences in peak latency do not necessarily correspond to changes in component timing.

In the vast majority of ERP experiments, the ERP waveforms are isolated from the EEG by means of signal-averaging procedures. It is tempting to think of signal averaging as a process that simply attenuates the nonspecific EEG, allowing us to see what the single-trial ERP waveforms look like. However, to the extent that the single-trial waveform varies from trial to trial, the averaged ERP may provide a distorted view of the single-trial waveforms, particularly when component latencies vary from trial to trial. Panels G and H of figure 2.1 illustrate this. Panel G shows three single-trial ERP waveforms (without any EEG noise), with significant latency variability across trials; panel H shows the average of those three single-trial waveforms. The averaged waveform differs from the single-trial waveforms in two significant ways. First, it is smaller in peak amplitude. Second, it is more spread out in time. In addition, even though the waveform in panel H is the average of the waveforms in panel G, the onset time of the averaged waveform in panel H reflects the onset time of the earliest single-trial waveform and not the average onset time. This leads to our next rule:

Rule #5 Never assume that an averaged ERP waveform accurately represents the single-trial waveforms.

Fortunately, it is often possible to measure ERPs in a way that avoids the distortions created by the signal-averaging process. For example, the area under the curve in the averaged waveform shown in panel H is equal to the average of the area under the single-trial curves in panel G. In most cases, measurements of area amplitude (i.e., mean amplitude over a fairly broad time interval) are superior to measurements of peak amplitude. Similarly, it is possible to find the time point that divides the area into two equal halves, which can be a better measurement of latency than peak measures (see Hansen & Hillyard, 1984; Luck, 1998).

It is worth mentioning that the five rules presented so far have been violated in a very large number of published ERP experiments. There is no point in cataloging the cases, especially given that some of my own papers would be included in the list. However, violations of these rules significantly undermine the strength of the conclusions that can be drawn from these experiments. For new students of the ERP technique, it would be worth reading a large set of ERP papers and trying to identify both violations of these rules and methods for avoiding the pitfalls that the rules address.

What Is an ERP Component?

So how can we accurately assess changes in latent components on the basis of the observed ERP waveforms? Ideally, we would like to be able to take an averaged ERP waveform and use some simple mathematical procedure to recover the actual waveforms corresponding to the components that sum together to create the recorded ERP waveform. We could then measure the amplitude and the latency of the isolated components, and changes in one component would not influence our measurement of the other components. Unfortunately, just as there are infinitely many generator configurations that could give rise to a given ERP scalp distribution, there are infinitely many possible sets of latent components that could be summed together to give rise to a given ERP waveform. In fact, this is the basis of Fourier analysis: any waveform can be decomposed into the sum of a set of sine waves. Similarly, techniques such as principal components analysis (PCA) and independent components analysis (ICA) use the correlational structure of a data set to derive a set of basic components that can be added together to create the observed waveforms. Localization techniques can also be used to compute component waveforms at the site of each ERP generator source. Unfortunately, these techniques have significant limitations, as we will discuss later in this section (see also chapters 7, 9, and 15).

All techniques for estimating the latent components are based on assumptions about what a component is. In the early days of ERP research, a component was defined primarily on the basis of its polarity, latency, and general scalp distribution. For example, the P3A and P3B components were differentiated on the basis of the earlier peak latency and more frontal distribution of the P3A component relative to the P3B component. However, polarity, latency, and scalp distribution do not really capture the essence of a component. For example, the peak latency of the P3B component may vary by hundreds of milliseconds, depending on the difficulty of the target-nontarget discrimination (Johnson, 1986), and the scalp distribution of the auditory N1 wave depends on the pitch of the eliciting stimulus in a manner that corresponds with the tonotopic map of auditory cortex (Bertrand, Perrin, & Pernier, 1991). Even polarity may vary: The C1 wave, generated in area V1 of visual cortex, is negative for upper-field stimuli and positive for lower-field stimuli due to the folding pattern of area V1 in the human brain (Clark, Fan, & Hillyard, 1995). Consequently, most investigators now define components in terms of a combination of computational function and neuro-anatomical generator site. Consistent with this approach, my own definition of the term ERP component is *scalp-recorded neural activity that is generated in a given neuro-anatomical module when a specific computational operation is performed.* By this definition, a component may occur at different times under different conditions, as long as it arises from the same module and represents the same cognitive function. The scalp distribution and polarity of a component may also vary according to this definition, because the same cognitive function may occur in different parts of a cortical module under different conditions.

Techniques such as PCA and ICA use the correlational structure of an ERP data set to define a set of components, and these techniques therefore derive components that are based on functional relationships. Specifically, different time points are grouped together as part of a single component to the extent they tend to vary in a correlated manner, as would be expected for time points that reflect a common cognitive process. The PCA technique, in particular, is problematic because it does not yield a single, unique set of underlying components without additional assumptions (see, e.g., Rosler & Manzey, 1981). That is, PCA really just provides a means of determining the possible set of latent component waveshapes, but additional assumptions are necessary to decide on one set of component waveshapes (and there is typically no way to verify that the assumptions are correct). The ICA technique appears to be a much better approach, because it uses both linear and nonlinear relationships to define the components. However, any correlation-based method will have significant limitations. One limitation is that when two separate cognitive processes covary, they may be captured as part of a single component even if they occur in very different brain areas and represent different computational functions. For example, if all the target stimuli in a given experimental paradigm are transferred into working memory, an ERP component associated with target detection may always be accompanied by a component associated with working memory encoding, and this may lead PCA or ICA to group them together as a single component. Another very important limitation is that, when a component varies in latency across conditions, both PCA and ICA will treat this single component as multiple components. Thus, correlation-based techniques may sometimes be useful for identifying latent ERP components, but they do not provide a magic bullet for determining which components an experimental manipulation influences.

Techniques for localizing ERPs can potentially provide measures of the time course of activity within anatomically defined regions. In fact, this aspect of ERP localization techniques might turn out to be as important as the ability to determine the neuro-anatomical locus of an ERP effect. However, there are no foolproof techniques for localizing ERPs at present, and we may never have techniques that allow direct and accurate ERP localization. Thus, this approach to identifying latent ERP components is not generally practical at present.

Avoiding Ambiguities in Interpreting ERP Components

The preceding sections of this chapter are rather depressing, because it seems that there is no perfect and general method for measuring latent components from observed ERP waveforms. This is a major problem, because many ERP experiments make predictions about the effects of some experimental manipulation on a given component, and the conclusions of these experiments are valid only if the observed effects really reflect changes in that component. For example, the N400 component is widely regarded as a sensitive index of the degree of mismatch between a word and a previously established semantic context, and it would be nice to use this component to determine which of two sets of words is perceived as being more incongruous. If two sets of words elicit different ERP waveforms, it is necessary to know whether this effect reflects a larger N400 for one set or a larger P3 for the other set; otherwise, it is impossible to determine whether the two sets of words differ in terms of semantic mismatch or some other variable (i.e., a variable to which the P3 wave is sensitive). Here I will describe six strategies for minimizing factors that lead to ambiguous relationships between the observed ERP waveforms and the latent components.

Strategy 1: Focus on a Specific Component

The first strategy is to focus a given experiment on only one or perhaps two ERP components, trying to keep as many other components as possible from varying across conditions. If 15 different components vary, you will have a mess, but variations in a single component are usually tractable. Of course, sometimes a "fishing expedition" is necessary when using a new paradigm, but don't count on obtaining easily interpretable results in such cases.

Strategy 2: Use Well-Studied Experimental Manipulations

It is usually helpful to examine a well-characterized ERP component under conditions that are as similar as possible to conditions in which that component has previously been studied. For example, the N400 wave was discovered in a paradigm that was intended to produce a P3 wave. The fact that the experiment was so closely related to previous P3 experiments made it easy to determine that the unexpected negative wave was a new component and not a reduction in the amplitude of the P3 wave.

Strategy 3: Focus on Large Components

When possible, it is helpful to study large components such as P3 and N400. When the component of interest is very large compared to the other components, it will dominate the observed ERP waveform, and measurements of the corresponding peak in the ERP waveform will be relatively insensitive to distortions from the other components.

Strategy 4: Isolate Components with Difference Waves

It is often possible to isolate the component of interest by creating difference waves. For example, imagine that you are interested in assessing the N400 for two different classes of nouns, class 1 and class 2. The simple approach to this might be to present one word per second, randomly choosing words from class 1 and class 2. This would yield two ERP waveforms, one for each class, but it would be difficult to know if any differences observed between the class 1 and class 2 waveforms were due to a change in N400 amplitude or due to changes in some other ERP component. To isolate the N400, one could redesign the experiment so that each trial contained a sequence of two words, a context word and a target word, with the target word selected from class 1 on some trials and from class 2 on others. In addition, the context and target words would sometimes be semantically related and sometimes be semantically unrelated. The N400 could then be isolated by constructing difference waves in which the ERP waveform elicited by a given word when it was preceded by a semantically related context word is subtracted from the ERP waveform elicited by that same word when preceded by a semantically unrelated context word. Separate difference waves would be constructed for class 1 targets and for class 2 targets. Because the N400 is much larger for words that are unrelated to a previously established semantic context, whereas most other ERP components are not sensitive to the degree of semantic mismatch, these difference waves would primarily reflect the N400 wave, and any differences between the class 1 and class 2 difference waves would primarily reflect differences in the N400 (for an extensive example of this approach, see Vogel, Luck, & Shapiro, 1998).

Although this approach is quite powerful, it has some limitations. First, differences waves constructed in this manner may contain more than one ERP component. For example, there may be more than one ERP component that is sensitive to the degree of semantic mismatch, so an unrelated-minus-related difference wave might consist of two or three components rather than just one. However, this is still a vast improvement over the raw ERP waveforms, which probably contain at least 10 different components. The second limitation of this approach is that it is sensitive to interactions between the variable of interest (e.g., class 1 versus class 2 nouns) and the factor that is varied to create the difference waves (e.g., semantically related versus unrelated word pairs). If, for example, the N400 amplitude is 1 µV larger for class 1 nouns than for class 2 nouns, regardless of the degree of semantic mismatch, then the unrelated-minus-related difference waves will be identical for class 1 and class 2 nouns. Fortunately, when two factors influence the same ERP component, they are likely to interact multiplicatively. For example, N400 amplitude might be 20 percent greater for class 1 than for class 2, leading to a larger absolute difference in N400 amplitude when the words are unrelated to the context word than when they are related. Of course, the interactions could take a more complex form that would lead to unexpected results. For example, class 1 words could elicit a larger N400 than class 2 words when the words are unrelated to the context word, but they might elicit a smaller N400 when the words are related to the context word. Thus, using difference waves can be very helpful in isolating specific ERP components, but care is still necessary when interpreting the results. It is also important to note that the signal-to-noise ratio of a difference wave will be lower than those of the original ERP waveforms.

Strategy 5: Focus on Components That Are Easily Isolated

The previous strategy advocated using difference waves to isolate ERP components. This strategy can be further refined by focusing on certain ERP components that are relatively easy to isolate. The best example of this is the lateralized readiness potential (LRP), which reflects movement preparation and is distinguished by its contralateral scalp distribution. Specifically, the LRP in a given hemisphere is more negative when a movement of the contralateral hand is being prepared than when a movement of the ipsilateral hand is being prepared, even if the movements are not executed. In an appropriately designed experiment, only the motor preparation will lead to lateralized ERP components, making it possible to form difference waves in which all ERPs are subtracted away except for those related to lateralized motor preparation (see Coles, 1989; Coles et al., 1995). Similarly, the N2pc component for a given hemisphere is more negative when attention is directed to the contralateral visual field than when it is directed to the ipsilateral field, even when the evoking stimulus is bilateral. Because most of the sensory and cognitive components are not lateralized in this manner, the N2pc can be readily isolated (see, e.g., Luck et al., 1997; Woodman & Luck, 2003).

Strategy 6: Component-Independent Experimental Designs

The best strategy is to design experiments in such a manner that it does not matter which latent ERP component is responsible for the observed changes in the ERP waveforms. For example, Thorpe, Fize, & Marlot (1996) conducted an experiment in which they asked how quickly the visual system can differentiate between different classes of objects. To answer this question, they presented subjects with two classes of photographs, pictures that contained animals and pictures that did not. They found that the ERPs these two classes of pictures elicited were identical until approximately 150 ms, at which point the waveforms diverged. From this experiment, it is possible to infer that the brain can detect the presence of an animal in a picture by 150 ms, at least for a subset of pictures (note that the onset latency represents the trials and subjects with the earliest onsets and not necessarily the average onset time). This experimental effect occurred in the time range of the N1 component, but it may or may not have been a modulation of that component. Importantly, the conclusions of this study do not depend at all on which latent component was influenced by the experimental manipulation. Unfortunately, it is rather unusual to be able to answer a significant question in cognitive neuroscience using ERPs in a component-independent manner, but one should use this approach whenever possible (for additional examples of this approach, see Hillyard et al., 1973; Luck, Vogel, & Shapiro, 1996; Miller & Hackley, 1992).

Avoiding Confounds and Misinterpretations

The problem of assessing latent components on the basis of observed ERP waveforms is usually the most difficult aspect of the design and interpretation of ERP experiments. There are other significant experimental design issues that are applicable to a wide spectrum of techniques but are particularly salient in ERP experiments; these will be the focus of this section.

One of the most fundamental principles of experimentation is to make sure that a given experimental effect has only a single possible cause. One part of this principle is to avoid confounds, but a subtler part is to make sure that the experimental manipulation doesn't have secondary effects that are ultimately responsible for the effect of interest. For example, imagine you observed that the mass of a heated beaker of water was greater than the mass of an unheated beaker. This might lead to the erroneous conclusion that hot water has a lower mass than cool water, even though the actual explanation is that some of the heated water turned to steam and escaped through the top of the beaker. To reach the correct conclusion, it is necessary to seal the beakers so that water does not escape. Similarly, it is important to ensure that experimental manipulations in ERP experiments do not have unintended side effects that lead to an incorrect conclusion.

To explore how this sort of problem may arise in ERP experiments, imagine an experiment that examines the effects of stimulus discriminability on P3 amplitude. This experiment presents letters of the alphabet foveally at a rate of one per second; the subject is required to press a button whenever the letter Q is presented. Ten percent of trials present a Q, whereas the other 90 percent present a randomly selected non-Q letter. In addition, the letter Q never occurs twice in succession. In one set of trial blocks, the stimuli are bright and therefore easy to discriminate (the bright condition); in another set of trial blocks, the stimuli are very dim and therefore difficult to discriminate (the dim condition).

There are several potential problems with this seemingly straightforward experimental design, mainly due to the fact that the target letter (Q) differs from the non-target letters in several ways. First, the target category occurs on 10 percent of trials, whereas the nontarget category occurs on 90 percent of trials. This is one of the two intended experimental manipulations (the other being target discriminability). Second, the target and nontarget letters are physically different from each other. Not only is the target letter a different shape from the nontarget letters—and might therefore elicit a somewhat different ERP waveform—the target letter also occurs more frequently than any of the individual nontarget letters. To the extent that the visual system exhibits long-lasting and shape-specific adaptation to repeated stimuli, it is possible that the response to the letter Q will become smaller than the response to the other letters. These physical stimulus differences probably won't have a significant effect on the P3 component, but they could potentially have a substantial effect on earlier components (for a detailed example, see experiment 4 of Luck & Hillyard, 1994).

A third difference between the target and nontarget letters is that subjects make a response to the targets and not to the nontargets. Consequently, any ERP differences between the targets and nontargets could be contaminated by motor-related ERP activity. A fourth difference between the targets and the nontargets is that because the target letter never occurred twice in succession, the target letter was always preceded by a nontarget letter, whereas nontarget letters could be preceded by either targets or nontargets. This is a common practice, because the P3 to the second of two targets tends to be reduced in amplitude. Eliminating target repetitions is usually a bad idea, however, because the response to a target is commonly very long-lasting and therefore influences the waveform recorded for the next stimulus. Thus, there may appear to be differences between the target and nontarget waveforms in the N1 or P2 latency ranges that actually reflect the offset of the P3 from the previous trial, which is present only in the nontarget waveforms under these conditions. This type of differential overlap occurs in many ERP experiments, and it can be rather subtle. For an extensive discussion of this issue, see Woldorff, 1988.

A fifth difference between the targets and the nontargets arises when one averages the data and uses a peak amplitude measure to assess the size of the P3 wave. Specifically, because there are many more nontarget trials than target trials, the signal-to-noise ratio is much better for the nontarget waveforms. The maximum amplitude of a noisy waveform will tend to be greater than the maximum amplitude of a clean waveform because the noise has not been "averaged away" as well. Consequently, a larger peak amplitude for the target waveform could be caused solely by its poorer signal-to-noise ratio even if the targets and nontargets elicited equally large responses.

The manipulation of stimulus brightness is also problematic, because this will influence several factors in addition to stimulus discriminability. First, the brighter stimuli are, well, brighter than the dim stimuli, which may create differences in the early components that are not directly related to stimulus discriminability. Second, the task will be more difficult with the dim stimuli than with the bright stimuli. This may induce a greater state of arousal during the dim blocks than during the bright blocks, and it may also induce strategy differences that lead to a completely different set of ERP components in the two conditions. A third and related problem is that reaction times will be longer in the dim condition than in the bright condition, and any differences in the ERP waveforms between these two conditions could be due to differences in the time course of motor-related ERP activity (which overlaps with the P3 wave).

There are two main ways to overcome problems such as these. First, one can avoid many of these problems by designing the experiment differently. Second, it is often possible to demonstrate that a potential confound is not actually responsible for the experimental effect; this may involve additional analyses of the data or additional experiments. As an illustration, let us consider several steps one could take to address the potential problems in the P3 experiment described above:

1. One could use a different letter as the target for each trial block, so that across the entire set of subjects, all letters are approximately equally likely to occur as targets or nontargets. This solves the problem of having different target and nontarget shapes.

2. To avoid differential visual adaptation to the target and nontarget letters, one could use a set of ten equiprobable letters, with one serving as the target and the other nine serving as nontargets. Each letter would therefore appear on 10 percent of trials. If it is absolutely necessary that one physical stimulus occurs more frequently than another, it is possible to conduct a sequential analysis of the data to demonstrate that differential adaptation was not present. Specifically, trials on which a target preceded nontarget can be compared with trials on which a nontarget preceded nontarget. If no difference is obtained—or if any observed differences are unlike the main experimental effect—then the effects of adaptation are probably negligible.

3. Rather than asking the subjects to respond only to the targets, the subjects can be instructed to make one response for targets and another for nontargets. Target and nontarget RTs are likely to be different, so some differential motor activity may still be present for targets versus nontargets, but this is still far better than having subjects respond to the targets and not to the nontargets.

4. It would be a simple matter to eliminate the restriction that two targets cannot occur in immediate succession, thus avoiding the possibility of differential overlap from the preceding trial. However, if it is necessary to avoid repeating the targets, it is possible to construct an average of the nontargets that excludes trials preceded by a target; then both the target and the nontarget waveforms will contain only trials on which the preceding trial was a nontarget.

5. There are two good ways to avoid the problem of peak amplitudes being larger when the signal-to-noise ratio is lower. First, as discussed above, the peak of an ERP waveform bears no special relationship to the corresponding latent component, so there is usually no reason to measure peak amplitude. Instead, component amplitude can be quantified by measuring the mean amplitude over a predefined latency range. Mean amplitude has many advantages over peak amplitude, one of which is that it is

not biased by the number of trials. If, for some reason, it is necessary to measure peak amplitude rather than mean amplitude, it is possible to avoid biased amplitude measures by creating the nontarget average from a randomly selected subset of the nontarget trials such that the target and nontarget waveforms reflect the same number of trials.

6. There is no simple way to compare the P3 elicited by bright stimuli versus dim stimuli without contributions from simple sensory differences. However, simple contributions can be ruled out by a control experiment in which the same stimuli are used but are viewed during a task that is unlikely to elicit a P3 wave (e.g., counting the total number of stimuli, regardless of the target-nontarget category). If the ERP waveforms for the bright and dim stimuli in this condition differ only in the 50–250 ms latency range, then the P3 differences observed from 300–600 ms in the main experiment cannot easily be explained by simple sensory effects and must instead reflect an interaction between sensory factors (e.g., discriminability) and cognitive factors (e.g., whatever is responsible for determining P3 amplitude).

7. The experiment should also be changed so that the bright and dim stimuli are randomly intermixed within trial blocks. In this way, the subject's state of arousal at stimulus onset will be exactly the same for the easy and difficult stimuli. This also tends to reduce the use of different strategies.

8. It is possible to use additional data analyses to test whether the different waveforms observed for the dim and bright conditions are due to differences in the timing of the concomitant motor potentials (which is plausible whenever RTs differ between two conditions). Specifically, if the trials are subdivided into those with fast RTs and those with slow RTs, it is possible to assess the size and scalp distribution of the motor potentials. If the difference between trials with fast and slow RTs is small compared to the main experimental effect, or if the scalp distribution of the difference is different from the scalp distribution of the main experimental effect, then this effect probably cannot be explained by differential motor potentials.

Most of these strategies are applicable in many experimental contexts, and they reflect a set of general principles that are very widely applicable. I will summarize these general principles in some additional rules:

Rule #6   Whenever possible, avoid physical stimulus confounds by using the same physical stimuli across different psychological conditions. This includes "context" confounds, such as differences in sequential order.

Rule #7   When physical stimulus confounds are unavoidable, conduct control experiments to assess their plausibility. Never assume that a small physical stimulus difference cannot explain an ERP effect (even at a long latency).

Rule #8   Be cautious when comparing averaged ERPs that are based on different numbers of trials.

Rule #9   Be cautious when the presence or timing of motor responses differs between conditions.

Rule #10   Whenever possible, vary experimental conditions within trial blocks rather than between trial blocks.

Number of Trials and Signal-to-Noise Ratio

One of the most basic parameters to set when designing an ERP experiment is the number of trials. When using conventional averaging, the size of the signal will remain constant as more and more trials are added together, but the size of the noise will decrease. Thus, the overall signal-to-noise ratio increases when the number of trials increases. The number of trials needed to obtain an acceptable signal-to-noise ratio will depend on the size of the signal you are attempting to record and the noise level of the data. If you are focusing on a large component such as the P3 wave, and you expect your experimental manipulation to change the amplitude or latency by a large proportion, then you will need relatively few trials. If, however, you are focusing on a small component such as the N1 wave or you expect your experimental effect to be small, then you will need a large number of trials. The noise level will also depend on the nature of the experiment and the characteristics of the subjects (e.g., young children and psychiatric patients typically have noisier signals than healthy young adults).

Experience is usually the best guide in selecting the number of trials. If you lack experience, then the literature can provide a guide (although you will want to see how clean the waveforms look in a given paper before deciding to adopt the same number of trials). Newcomers to the ERP technique usually dramatically underestimate the number of trials needed to obtain a reasonable signal-to-noise ratio.

In my own lab, the rule of thumb is that we need 30–60 trials per condition when looking at a large component such as the P3 wave, 150–200 trials per condition when looking at a medium-sized component such as the N2 wave, and 400–800 trials per condition when looking at a small component such as the P1 wave. When recording from young children or psychiatric patients, you should try to double or triple these numbers.

It is important to realize that the relationship between the number of trials and the signal-to-noise ratio is a negatively accelerated function. To be precise, if R is the amount of noise on a single trial and N is the number of trials, the size of the noise in an average of the N trials is equal to $(1/\sqrt{N}) \times R$. In other words, the remaining noise in an average decreases as a function of the square root of the number of trials. Moreover, because the signal is assumed to be unaffected by the averaging process, the signal-to-noise (S/N) ratio increases as a function of the square root of the number of trials.

As an example, imagine an experiment in which you are measuring the amplitude of the P3 wave, and the actual amplitude of the P3 wave is 20 µV (i.e., if you could measure it without any EEG noise). If the EEG noise is 50 µV on a single trial, then the S/N ratio on a single trial will be 20:50, or 0.4 (which is not very good). If you average two trials together, then the S/N ratio will increase by a factor of 1.4 (because $\sqrt{2} = 1.4$). To double the S/N ratio from .4 to .8, it is necessary to average together four trials (because $\sqrt{4} = 2$). To quadruple the S/N ratio from .4 to 1.6, it is necessary to average together 16 trials (because $\sqrt{16} = 4$). Thus, doubling the S/N ratio requires four times as many trials, and quadrupling the S/N ratio requires 16 times as many trials. To get from a single-trial S/N ratio of 0.4 to a reasonable S/N ratio of 10.0 would require 625 trials. This relationship between the number of trials and the S/N ratio is rather sobering, because it means that achieving a substantial increase in S/N ratio requires a very large increase in the number of trials. This is why most ERP experiments need so many trials.

It is also important to do whatever you can to reduce the size of the noise in the raw EEG. There are four main sources of noise. The first is EEG activity that is not elicited by the stimuli (e.g., alpha waves). This source of noise can often be reduced by making sure that the subjects are relaxed but alert. The second source is trial-to-trial variability in the actual ERP components due to variations in neural and cognitive activity; this is probably a minor source of variability in most cases, and it may be reduced by changing the task in ways that ensure trial-by-trial consistency.

The third source of noise is artifactual bioelectric activity, such as blinks, eye movements, muscle activity, and skin potentials. Blinks and eye movements can be detected and rejected during averaging, so they are not a large problem (unless a large proportion of trials is rejected). Of the remaining sources of bioelectric noise, skin potentials are probably the most significant problem. These potentials arise when the conductance of the skin changes (often due to perspiration) or the impedance of the electrode suddenly changes (often due to head movements). These can be minimized by keeping the recording environment cool and keeping electrode impedances low (high impedance amplifiers will not help reduce this type of artifact). The final source of noise is environmental electrical activity, such as line-frequency noise from video monitors and other electrical devices. This can be minimized by means of extensive shielding (e.g., video monitors can be placed inside shielded boxes). In general, it is worth spending considerable time and effort to set up the recording environment in a way that minimizes these sources of noise, because this can decrease the number of trials and/or subjects in a given experiment by 30–50 percent.

References

Bertrand, O., Perrin, F., & Pernier, J. (1991). Evidence for a tonotopic organization of the auditory cortex with auditory evoked potentials. *Acta Otolaryngologica, 491*, 116–123.

Clark, V. P., Fan, S., & Hillyard, S. A. (1995). Identification of early visually evoked potential generators by retinotopic and topographic analyses. *Human Brain Mapping, 2*, 170–187.

Coles, M. G. H. (1989). Modern mind-brain reading: Psychophysiology, physiology and cognition. *Psychophysiology, 26*, 251–269.

Coles, M. G. H., Smid, H., Scheffers, M. K., & Otten, L. J. (1995). Mental chronometry and the study of human information processing. In M. D. Rugg & M. G. H. Coles (Eds.), *Electrophysiology of mind: Event-related brain potentials and cognition* (pp. 86–131). Oxford: Oxford University Press.

Hansen, J. C., & Hillyard, S. A. (1984). Effects of stimulation rate and attribute cuing one event-related potentials during selective auditory attention. *Psychophysiology, 21*, 394–405.

Hillyard, S. A., Hink, R. F., Schwent, V. L., & Picton, T. W. (1973). Electrical signs of selective attention in the human brain. *Science, 182*, 177–179.

Johnson, R., Jr. (1986). A triarchic model of P300 amplitude. *Psychophysiology, 23*, 367–384.

Luck, S. J. (1998). Sources of dual-task interference: Evidence from human electrophysiology. *Psychological Science, 9*, 223–227.

Luck, S. J., Girelli, M., McDermott, M. T., & Ford, M. A. (1997). Bridging the gap between monkey neurophysiology and human perception: An ambiguity resolution theory of visual selective attention. *Cognitive Psychology, 33*, 64–87.

Luck, S. J., & Hillyard, S. A. (1994). Electrophysiological correlates of feature analysis during visual search. *Psychophysiology, 31*, 291–308.

Luck, S. J., Vogel, E. K., & Shapiro, K. L. (1996). Word meanings can be accessed but not reported during the attentional blink. *Nature, 382*, 616–618.

Miller, J., & Hackley, S. A. (1992). Electrophysiological evidence for temporal overlap among contingent mental processes. *Journal of Experimental Psychology: General, 121*, 195–209.

Rosler, F., & Manzey, D. (1981). Principal components and varimax-rotated components in event-related potential research: Some remarks on their interpretation. *Biological Psychology, 13*, 3–26.

Thorpe, S., Fize, D., & Marlot, C. (1996). Speed of processing in the human visual system. *Nature, 381*, 520–522.

Vogel, E. K., Luck, S. J., & Shapiro, K. L. (1998). Electrophysiological evidence for a postperceptual locus of suppression during the attentional blink. *Journal of Experimental Psychology: Human Perception and Performance, 24*, 1656–1674.

Woldorff, M. (1988). Adjacent response overlap during the ERP averaging process and a technique (Adjar) for its estimation and removal. *Psychophysiology, 25*, 490.

Woodman, G. F., & Luck, S. J. (2003). Serial deployment of attention during visual search. *Journal of Experimental Psychology: Human Perception and Performance, 29*, 121–138.

3   Basic Principles of ERP Quantification

Todd C. Handy

This chapter is an elementary introduction to the statistical quantification of event-related potentials (ERPs). ERPs are signal-averaged epochs of EEG that are time-locked to the onset of a stimulus or motor event. An ERP waveform is thus a time series that plots scalp voltage (in microvolts) over time (in milliseconds), where fluctuations in voltage inform regarding the internal state of the given subject. However, contemporary ERP studies typically record EEG from multiple scalp electrode sites, thereby giving ERP data a spatial parameter that directly compliments the temporal and frequency information intrinsic to time-series data. As a result, the statistical interrogation of ERP waveforms can be organized into three general—but often overlapping—categories, depending on whether the goal of analysis is to quantify the temporal, spatial, or temporospatial properties of the data.

Temporal Analysis

When ERPs are treated as time series data, analysis centers on examining how the waveforms recorded at individual electrode sites vary over time across one or more experimental conditions. This approach includes the most common form of ERP analysis, where the amplitude and latency characteristics of specific ERP components—defined here as positive- and negative-going deflections in the ERP waveform, such as the P1, P300, or N400—are quantified as a function of the specific experimental condition (e.g., Gratton et al., 1989; Hall et al., 1973). Canonical time series analyses can also be performed on ERP waveforms, which transforms data from the time domain into the frequency domain. In this manner, one can correlate changes in the frequency power spectra of ERP waveforms with changes in one or more independent variables (e.g., Basar et al., 1999).

Spatial Analysis

When one examines ERP data in relation to their spatial (or topographic) characteristics, analysis is predicated on quantifying variation in voltage across the scalp electrode array at a single timepoint or time window. The most basic form of spatial analysis is *topographic mapping*, which allows one to consider spatial variation in scalp voltage as an informative factor that may vary between conditions (e.g., Lehmann, 1986). For example, although an ERP component is typically focused over a spatially restricted subset of electrode sites on the scalp, each component is always associated with an idiosyncratic scalp topography, as measured across all electrode sites in the time window of that component. As a consequence, whether or not two different experimental conditions lead to generation of the same ERP component can be assessed by determining the extent to which the two components generate a similar topographic pattern; the greater the difference in the scalp topography, the greater the likelihood that different components may be involved. Spatial-based analyses can also be used for localizing ERP signal sources in cortex (see chapters 7 and 8).

Spatiotemporal Analysis

Finally, one can quantify ERP data in the spatiotemporal domain, premising analyses on how scalp topographic patterns vary across time. Researchers typically adopt the spatiotemporal approach when questions of interest concern how cognitive and electrophysiological states change over time. For example, principle and independent component analyses are methods of linearly decomposing ERP waveforms in order to identify the temporal and spatial characteristics of different signal sources contributing to the recorded waveforms (e.g., Dien, 2003). Likewise, by correlating topographic maps at successive points in time, one can infer how perceptual, cognitive, and motor states may transition in sequence over time; periods of high correlation values indicate relatively stable internal states, whereas periods of low correlation indicate a transition between states (e.g., Ducommun et al., 2002; Janata, 2001; Pegna et al., 1997).

Scope of the Chapter

Given these different domains of ERP quantification, the remainder of this chapter will focus on issues associated with quantifying individual ERP components, a topic that is essential to consider during the design phase of any ERP experiment. Importantly, there is much debate over how to define and functionally interpret ERP components (e.g., van Boxtel, 1998), a topic discussed in the two preceding chapters of this volume. Fortunately, however, although these issues may directly influence what waveforms are selected for analysis, they do not concern how a specific waveform feature—once selected—is quantified. We will use the term *ERP component* in this chapter to refer to positive- and negative-going deflections in a given waveform without consideration of how the component may be interpreted at a functional level.

Hypotheses and Analysis

When considering how to proceed with component analysis, the first question to ask is whether the hypothesis being tested makes predictions about how a specific component should vary between experimental conditions. For example, the hypothesis might predict that a component should be present in one condition and not the other, or that the component should occur in different time windows between the two conditions. If so, analysis will typically be restricted a priori to the set of electrode sites where the component of interest is maximal, and to a restricted time window in the waveform (i.e., the set of timepoints where the component occurs). For the purposes of this chapter, we will use the term *effect-specific hypothesis* for situations where the hypothesis under study makes a priori predictions about (1) what ERP components will be affected by the experimental manipulation, and (2) how those components will be affected, in terms of both amplitude modulations and latency characteristics.

The alternative to an effect-specific hypothesis is the hypothesis that remains non-committal regarding when and where in the ERP data an effect will be manifest. For instance, a hypothesis might predict that neural processing will differ between two experimental conditions, but exactly how those effects may be manifest in the ERP waveforms remains unspecified. Under these conditions, the goal is to perform a more comprehensive or exploratory analysis that considers the entire span of the waveform. As a result, relative to procedures associated with an effect-specific hypothesis, a broader selection of electrode sites and time windows is taken into consideration. By adopting a more comprehensive approach for quantification, it allows the investigator to make a thorough description of any and all effects that may be present in the data. Continuing the convention established above, we will refer to any hypothesis falling into this prediction-unspecific category as an *effect-unspecific hypothesis*.

The importance of distinguishing between effect-specific and effect-unspecific hypotheses transcends the practicalities of waveform analysis. As Picton et al. (2000) outline, a superordinate issue concerns the validity of interpreting post hoc results generated from an effect-unspecific hypothesis. On the one hand, the behavior of the ERP component of interest supports an effect-specific hypothesis. The component either shows or fails to show the predicted change between conditions, and appropriate conclusions are then made regarding the validity of the hypothesis. On the other hand, an effect-unspecific hypothesis can be accepted based on *any* significant difference observed in the ERP waveforms. As a consequence, the broader the scope of the analysis, the greater the chance of supporting the effect-unspecific hypothesis. Although results obtained in this manner may be descriptive of how the ERP waveforms differed between conditions, the effects have been documented in the absence of an a priori prediction that the effects should in fact be observed. Importantly, this is not to say that studies employing effect-unspecific hypotheses are flawed relative to studies adopting effect-specific hypotheses. Rather, the critical point is that the qualitative form a hypothesis takes not only constrains the quantitative procedures that are undertaken, but that it affects the subsequent interpretations that one can make regarding the data as well. Ideally, if one makes a post hoc theoretical interpretation regarding an unpredicted ERP effect, one should test that theoretical interpretation in a follow-up study using an effect-specific hypothesis, a point elaborated below.

With these considerations in mind, the following two sections of the chapter address analysis procedures optimal for effect-specific and effect-unspecific hypotheses, respectively. The former concerns quantifying specific ERP components, and the later quantifying waveforms in their entirety. For ease of discussion, we present these procedures as mutually exclusive options for analysis. In practice, however, studies may adopt elements of both analytic approaches (see, e.g., Friederici, Steinhauer, & Pfeifer, 2002).

Quantifying Waveform Components

An effect-specific hypothesis constrains component analysis in two essential ways. First, the electrode sites chosen for analysis should accurately reflect where the component of interest manifests its maximum (or minimum) amplitude. Ideally, the appropriate electrode sites are determined as part of the a priori prediction. For example, the P300 elicited by visual targets tends to have an amplitude maximum over midline parietal scalp sites. As a consequence, analysis of the P300 will often be limited to electrode sites PZ and its proximal neighbors. In practice, however, given the potential for extensive individual and group differences in ERP scalp topography, it may not always be the case that a component of interest will be maximal over the expected scalp sites. This possibility increases as one moves from considering sensory-evoked ERP components—which tend to have less individual variability in their scalp distribution—to components reflective of more cognitive or strategic processes, which tend to have greater spatial variability across subjects. Thus, although an effect-specific hypothesis may point toward the appropriate electrode sites to analyze a priori, it may be necessary to adjust the electrode sites of interest if post hoc inspection of a component's scalp topography reveals an unexpected pattern.

Second, in light of an effect-specific hypothesis, the property measured in the ERP component of interest should be able to accurately capture the predicted effect in that component. As figure 3.1a shows, one can quantify individual ERP components in relation to the amplitude *or peak* of the component (in μv), the latency of the peak (in ms), and in some cases the latency of the onset of component (in ms) as well (e.g., notice in figure 3.1a there is a clear onset latency for peak A but not peak B). The most common measures of ERP components center on identifying whether there is a difference in amplitude between conditions (figure 3.1b), a difference in peak latency (figure 3.1c), a difference in onset latency (figure 3.1d), a difference in peak-to-peak amplitude (figure 3.1e), or some combination thereof (figure 3.1f). Which analysis one performs depends on the predictions of the given hypothesis. For example, if the prediction is that the P300 component will vary in amplitude between conditions, then measuring amplitude is the relevant quantification. Alternatively, if the hypothesis predicts that

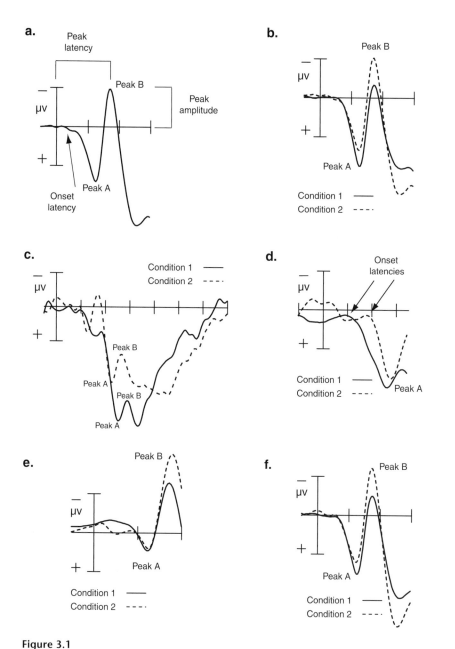

Figure 3.1

ERP components and the basic differences that are quantified. (*a*) Peak latency and peak amplitude shown for peak B, onset latency shown for peak A. (*b*) Differences in peak amplitude between conditions. (*c*) Differences in peak latency between conditions, with peaks A and B occurring earlier in condition 2 relative to condition 1. (*d*) Difference in onset latency of peak A between conditions 1 and 2. (*e*) A difference in peak-to-peak measures between peaks A and B, with a larger peak-to-peak distance in condition 2. (*f*) A combination of differences, showing an effect of condition on both peak amplitude and peak-to-peak measures for peaks A and B.

P300 will occur later in one condition relative to another, then measuring peak or onset latency is the appropriate action.

Measures

Given the constraints an effect-specific hypothesis places on ERP analysis, we now turn to a compendium of measures most often applied to individual ERP components. For simplification, the discussion assumes that the measures are being taken on group-averaged data. However, component measurement is often performed at the single-subject level for the purpose of testing the statistical significance of data patterns observed in the group-averaged waveforms. In this regard, there are important caveats unique to amplitude and latency measures, respectively, that one must consider when quantifying single-subject components. We detail these caveats following this compendium.

Amplitude   There are two common ways to measure the amplitude of an ERP component. The first is to measure amplitude at the time point where the component reaches its maximum (or minimum) amplitude—that is, measure the amplitude at the *peak latency*. This is referred to as a *peak amplitude measure*. The second approach is to compute an average amplitude over a time window that contains the component of interest, such that the resulting value is simply the arithmetic average of all time points within the defined time window. This is referred to as a *mean amplitude measure*. When making a mean amplitude measure, the time window typically centers on the peak latency. Further, the temporal extent of the window—or the number of time points included in the average—will be sufficiently restricted so as to avoid including time points from adjacent components in the waveform. Importantly, deciding whether a peak or mean amplitude measure is most appropriate for the given situation depends on understanding the strengths and weaknesses of each.

One issue to consider is whether or not a component has a well-defined peak. In figure 3.2a, for example, the ERP waveform has a clear positive-going peak. In this situation, a peak amplitude measure can be taken with little ambiguity as to whether it accurately captures the component peak. However, as figure 3.2b shows, ERP components can often have a flatter or more heterogeneous morphology, providing no definitive point at which to measure peak amplitude. In this case, it may be preferable to take a mean amplitude measure that spans the temporal breadth of the component. Mean amplitude measures are also commonly applied to ERP components that have sharply defined peaks. However, this can be problematic if there is a change between conditions in the component's basic shape. For instance, if there is a slight delay in the onset latency between two experimental conditions but the peak amplitude remains the same, this can produce a difference in a mean amplitude measure that one would not observe in a peak amplitude measure (figure 3.2c). If one uses a mean amplitude

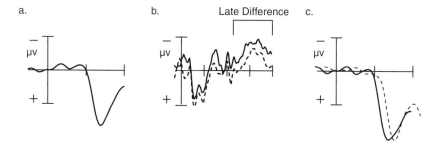

Figure 3.2
Component morphology and amplitude measures. (*a*) A well-defined positive-going peak that can be quantified using a peak or mean amplitude measure. (*b*) A mean amplitude measure is optimal for quantifying the late difference effect highlighted in the waveform, due to the broader, less-distinct shape of the component. (*c*) An equivalent peak amplitude between conditions, but with an onset latency shift that would produce a difference in a mean amplitude measure.

measure in this situation but the hypothesis of the given study concerns absolute differences in peak amplitude, then the mean amplitude measure would provide a misleading quantification of the data. Alternatively, peak amplitude measures are more sensitive to noise in ERP waveforms, making a mean amplitude measure more preferable when noise is a concern—especially if making comparisons between conditions with unequal trial numbers (see chapter 2).

A second point to consider is the baseline against which an amplitude will be measured. In short, independent of whether one quantifies peak or mean amplitude, amplitude must be measured relative to some zero point. In most situations the baseline is based on the mean of the waveform computed across some prestimulus time window in that same waveform (e.g., from −200 to 0 ms prestimulus). The procedure is to scale the waveform such that the mean across the baseline window is equal to 0 µv. Importantly, however, this makes amplitude measures sensitive to noise (or nonlinear fluctuations) in the baseline time window. If the noise structure differs between conditions, this can result in amplitude differences between conditions that vary with the size of the baseline time window. For example, figure 3.3 plots the same two waveforms as a function of the duration of the baseline. When using a 25-ms baseline (figure 3.3a), there is a difference in peak amplitude between conditions in peak C, but not peaks A and B. However, as the baseline duration is increased (figure 3.3b–d), the difference in amplitude in peak C disappears, and differences emerge in peaks A and B. This effect of baseline duration on amplitude differences in the ERP components arises because shorter baselines are more sensitive to residual voltage fluctuations than if the baseline is scaled over a larger number of time points. For this reason, the use of longer (e.g., 200+ ms) rather than shorter baseline time windows is recommended.

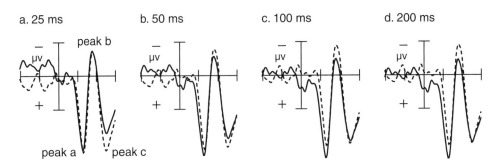

Figure 3.3
The effect of baseline duration on the scaling and measure of ERP components. As the baseline is increased from 25 ms to 200 ms of the pre-stimulus portion of the waveforms (*a–d*), differences in peak amplitude emerge for peaks A and B, and an initial difference in peak amplitude for peak C disappears. These effects of baseline duration are due to the variance in the pre-stimulus portion of the waveforms.

Peak-to-Peak Amplitude   An alternative approach to quantifying a component's amplitude is to measure the peak relative to an adjacent peak (or trough) in the wave-form. In this manner one can obtain an amplitude measure that remains free from residual noise, DC shifts, and other confounding artifacts that may exist in a pre-stimulus baseline (see Picton et al., 2000). However, when employing a peak-to-peak measure, one must consider the degree to which the comparison landmark in the waveform (i.e., the adjacent peak or trough) remains stable or constant across experi-mental conditions. If the peak or trough reflects an underlying electrophysiological process that is (1) uninfluenced by the experimental manipulation, or (2) reflects the same underlying process as the component of interest, then the waveform landmark may provide a valid reference from which to measure the peak of interest. In other words, the processes generating the reference landmark in each condition must covary together between conditions. If not, any difference in the peak-to-peak measure be-tween conditions cannot be unambiguously attributed to an effect in the actual peak of interest. That is, it remains unclear whether a difference was driven by a change only in the peak, a change only in the reference landmark, or a change in both (see figure 3.1f).

Peak Latency   When measuring the peak amplitude of an ERP component, the goal is to identify the latency (or time point) at which the component reaches its maximum or minimum. However, a measure of peak latency is often desirable in its own right, serving as an identifier of when the given component occurred in time. Quantifying peak latency allows one to determine whether a component showed a significant tem-poral lag between two experimental conditions of interest. The result is a measure that can inform on factors influencing the speed and relative timing of perceptual, cognitive, and motor processes. For example, the P600 ERP component is associated with language processing and is elicited in response to violations of grammar or syntax. Comparisons in P600 latency between two groups of subjects—for example, adolescent readers with good versus poor reading comprehension skills—could be used to determine whether readers with good comprehension are faster to detect syntactical violations than readers with poor comprehension. The prediction would be that the peak latency of the P600 should occur earlier for those adolescents with better reading skills.

One can measure peak latency in at least two different ways, both associated with signal detection. First, as described above, one can identify the peak latency by determining the time point at which the waveform reaches a maximum (or minimum) within a prespecified time window surrounding the component of interest. This method of peak latency identification is referred to as *peak-picking*. Second, one can use cross-correlation procedures to compare successive segments of a recorded waveform with a template of the component expected to be in that waveform. To estimate the component latency, the template is cross-correlated with successive segments of the averaged waveform. The latency estimate is then taken to be the middle time point of the ERP segment that had the highest cross-correlation value with the component template. Cross-correlations can also be performed in an iterative manner, such as a *Woody filter* (Woody, 1967), where the aim is to use characteristics in the average waveform to help constrain the shape of the component template and improve the accuracy of the latency estimation; for details of this method, see John, Ruchkin, & Vidal, 1978.

Toward understanding the relative effectiveness of peak-picking and cross-correlation, Gratton et al. (1989) directly compared these two measures by applying them to common sets of data. The accuracy of latency estimates for each measure were examined as a function of the level of background EEG noise in the waveforms (or signal-to-noise ratio), the use of frequency and spatial filtering prior to computing the latency estimate, and whether or not additional ERP components were overlapping with the component (or signal) of interest. When considered across all simulations performed, the cross-correlation procedure provided a more accurate measure of peak latency relative to peak-picking. However, as might be expected, both methods performed better as the signal-to-noise ratio in the waveforms increased.

Onset Latency Although measuring peak latency can be an effective method for quantifying differences in the timing of ERP components, it is only informative regarding the timing of the component maximum (or minimum). Alternatively, for some hypotheses it may be essential to determine the latency at which the component began, a property of ERP components that can vary between conditions without necessarily translating into a difference in peak latency. Developing measures of onset latency has been particularly relevant for studies examining the lateralized readiness potential (or LRP), a response-locked ERP component that indexes motor preparatory activity at centrolateral scalp electrode sites overlaying motor areas in cortex. The LRP is thus an effective approach for elucidating when preparation began for making a motor response, an event that is directly signaled in the onset latency of the LRP. In other words, demonstrating a significant difference in LRP onset latency between two experimental conditions can be evidence that the initiation of response programming was later in one condition relative to the other.

Procedures for identifying LRP onset latency all center on detecting the timepoint at which the waveform begins to deviate from some baseline or pre-LRP state. As Mordkoff and Gianaros (2000) reviewed, detection algorithms fall into three basic categories. Criterion methods establish an absolute threshold value (in μv), where the onset latency of the LRP is then taken to be the timepoint at which the threshold value was first exceeded for a prespecified number of timepoints (e.g., Smulders, Kenemans, & Kok, 1996). Deviation methods are similar, but instead of an absolute threshold, the threshold is made proportional to the variance in the pre-LRP baseline. If the waveform exceeds this value—for example, 2 standard deviations above the baseline variance—across a prespecified number of time points, then the onset latency is again taken as the first timepoint at which the threshold was exceeded (e.g., Osman et al., 1992). Finally, regression methods are premised on fitting straight lines to adjoining segments of the waveform, one line being fit across timepoints in the baseline, and one line being fit across time points where the LRP rises to its peak (e.g., Schwarzenau et al., 1998). In this manner the first line represents the baseline and the second represents the rise of the LRP; onset latency is then taken as the time point where the two lines intersect. In a direct comparison of these different detection algorithms, Mordkoff and Gianaros (2000) concluded that relative to threshold and deviation methods, the regression approach is less prone to estimation errors of the LRP onset.

Applying Component Measures

The foregoing has discussed the most common ways to quantify individual ERP components, in terms of amplitude and latency. What remains to consider are the practical issues that arise when applying these measures to ERP data sets. Here I detail two points. The first concerns whether or not a given subject should be included in an ERP data set; the second concerns the idiosyncrasies of quantifying a component across subjects for the purpose of group statistical analyses.

Exclusion Criteria Critical to any behavioral study is the question of whether or not each subject tested actually shows behavioral evidence that the task was in fact performed. If a subject fails to perform to some predetermined criterion performance level—for example, performing above chance levels in a discrimination task where accuracy is the dependent measure—then that subject may be excluded from analysis

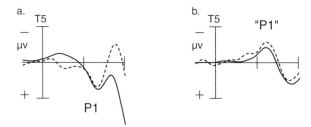

Figure 3.4
An atypical pattern for a sensory-evoked ERP component. (*a*) The visually evoked P1 is a component observed over lateral occipitotemporal electrode sites that has a peak latency in the 90–
140 ms range. (*b*) In some individuals, the P1 may be negative-going, an atypical pattern for this
component that could result in exclusion of that subject from a study exploring an effect-specific
hypothesis addressing the P1.

on the grounds that his or her data do not accurately reflect the mental processes
under study. Behavioral *exclusion criterion* are equally applicable to ERP studies, yet ERP
studies have the additional consideration of whether each subject's waveforms manifest the component of interest, in terms of whether or not (1) the component is present, (2) it occurs within an expected latency range, and (3) it is maximal over the
expected scalp region. For some studies it may be both valid and essential to exclude
subjects from analysis if there are unexpected abnormalities in their waveforms. However, in other situations it may be entirely inappropriate to adopt a component-based
exclusion criteria. The question depends on whether or not the "abnormal" pattern is
informative regarding the hypothesis under investigation.

For example, consider a study testing a hypothesis about a cognitive component
such as the P300. If the P300 is absent in a particular subject, this result may indicate
that even though the task was adequately performed, the subject nevertheless did not
engage strategic processes associated with P300 generation. If so, this is highly relevant
to the hypothesis of the study and it is imperative that the subject be included in
analysis. On the other hand, some subjects may show an atypical pattern in one or
more sensory-evoked ERP components, such as a negative-going component in the
typical time window and scalp location of the positive-going visual P1 (figure 3.4). Because the polarity of a sensory-evoked component should not vary with changes in
mental states, the negative-going P1 pattern more likely reflects an atypical anatomical
orientation of the P1 generating dipole in that subject. In this situation, it may be valid
to exclude that subject from analysis on the grounds that the data pattern reflects a
statistical outlier.

If one employs an exclusion criterion, it is essential (1) to establish it *a priori*, (2) to
clearly explicate it in any reporting of the results, and (3) to provide details regarding

specific subjects excluded from analysis based on the criterion. Moreover, one must apply the criterion in a manner that does not systematically eliminate subjects based on whether or not the effect of interest is manifest in the given waveforms. Toward alleviating these concerns, one reasonable approach would be to present the waveforms from excluded subjects to objectively show the validity of the exclusion criteria.

Measuring Multiple Waveforms   The quantification procedures discussed thus far describe how to accurately quantify amplitude and latency in a single ERP waveform. In most cases, however, analysis will include quantifying these properties in multiple waveforms, requiring an additional level of consideration. In particular, a time window that accurately quantifies a component's amplitude or latency in one waveform may inaccurately quantify that same property in a second waveform. The problem stems from the fact that the component of interest will invariably show some degree of shift in peak latency between the waveforms to be quantified. If latency is the measure of interest, the goal is to quantify this latency variability, which requires confirming the validity of the time window for capturing component latency in each waveform measured. If amplitude is the measure of interest, latency variance can be more problematic for both group-average and single-subject quantifications.

When generating descriptive statistics in group-averaged waveforms, the amplitude of a component will typically be measured at one or more electrode sites in two or more conditions. Each of these factors paired together—an electrode site and a condition—represents a single waveform and the potential for a shift in the peak latency of the component of interest. Given this, the question to consider is whether it is valid to shift the timepoint or time window used for quantifying amplitude between waveforms, based on where the peak latency occurs in each waveform. For example, the lateral occipital P1 is a sensory-evoked component that, when elicited by a lateralized visual stimulus, will show a latency shift between electrode sites contralateral versus ipsilateral to the visual field of the stimulus, due to the time it takes to transfer visual information from the contralateral to ipsilateral cerebral hemisphere (figure 3.5). In such situations, measuring the amplitude of the P1 at ipsilateral sites based on a peak latency identified from contralateral sites will underestimate the actual amplitude, because the latency used to quantify the ipsilateral P1 occurs prior to its actual peak latency. To account for such problems, one approach has been to establish a separate timepoint or time window for each waveform included in the analysis, based on the peak latencies in the grand-averaged waveforms (e.g., Handy et al., 2003; Handy & Mangun, 2000).

When quantifying amplitude across subjects, the central question to consider is whether to measure amplitude at a fixed latency determined from the grand-averaged data, or whether to use peak-picking within each subject. Although highly similar at a superficial level, these approaches capture distinctly different aspects of the group data

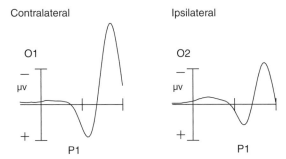

Figure 3.5
The lateral occipitotemporal P1 will show a difference in peak latency as a function of the visual field of the ERP-eliciting stimulus and the electrode site of recording. The peak latency is earlier at electrode sites contralateral to the visual field of the stimulus (*left*), relative to sites that are ipsilateral to the stimulus (*right*). A mean amplitude measure taken at the ipsilateral electrode site would underestimate amplitude if the time window were based on the peak latency of the component at the contralateral site.

pattern, as figure 3.6 illustrates. When a fixed latency is used to quantify the amplitude of a component in a given experimental condition, it will typically be the time point of the peak amplitude in the grand-averaged waveform. This allows one to make a direct statistical test of effects shown in the grand-averaged data—within each condition, the amplitude of each subject's waveform is measured at the peak latency of the component identified in the grand average (figure 3.6a). The alternative is to use peak-picking (described above) to identify peak latencies at the single-subject level. In this case the amplitude measured in each subject will occur—more often than not—at different latencies, based on the peak latency measured for each subject (figure 3.6b). This is an equally valid way to statistically test amplitude differences between conditions at the group level, but there are two points to consider that differ from a fixed-latency approach. One, because the peak amplitudes measured in each subject in each condition will come from a variety of different time points, the quantification does not correspond to what is observed in the grand-averaged waveforms. Two, peak-picking—with its use of a time window approach—requires one to verify that each peak latency in the statistical test was accurately quantified.

Quantifying Entire Waveforms

Thus far we have considered ERP quantification in relation to measuring specific features of ERP waveforms, and in particular, the latency and amplitude of discrete components. These methods of component quantification are ideally suited for effect-specific hypotheses, where the ERP component and measure of interest are determined

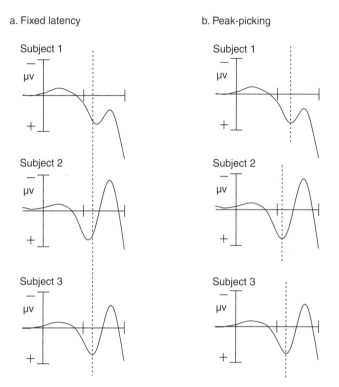

Figure 3.6
Measuring peak amplitude across subjects. (*a*) When a fixed latency procedure is used, each subject's waveform is measured at the same timepoint, as designated by the vertical dashed line. This method of measure retains correspondence with group-averaged waveforms. (*b*) When a peak-picking procedure is used, each subject's waveform is measured at the latency of the individual peaks. As a result, measures will be taken across different timepoints between subjects, and the quantification is not in correspondence with group-averaged waveforms.

a priori. However, the goal for some studies may be more descriptive or comprehensive in nature, where the investigation is driven by an effect-unspecific hypothesis. For example, perhaps a researcher suspects that cortical processing may differ between two different conditions, but remains unsure how and where those differences manifest in the ERP waveforms recorded in each condition (see above). In such cases, analysis will be predicated on quantifying a broader temporal spectrum of the ERP waveform morphology, rather than isolating and measuring a specific component feature. The following section outlines the basic approach for conducting comprehensive waveform analyses, and the role this methodology plays in promoting theory-based hypothesis testing in ERP research.

a. Waveforms and Windows

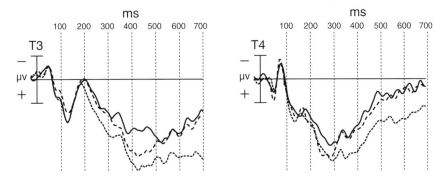

b. Statistical Results by Window

				ms		
	100-200	200-300	300-400	400-500	500-600	600-700
Effect A	---	---	---	0.001	---	---
Effect B	---	0.05	0.01	0.01	0.05	0.01
A x B	---	---	0.01	0.001	---	---

Figure 3.7
Quantifying an entire waveform. (*a*) The basic procedure is to divide waveforms into a series of time windows, with a separate statistical analysis done on mean amplitude measures within each time window. (*b*) Statistical results can then be displayed as a function of the time window and the *p* value of the particular effect. In this manner, the latency and duration of specific effects are determined via the windows over which the effects are significant.

Basic Approach

The methodology described here concerns quantifying differences between two or more group-averaged waveforms in the absence of any a priori predictions about when and where in the time series data these differences may—or may not—arise. The basic procedure is to test the statistical significance of differences in mean amplitude (1) between two or more conditions, and (2) across a sequential series of time windows that span the desired breadth of the waveforms (e.g., John et al., 1977; John, Ruchkin, & Vidal, 1978). Consider the waveforms in figure 3.7, representing three conditions recorded at two electrode sites. The size (in milliseconds) of the sliding time window is selected for quantifying mean amplitude—in this case 100 ms—and then it is applied within each subject to successive windows of each of the waveforms. The mean amplitudes measured in each window are then entered into a statistical test such as an ANOVA. The end result is a set of separate statistical analyses across contiguous windows of the ERP waveforms. Differences between the two waveforms are then quantified in relation to the windows showing *p*-values that fall below some predetermined threshold. The smaller the size of the sliding *analysis window*, the greater the temporal resolution in identifying when differences began to emerge in the waveform.

Given this basic framework, several points warrant consideration. First, one can perform analyses using a variety of statistical tests, incorporating any number of additional variables, including multiple conditions and electrode sites. Tests such as ANOVAs also allow one to categorize analysis windows in relation to both main effects and interactions between factors. In addition, it may also be useful to consider including analysis window as a factor in a single statistical test, rather than performing a series of independent tests. Second, the size of analysis windows does not necessarily need to remain constant across the temporal span of the waveform. In some cases it may be preferable to tailor the size of the windows to the frequency structure of the waveform morphology, which may have shorter latency, sensory-related components early in the waveform and longer latency, cognitive-related components later in the waveform (see, e.g., figure 3.7a, right). Finally, the use of multiple analysis windows relies on performing a number of statistical tests. Accordingly, it may be both appropriate and necessary to adopt a correction for multiple comparisons in order to protect against type I errors.

Hypothesis Testing

If the goal of the given study is to simply describe any and all differences between two conditions, then the multiple time windows approach to analysis can be quite effective. However, as discussed above and elsewhere (e.g., Picton et al., 2000), testing hypotheses in the ERP domain may have reduced or absent theoretical value when there is no a priori prediction regarding how an ERP waveform should be affected between experimental conditions. The problem arises because *any* difference observed in the waveform can be interpreted as support for the effect-unspecific hypothesis— that is, a hypothesis that predicts some difference will be observed between conditions without specifying exactly how the effect will be manifest. Any theoretical interpretations made in this context are thus post hoc in nature, in that the observed effect was not specifically predicted. This necessarily limits the utility of a comprehensive waveform analysis on its own, from the standpoint of theory-driven hypothesis testing. To make a true theoretical advance, the validity of any post hoc interpretation stemming from an effect-unspecific hypothesis must itself be directly tested within the confines of an effect-specific hypothesis.

Quantifying Noise

ERPs are predicated on extracting a signal source—the event-related response, or ERR—from noise sources in the EEG. As a consequence, an ERP waveform is a valid representation of the ERR only to the extent that noise has been removed from the averaged waveform (e.g., Glaser & Ruchkin, 1976; Perry, 1966). Importantly, we can make a distinction between noise sources in the EEG recording that are random and noise sources that are systematic. The former concerns ambient noise that is uncorrelated with the event of interest and that, in theory, will average to a flat line—or zero value at each time point—in the ERP waveform. Random noise includes sources intrinsic to the subject, such as heartbeats and task-unrelated EEG signals, as well as sources extrinsic to the subject, such as EMF interference from adjacent electrical equipment and noisy recording systems. Conversely, systematic noise concerns signals in the EEG that have some degree of correlation with the event of interest and that will therefore not average to zero in the ERP waveform. For example, a subject may frequently blink following the event of interest (introducing systematic EOG and EMG artifacts into the ERP), or the event of interest may always occur immediately following or preceding a different event type (introducing response overlap into the ERP). This final section of the chapter discusses several different methods of quantifying residual random noise in ERP waveforms. Procedures for estimating and removing systematic noise in ERPs are detailed elsewhere (e.g., Gratton, 1998; Woldorff, 1993, and by Talsma and Woldorff, chapter 6 of this volume).

Perhaps the simplest way to examine random noise in an ERP waveform is to examine the amount of nonlinear variance in the segment of the waveform that precedes event onset. To the extent that averaging has reduced the magnitude of residual noise, the pre-event segment will approximate a straight line, at least in the absence of additional systematic noise. Indeed, ERP plots frequently show the baseline portion of an ERP waveform in order to allow cursory analysis of residual noise in the data presented. Examination of the pre-event baseline is also an efficient way to assess the effectiveness of digital filtering as a means of reducing residual noise in the ERP waveform—effective filtering will reduce baseline variance. However, one cannot filter out random noise that occurs in the same frequency band as the signal of interest (for more details on filtering, see Edgar, Stewart, & Miller, 2004). Filtering issues aside, even if baseline variance is computed as a means of comparing noise between two conditions of interest (e.g., Handy et al., 2003), noise variance will not necessarily remain constant across post-event portions of the waveform (e.g., Gratton et al., 1989). This can be visualized, for example, by plotting the standard deviation of each timepoint in a waveform, rather than the time point mean (e.g., John, Ruchkin, & Vidal, 1978). Assuming a constant ERR, increases or spikes in the standard deviation plot indicate those portions of the ERP waveform having greater noise variance.

The foregoing suggests the importance of quantifying noise not just in the pre-event baseline of a waveform, but of quantifying as well the structure of residual noise that may be superimposed upon the ERR itself. We consider three procedures for conducting such analysis here (for additional discussion, see Glaser & Ruchkin, 1976; Picton, Lins, & Scherg, 1995).

± Reference

Developed by Schimmel (1967), the ± reference is a method that allows one to estimate the structure of noise in an averaged waveform that has had the ERR removed. To derive a "normal" ERP, epochs of EEG time-locked to the onset of the event of interest are simply averaged together, preserving the structure of the ERR while decreasing the amplitude of the random noise as a square-root function of the number of epochs in the average (e.g., Hillyard & Picton, 1987). In contrast, the ± reference is derived by making an average that adds and subtracts epochs in an alternating fashion, such that even numbered epochs are summated and odd number epochs are subtracted. The logic of the procedure is that if each epoch has a relatively invariant ERR, the ERR will summate to zero in the derived waveform, leaving only the amount of residual noise remaining. The underlying assumption is that because the noise is stochastic, its magnitude and structure will be comparable independent of whether one employs normal summation averaging, or adopts the addition/subtraction procedure. The resulting ± reference thus allows one to visualize the noise structure superimposed onto an ERP waveform, with the ERR in that ERP removed. Should the frequency range of the noise be of interest, for example, one can then apply a spectral analysis (or Fourier transform) to the ± reference waveform.

Split-Epoch Averages

A second approach for quantifying noise is predicated on comparing two ERP waveforms that contain estimates of the same ERR. In essence, the EEG epochs from a condition of interest that would normally be averaged into a single ERP waveform (figure 3.8a) are instead divided into two separate groups for averaging, thereby producing two ERP waveforms (figure 3.8b). When the two waveforms are compared, the degree to which they differ is presumed to be a reflection of the amount of residual noise superimposed on the same invariant signal in the two waveforms; the closer the resemblance, the less noise that is obscuring the signal. Of course, when using the split-epoch method, one must consider that noise analysis is based on ERP averages that have been generated using half of the actual EEG epochs associated with the given condition. This means that the magnitude of noise in the split-epoch averages will be larger than in the actual ERPs of interest. If the split averages nevertheless show a strong correspondence, this offers strong evidence of an adequate signal-to-noise ratio in the given data. However, if the split averages have some degree of dissimilarity, one

a. ERR Estimate: 100 epochs

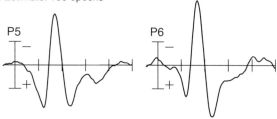

b. Split-Epoch Averages (50 epochs each)

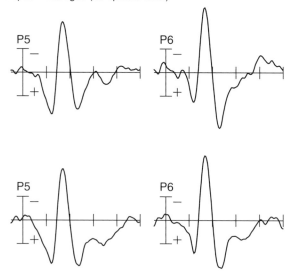

Figure 3.8

Quantifying noise via a split-epoch procedure. (*a*) The ERP waveform averaged from the total number of epochs containing the event-related response (ERR) of interest. (*b*) The magnitude of noise superimposed on the ERR can be gauged by comparing the degree to which the split-epoch averages resemble each other. In this case, variance between averages is most prominent in the later portion of the waveforms.

a. Noise Estimate: 10 epochs

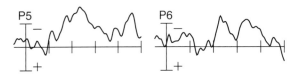

b. Noise Estimate: 50 epochs

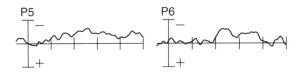

c. Noise Estimate: 100 epochs

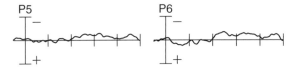

Figure 3.9
Quantifying noise via a nonevent procedure. As the number of epochs containing no ERR are
included in the average (*a–c*), the amplitude of residual noise in the waveform decreases.

must consider whether an acceptable signal-to-noise ratio would be obtained if the
number of epochs were doubled, as in the case of the actual ERP waveform of interest.

Nonevents

A final method for quantifying the structure of random noise is based on recording
EEG epochs that have no ERR. In essence, one includes "nonevents" as a condition of
interest in the given paradigm, where an event marker is recorded onto the EEG (to
allow subsequent signal averaging) but no stimulus or event is actually presented. The
goal is to present these nonevents such that there is no overlapping response from any
actual events preceding or following the nonevent epoch. If so, then the nonevent
epochs can be averaged together in the same manner as a normal ERP waveform.
The greater the number of nonevent epochs averaged together, the lower the amount
of residual noise (or variance) in the resulting waveform (figure 3.9). As with the ±
reference, one can interpret the variance observed in the nonevent average as the
magnitude of residual noise that would be superimposed upon the ERR in an ERP with
a similar number of averaged epochs. Figure 3.10 demonstrates this principle, showing

a. ERR Estimate: 100 epochs

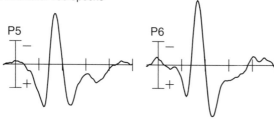

b. ERR Estimate: 10 epochs

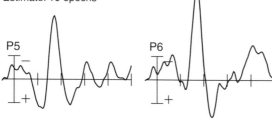

c. Noise Estimate: 10 epochs

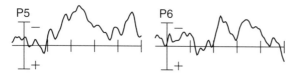

d. ERR (100 epochs) + Noise (10 epochs)

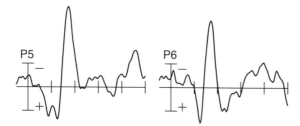

Figure 3.10

Demonstrating the additivity of random noise in an ERP waveform. (*a*) An estimate of the event-related response (ERR), based on an average of 100 epochs. (*b*) An estimate of the same ERR based on an average of only 10 epochs, thereby increasing the amount of residual noise relative to (*a*). (*c*) An estimate of residual noise using the nonevent procedure, based on an average of 10 non-event epochs. (*d*) When the noise estimate in (*c*) is added to the 100-epoch ERR estimate from (*a*), the result is a waveform that resembles the 10-epoch ERR estimate in (*b*).

how adding a residual noise estimate of N epochs to an ERR estimate of 10N epochs (i.e., an ERR estimate with very low noise) actually resembles an ERR estimate from N epochs. Importantly, the nonevent method of quantifying noise structure assumes that random noise variance remains constant between EEG epochs that contain and EEG epochs that do not contain ERRs. As mentioned above, this may not always be a valid assumption (e.g., Gratton et al., 1989). Nevertheless, it is a relatively simple way to include noise quantification into an ERP study, with the idea that one can equate the number of epochs averaged into an ERP and nonevent average in order to estimate the amount of residual noise specific to an average of that number of epochs.

References

Basar, E., Basar-Eroglu, C., Karakas, S., & Schürmann, M. (1999). Oscillatory brain theory: A new trend in neuroscience. *IEEE Engineering in Medicine and Biology*, May/June, 56–66.

Ducommun, C. Y., Murray, M. M., Thut, G., Bellmann, A., Viaud-Delmon, I., Clarke, S., & Michel, C. M. (2002). Segregated processing of auditory motion and auditory location: An ERP mapping study. *NeuroImage, 16*, 76–88.

Friederici, A. D., Steinhauer, K., & Pfeifer, E. (2002). Brain signatures of artificial language processing: Evidence challenging the critical period hypothesis. *Proceedings of the National Academy of Sciences, 99*, 529–534.

Glaser, E. M., & Ruchkin, D. S. (1976). *Principles of neurobiological signal analysis*. New York: Academic Press.

Gratton, G. (1998). Dealing with artifacts: The EOG contamination of the event-related potential. *Behavior Research Methods, Instruments and Computers, 30*, 44–53.

Gratton, G., Kramer, A. F., Coles, M. G. H., & Donchin, E. (1989). Simulation studies of latency measures of components of the event-related brain potential. *Psychophysiology, 26*, 233–248.

Hall, R. A., Rappaport, M., Hopkins, H. K., & Griffin, R. B. (1973). Peak identification in visual evoked potentials. *Psychophysiology, 10*, 52–60.

Handy, T. C., Grafton, S. T., Shroff, N. M., Ketay, S. B., & Gazzaniga, M. S. (2003). Graspable objects grab attention when the potential for action is recognized. *Nature Neuroscience, 6*, 421–427.

Handy, T. C., & Mangun, G. R. (2000). Attention and spatial selection: Electrophysiological evidence for modulation by perceptual load. *Perception & Psychophysics, 62*, 175–186.

Hillyard, S. A., & Picton, T. W. (1987). Electrophysiology of cognition. In F. Plum (Ed.), *Handbook of physiology: The nervous system V* (pp. 519–584). Bethesda, MD: American Physiological Society.

Janata, P. (2001). Brain electrical activity evoked by mental formation of auditory expectations and images. *Brain Topography, 13*, 169–193.

John, E. R., Karmel, B. Z., Corning, W. C., Easton, P., Brown, D., Ahn, H., John, M., et al. (1977). Neurometrics. *Science, 196*, 1393–1410.

John, E. R., Ruchkin, D. S., & Vidal, J. J. (1978). Measurement of event-related potentials. In E. Callaway, P. Tueting, & S. H. Koslow (Eds.), *Event-related brain potentials in man* (pp. 93–138). New York: Academic Press.

Lehmann, D. (1986). Spatial analysis of human evoked potentials. In R. Q. Cracco & I. Bodis-Wollner (Eds.), *Evoked potentials* (pp. 3–14). New York: Alan R. Liss, Inc.

Mordkoff, J. T., & Gianaros, P. J. (2000). Detecting the onset of the lateralized readiness potential: A comparison of available methods and procedures. *Psychophysiology, 37*, 347–360.

Osman, A. M., Bashore, T. R., Coles, M. G. H., Donchin, E., & Meyer, D. E. (1992). On the transmission of partial information: Inferences from movement-related brain potentials. *Journal of Experimental Psychology: Human Perception and Performance, 18*, 217–232.

Pegna, A. J., Khateb, A., Spinelli, L., Seeck, M., Landis, T., & Michel, C. M. (1997). Unraveling the cerebral dynamic of mental imagery. *Human Brain Mapping, 5*, 410–421.

Perry, N. W. (1966). Signal versus noise in the evoked potential. *Science, 153*, 1022.

Picton, T. W., Benton, S., Berg, P., Donchin, E., Hillyard, S. A., Johnson, R. Jr., Miller, G. A., et al. (2000). Guidelines for using human event-related potentials to study cognition: Recording standards and publication criteria. *Psychophysiology, 37*, 127–152.

Picton, T. W., Lins, O., & Scherg, M. (1995). The recording and analysis of event-related potentials. In R. Johnston, Jr. (Ed.), *Handbook of neuropsychology, Vol. 10* (pp. 3–73). Amsterdam: Elsevier.

Schimmel, H. (1967). The ($\pm$) reference: Accuracy of estimated mean components in average response studies. *Science, 157*, 92–93.

Schwarzenau, P., Falkenstein, M., Hoorman, J., & Hohnsbein, J. (1998). A new method of the estimation of the onset of the lateralized readiness potential (LRP). *Behavior Research Methods, Instruments, & Computers, 30*, 110–117.

Smulders, F. T. Y., Kenemans, J. L., & Kok, A. (1996). Effects of task variables on measures of the mean onset latency of the LRP depend on the scoring method. *Psychophysiology, 33*, 194–205.

van Boxtel, G. J. M. (1998). Computational and statistical methods for analyzing event-related potential data. *Behavior Research Methods, Instruments, & Computers, 30*, 87–102.

Woldorff, M. G. (1993). Distortion of ERP averages due to overlap from adjacent ERPs: Analysis and correction. *Psychophysiology, 30*, 98–119.

Woody, C. D. (1967). Characterization of an adaptive filter for the analysis of variable latency neuroelectrical signals. *Medical and Biological Engineering, 5*, 539–553.

4   Application of Repeated Measures ANOVA to High-Density ERP Datasets: A Review and Tutorial

Joseph Dien and Alecia M. Santuzzi

Repeated measures analysis of variance (ANOVA) is the statistical tool most commonly applied to the analysis of event-related potentials (ERPs). Although most, if not all, advanced statistics textbooks cover ANOVA, the application of ANOVA models to ERP data involves nuances that most available treatments do not address. Moreover, the increased use of high-density electrode montages for contemporary ERP data collection has introduced issues that were not consequential in the past when most laboratories recorded only three electrodes.

This chapter is divided into three parts: (1) a general review of repeated measures, focused on the aspects relevant to ERP analysis; (2) a suggested protocol for ANOVA of high-density ERP data that expands on existing guidelines (cf., Picton et al. 2000); and (3) analysis of example datasets. In sum, the suggested strategy for ERP data analysis involves (1) organizing electrodes into two-level regional factors to facilitate analysis, and (2) applying both multivariate and univariate test statistics to improve statistical power.

Univariate Between-Groups Factors

To set the stage for the suggested protocol, let us review the defining characteristics of univariate ANOVA, beginning with a simple two-group design. Readers who would not find such a review helpful may skip to the *Application to ERP Data* sections that discuss the relevance of these principles to ERP datasets and thence to the succeeding section outlining the proposed ERP analysis protocol.

As an illustration, the numbers below represent the P300 scores (which are typically reduced in depressed patients) of 20 depressed subjects that were measured after either no treatment (Control) or receiving treatment (Treatment). The within-group variance is presented in parentheses.

Treatment	Control
1.8, 1.9, 2.1, 2.0, 2.2, 1.1, 1.2, 1.1, 1.3, 1.4 (.19)	1.7, 1.6, 1.6, 1.8, 1.5, .9, .9, 1.1, .8, .7 (.18)

The two groups represent two levels of a grouping factor, and thus a potential source of differences to test. The means for each condition are 1.6 for the Control group and 1.3 for the Treatment group. The question of interest is whether the difference between the groups is large enough to plausibly attribute it to the treatment, above and beyond random fluctuations.

The total amount of variance to explain is a function of the amount of fluctuation among the individual scores on the dependent variable. There are two sources of this variance. The first comprises the unattributed fluctuations due to measurement error, individual differences, random chance, and other unmeasured effects. This is designated as error, e. The second source of variance is the effect that can be attributed to the treatment, designated a. Within each group, the only source of variance in the form of a mean sum of squares (MS_w) should be e. The variance representing the difference between the two groups (MS_{bet}), on the other hand, should be due to both sources, e as well as a. The ratio between these two sources of variance is the F-statistic:

$$F = \frac{MS_{be}}{MS_w} = \frac{e + a}{e}$$

If there is no treatment effect between the groups ($a = 0$), then F is expected to approximate 1 plus or minus some chance variation. Large F-values increase the likelihood of a statistically significant treatment effect. In this example, the between-groups variance is not quite large enough to declare statistical significance, $F(1, 18) = 3.37$, $p = .083$.

This approach can be extended to fit designs with more than one factor. For instance, in the case of an analysis with an additional two-level grouping factor (gender), four sources of variance can be identified:

e—random error
a—effect of treatment
b—effect of gender
ab—interaction of gender with treatment beyond main effects

In this case there would be three effects to test: Gender, Treatment, and the interaction (Gender $\times$ Treatment). Each test would use the same MS_w as an estimate of the within-cell variance in the denominator of the F-ratio.

	Treatment	Control
Men	1.8, 1.9, 2.1, 2.0, 2.2 (.025)	1.7, 1.6, 1.6, 1.8, 1.5 (.013)
Women	1.1, 1.2, 1.1, 1.3, 1.4 (.017)	.9, .9, 1.1, .8, .7 (.022)

The addition of a grouping factor can improve the sensitivity of the treatment factor by accounting for a potentially large source of individual differences that would otherwise be included in the error variance. For example, when the aforementioned scores are segregated by both treatment and gender, the within-group variances drop dramatically. Whereas the previous MS_w was the average of .188 and .176, or .182, the new MS_w is .019. The error, e, has dropped dramatically because the grouping factor accounted for a major source of previously unexplained variance. As a result, this change in the MS_w has produced changes in the test for treatment effect, such that Treatment is closer to statistical significance, $F(1, 16) = 3.75$, $p = .07$.

Another major benefit of adding factors is the additional information provided by interactions. Interaction effects occur when the effect of one factor is dependent on the level of the other factor. For example, in the above case there would have been an interaction if the men do poorly with treatment but women do well. When an interaction is present, the tests of the individual factors (the main effects) become irrelevant. Consider the following dataset:

	Treatment	Control
Men	2.0, 2.1, 2.2, 2.3, 2.4	1.0, 1.1, 1.2, 1.3, 1.4
Women	1.0, 1.1, 1.2, 1.3, 1.4	2.0, 2.1, 2.2, 2.3, 2.4

When the main effect of Treatment is examined, collapsing across Gender, no difference is detected between the treatment groups.

	Treatment	Control
Men and Women	1.0, 1.1, 1.2, 1.3, 1.4, 2.0, 2.1, 2.2, 2.3, 2.4	1.0, 1.1, 1.2, 1.3, 1.4, 2.0, 2.1, 2.2, 2.3, 2.4

A similar result occurs for the Gender effect, such that no difference is detected between men and women when collapsing across Treatment. Yet there appears to be real differences among the four groups when we take both Treatment and Gender into consideration. Examining the full ANOVA model, we find that Gender and Treatment have no significant main effects; however, the Gender × Treatment interaction is clearly significant, $F(1, 16) = 200$, $p < 0.0001$. Of course, ERP studies normally use more than one electrode and more than one cell per subject, leading us to the next section.

Univariate Within-Group Factors

As opposed to the previously described between-groups factors, a univariate repeated measures ANOVA involves within-group factors. A within-group factor is used when the levels of the factor are not statistically independent. For example, if the levels are repeated measurements on the same subjects, people who score high on the first level are likely to continue to score high on subsequent levels. A within-group factor takes this correlation among levels into account by controlling for it in the analysis. Each subject providing repeated measurements is treated as a level in a subject factor. Although the statistical significance of the subject factor is usually not of theoretical interest, the benefit is comparable to the situations previously described in that it accounts for variance that would otherwise be treated as error variance.

The chief difference between the within-groups factors and the between-groups factors discussed above is the involvement of subject factors. Subject factors are normally *random* factors, which are fundamentally different from the *fixed* factors discussed thus far. For fixed factors, the assumption is that the levels included in the analysis represent the factor in its entirety. Thus, if one is interested in comparing a set of five types of treatment, one might make each treatment a level in a Treatment factor. A random factor treats the set of levels as a random sample of all possible levels of a factor. Thus, five levels of Treatment may be selected and examined as representative of all available treatments. The advantage of this procedure is that one may then generalize beyond the set of levels in the analysis. The disadvantage is that this reduces the power of the statistical test.

As researchers do not usually determine the significance of the subject factor, it may seem odd to examine whether it is fixed or random in nature. Certainly, a subject factor should normally be treated as random, as subjects are usually assumed to be a random sample of a population. More importantly, the use of subjects in a random factor also has implications for the statistical calculations. The other factors in the analysis cannot be calculated properly when the subject factor is defined as fixed. With a fixed subject factor, each cell in the ANOVA matrix contains only a single value (e.g., the single reading of electrode 5 in task 1 for subject 1). With only a single value in each cell, the within-group variance, e, equals zero; in effect, all error variance has been attributed to individual difference. As division by zero is not possible, one cannot calculate an F-ratio with this within-group variance. When we include a random factor in the design, we use the interaction term between each fixed factor and the random factor in place of the within-groups variance. These interaction terms reflect the extent to which the content of each cell cannot be modeled as simply the sum of a main effect for each individual plus a main effect of the fixed factor. Therefore, examining subjects as levels of a random factor allows for the mathematical computation of the F-ratio with an MS_w that is adjusted for deviation from the sum of the main effects.

Another counterintuitive characteristic is that including a random effect, such as a subjects factor, may yield substantial changes in the tests for the remaining factors in a design. The following example illustrates the reason that the tests for the fixed factors are changed in the presence of a random factor (adapted from Maxwell & Delaney, 1990). Consider a population of 18 undergraduate participants in a Novelty P3 paradigm, each with an auditory N1 evoked by frequent tones, rare tones, and novel environmental sounds, thus comprising two fixed factors, Stimulus (3 levels) and Subject (18 levels).

	Subjects																		
Stimulus	a	b	c	d	e	f	g	h	i	j	k	l	m	n	o	p	q	r	Mean
Standard	.7	.6	.5	.7	.6	.5	.4	.4	.4	.1	.2	.3	.4	.4	.4	.1	.2	.3	**.4**
Rare	.4	.4	.4	.1	.2	.3	.7	.6	.5	.7	.6	.5	.1	.2	.3	.4	.4	.4	**.4**
Novel	.1	.2	.3	.4	.4	.4	.1	.2	.3	.4	.4	.4	.7	.6	.5	.7	.6	.5	**.4**
Mean	**.4**	**.4**	**.4**	**.4**	**.4**	**.4**	**.4**	**.4**	**.4**	**.4**	**.4**	**.4**	**.4**	**.4**	**.4**	**.4**	**.4**	**.4**	.4

In this dataset there are no main effects for either stimulus type or subject. Consider the situation when only three subjects are examined as a random sample of the program, thus analyzing one fixed factor, Stimulus (3 levels), and one random factor, Subject (3 levels).

	Subjects			
Stimulus	g	k	r	mean
Standard	.4	.2	.3	.300
Rare	.7	.6	.4	.567
Novel	.1	.4	.5	.333
Mean	.4	.4	.4	.4

Although the effect of Subject remains null, the variability of the Stimulus factor has been increased. Mathematically, the F-ratio of the fixed effect

$$F = \frac{MS_{bet}}{MS_w} = \frac{e + a}{e}$$

has changed to

$$F = \frac{MS_{bet}}{MS_w} = \frac{e + a + r}{e}$$

in which r is the increased variance added by the random factor. The addition of this variance has artificially inflated the F-ratio, creating a positive bias. Using the MS of the interaction between the fixed factor and random factor as the denominator corrects the bias. As there is only one value in each cell, there is no within-cell variability and, thus, e equals zero. Thus, we omit e from the equation,

$$F = \frac{MS_{bet}}{MS_w} = \frac{r + a}{r}$$

yielding an equation that is equivalent to the usual test of a fixed effect, such that the numerator differs from the denominator by only the magnitude of the effect of interest.

A repeated measures analysis of this type is called a *mixed model*, as it contains both fixed and random factors. If, in addition, the design contains a between-groups factor, such as gender, it is often called a *split-plot* analysis. The between-groups factor splits the sample into groups and the mixed model is computed and compared across groups.

Univariate ANOVA Assumptions

Univariate repeated measures ANOVA requires three assumptions (Stevens, 1999):

1. Multivariate normality
2. Multisample sphericity
3. Independence

Two examples of how *univariate* normality may be violated is the presence of non-normal skew and kurtosis. Skew refers to the extent to which the distribution mode tends toward one side of the median or the other. Kurtosis refers to the extent to which the curve is too flat or too peaked relative to a normal distribution. Researchers have long thought ANOVAs to be robust to violations of univariate normality (Glass, Peckham, & Sanders, 1972), although more current studies suggest that this is not the case (Wilcox, 2001).

Multivariate normality means that not only individual variables but also all possible linear combinations of these variables have normal distributions. In this context, the variables are the cell values. As explained later, one can compute univariate ANOVAs with multivariate calculations as well as univariate calculations. The following table (adapted from Jackson, 1991) depicts a set of values that has univariate normality but not multivariate normality.

0	1	3	6	9	12	12	9	6	3	1	0	62
1	3	7	15	25	32	32	25	15	7	3	1	166
3	7	19	40	66	84	84	66	40	19	7	3	438
6	15	40	**0**	138	176	176	138	**168**	40	15	6	918
9	25	66	138	225	287	287	225	138	66	25	9	1500
12	32	84	176	287	367	367	287	176	84	32	12	1916
12	32	84	176	287	367	367	287	176	84	32	12	1916
9	25	66	138	225	287	287	225	138	66	25	9	1500
6	15	40	**168**	138	176	176	138	**0**	40	15	6	918
3	7	19	40	66	84	84	66	40	19	7	3	438
1	3	7	15	25	32	32	25	15	7	3	1	166
0	1	3	6	9	12	12	9	6	3	1	0	62
62	166	438	918	1500	1916	1916	1500	918	438	166	62	

Note that the marginal values have a normal distribution, whereas the table as a whole does not, due to the four values in the middle (highlighted in bold). This example violates multivariate normality, as there appears to be an interaction effect between the variable distributions. In other words, the distribution of one variable is different at particular points in the distribution of another variable. Multivariate normality requires that individual variable distributions (marginal values) and combinations of these values (cell values) be normal distributions.

Multisample sphericity (Huynh, 1978) is an important consideration as psychophysiological experiments are especially prone to violating the assumption (Vasey & Thayer, 1987). Sphericity requires that the variances of the difference scores between all possible pairs of variables be equal. To calculate sphericity, one may calculate the variance of the difference scores from the covariance matrix. The following is an example of a covariance matrix (S) with sphericity (Stevens, 1990). The cells on the diagonal contain the variances of the three variables ($y1$, $y2$, and $y3$), and the off-diagonal cells contain the covariances for each pairwise combination of the three variables.

	$y1$	$y2$	$y3$
$y1$	1.0	.5	1.5
$y2$	.5	3.0	2.5
$y3$	1.5	2.5	5.0

The formula for the variance of the difference scores is

$$s_{i-j}^2 = s_i^2 + s_j^2 - 2s_{ij}$$

where s is the standard deviation of a variable, i is the first variable of the difference score, and j is the second variable of the difference score. The variances for the differences for each pair of variables is

$$s_{1-2}^2 = s_1^2 + s_2^2 - 2S_{12} = 1 + 3 - 2(.5) = 3$$

$$s_{1-3}^2 = 1 + 5 - 2(1.5) = 3$$

$$s_{2-3}^2 = 3 + 5 - 2(2.5) = 3$$

A special case of sphericity, when the variances of difference scores are all equal to each other and the covariances of difference scores are all equal to each other, is called *compound symmetry*. Compound symmetry is unlikely for scalp electrodes because neighboring sites will likely covary more than distant sites. A similar situation arises when considering time intervals between repeated measurements; smaller time intervals will result in higher covariances, leading to a violation of compound symmetry and, likely, a violation of sphericity in general.

Statisticians currently agree that available tests for sphericity, such as Mauchly's W, are not very useful (Keselman et al., 1980). One major problem is that they are overly sensitive to departures from normality. Therefore, they might indicate a violation of sphericity when in fact there is a minor violation of normality instead. Additionally, these indexes provide no additional information beyond what the corrected univariate and multivariate tests already provide. Instead, epsilon indexes, as described next, are more often used to assess sphericity.

Epsilon indexes represent departures from sphericity. The epsilon index ranges from 1.0 (no departure) to the reciprocal of the number of levels in the factor minus 1 (maximum heterogeneity). In equation form, the lower bound for epsilon is

$$\frac{1}{(a-1)}$$

where a is the number of levels in the repeated measures factor. The epsilon value is multiplied with the degrees of freedom of the numerator and denominator of the F-value. Note that this correction factor may be used as a direct measure of sphericity. Each factor will have a separate epsilon value.

In effect, epsilon reflects the amount of statistical power that is sacrificed due to the deviation from sphericity. A problem is that in a dataset with heterogeneous error terms, a pooled (or averaged) error term will be too high for some tests and too low for others. The original Greenhouse-Geisser lower bound epsilon estimate adjusts the F-tests as if the error term is too low for all factors. Thus, this epsilon correction tends to overcorrect the degrees of freedom and yields statistically conservative estimates.

Two corrections to the original epsilon computation have been proposed. The Greenhouse-Geisser (or Box) epsilon-hat is an improvement but tends to be too conservative. For a true e of 1.00 with two groups and 15 subjects, Maxwell and Arvey

(1982) found that the Greenhouse-Geisser calculation gave an estimate of .688. The Huynh-Feldt epsilon-tilde tends to be too liberal to the extent that it can actually exceed 1.0 (in which case it is treated as 1.0 in practice). There is a lack of a consensus on which index to use. One recommendation that we tentatively endorse is to use the average of the two epsilon estimates (Stevens, 1996). Unfortunately, commercial statistics packages do not currently offer this as an output option, so it is not readily available, short of manually calculating the corrected degrees of freedom and then consulting a significance table.

Studies with between-groups factors require *multisample sphericity* (Huynh, 1978), meaning that the covariance matrices across the different levels of the between-groups factor should be identical. To minimize the negative effects of heterogeneous matrices, ANOVA designs should be balanced for the between-groups factors, such as gender. Glass (1972) emphasized that ANOVAs are especially sensitive to violations of assumptions in cases with unequal sample sizes. Effective corrections for testing contrasts are available in the case of such violations (Keselman, Keselman, & Shaffer, 1991).

Independence means that each of the observations is uncorrelated with the others. Lack of independence can impose a large amount of bias in statistical analysis. For example, in an analysis of three groups with 30 subjects in each, a mere .10 intraclass correlation results in a type I error rate of .4917, almost ten times the expected rate of .05 (Scariano & Davenport, 1987). The problem exacerbates with larger sample sizes. Repeated measures methodology does not protect against violations of this assumption because it corrects only lack of independence in main effects due to individual differences, not variance due to error. Therefore, statistical analyses that better account for correlated error variances across repeated measures (such as time series analysis) would be more appropriate. Epsilon correction factors do not correct for lack of independence as some assert (e.g., Hamm, Johnson, & Kirk, 2002).

Multivariate Between-Groups Factors

A multivariate analysis of variance (MANOVA) may be described as an ANOVA that is generalized to handle a set of dependent variables simultaneously. The computation of MANOVA effects with a set of dependent measures is similar to that for ANOVA with a single dependent measure. MANOVA computations use the best linear composite of the dependent measures on each level of an independent variable. The advantage of analyzing the dependent measures as a set is that it may detect subtle effects that are consistent across the set of variables that might not be noted when one tests the variables singly (Davidson, 1972). The presence of multiple dependent variables makes the mathematics of a MANOVA much more complex.

Let us first consider a MANOVA without any within factors. Whereas an ANOVA has a single score for each observation, a MANOVA has a matrix of scores. We may observe the parallel by proceeding through step-by-step in a hypothetical ERP example (adapted from a discussion in Tabachnick & Fidell, 1989). The analysis compares the effects of two between-groups factors (treatment and symptom severity) on the peak microvolt amplitude of the Novelty P3 and the P300. There are three subjects in each of the six cells, for a total of 18 observations.

	Mild		Moderate		Severe	
	nP3	P3	nP3	P3	nP3	P3
Treatment	4	4	3	3	2	2
	2	4	3	2	3	3
	3	2	2	2	2	2
Control	2	2	1	2	1	1
	1	2	2	1	2	1
	1	1	1	2	1	1

We shall compare an ANOVA of this data using the Novelty P3 to a MANOVA using both Novelty P3 and P300 scores. The data for the first cell (mild disability with treatment) in the ANOVA would be 4, 2, and 3. For the MANOVA, the data for these three subjects are [4 4], [2 4], and [3 2] for the Novelty P3 and the P300, respectively. The brackets denote an array, an ordered set of numbers that are manipulated in parallel. When computing an ANOVA, one calculates the within and between sums of squares (SS). The within SS for the first cell would require first taking its mean ($M = 3$), subtracting it from each score, yielding 1, -1, and 0, respectively. To form the within variance for the first cell, square and sum these numbers ($1 + 1 + 0 = 2$). To form the total within SS for the dataset, calculate and then sum the within variance for every cell (5.33). Convert the total within SS to a mean square variance (MS) by dividing it by the within degrees of freedom ($5.33/14 = .38$). Then compare the within MS to the between MS in the form of an F-ratio. For the Novelty P3, the treatment factor yields a significant effect: $F(1, 14) = 21.0$, $p = .0004$.

In a MANOVA, the procedure is similar. The within matrix for the first cell is computed by taking the means for both dependent variables ($M = 3$ and 3.3, for nP3 and P3, respectively) and subtracting them from each score, yielding [1 .7], [-1 .7], and [0 -1.3]. The matrix of scores is squared (i.e., premultiplied by its transposed matrix). For the first child, the resulting sums of squares and cross-products are

|1.0 .70|

|.70 .49|

Add the squared matrices for each subject together to produce the multivariate equivalent of the univariate *SS* value. Finally, to conduct the significance test, measure the variance of each matrix using a *determinant*, a single number that represents the extent to which the data vary in a multivariate context. A determinant can be utilized in one of several multivariate statistics that tests significance and is comparable to the univariate *F*-test.

Researchers have developed specialized *F*-tests for testing the multiple dimensions considered in MANOVA. The four common ways of testing these multiple numbers are Wilks' Lambda, Roy's Greatest Root, the Hotelling-Lawley Trace, and the Pillai-Bartlett Trace. Extensive comparisons among these computations have shown that for both optimal power and robustness to violations of assumptions the Pillai-Bartlett trace is recommended, although the Wilks' Lambda historically has been the most utilized (Olson, 1976, 1979; but see Stevens, 1979). Note that when comparing only two groups, all four methods produce the same result (all are identical to Hotelling's T^2). A complication of the MANOVA process arises when comparing more than two groups. Given three groups, for instance, comparisons of interest may be between group 1 vs. groups 2 and 3, or between group 2 vs. groups 1 and 3, or so on. Given k groups and p predictors, there will be a number of combinations equal to the lesser of $k - 1$ and p. Each combination represents a potential dimension of difference between the groups.

Multivariate Within-Groups Factors

The multivariate analog of a repeated measures ANOVA is a *profile analysis*. Profile analysis is similar to the previously described MANOVA in that it incorporates more than one dependent measure and rests on the same assumptions. Profile analysis differs from the general MANOVA in that within-group factors are also analyzed. Thus, profile analysis is a more specialized type of MANOVA with the goal of testing the relations among the dependent measures as well as grouping factors. This goal is accomplished through the testing of three hypotheses: levels (main effect of grouping factor), flatness (main effect of within-groups factor), and parallelism (interaction).

Profile analysis requires an additional step of transforming the p variables into $p - 1$ linear combinations. One can compute the linear combinations in any number of ways as long as the resulting dataset comprises orthogonal scores. This step is normally invisible to the statistics user unless they wish to use specific linear combinations (e.g., polynomial series) and examine the results. The linear combinations are used to perform interaction tests. For example, consider the cell means in the following hypothetical Novelty P3 dataset with two within-groups factors, Stimulus (three levels) and Treatment (two levels), using Novelty P3 microvolt amplitude as the dependent variable.

	Standard	Rare	Novel
Control	3	4	5
Treatment	6	7	8

Tests of main effects for Treatment are expected to be significant; there is a difference of $+3$ between the two levels of Treatment for all three levels of Stimulus. The same process would be used for the effect of Stimulus (flatness).

For the interaction test, the scores might be converted into the following difference scores (the exact set of difference scores is arbitrary, as long as they represent an orthogonal set of $p - 1$ linear combinations, where p is the number of levels in the within factor): $D1 = $ Rare $-$ Standard and $D2 = $ Novel $-$ Rare.

	D1	D2
Control	+1	+1
Treatment	+1	+1

A test of these linear combinations using MANOVA (i.e., a profile analysis) is equivalent to performing a test of the interaction effect when using individual scores, rather than forming linear combinations. Clearly, in this case, there is no interaction among the differences because they are all the same value. Thus, the interaction effects that are derived in profile analysis may be computed using MANOVA with difference scores between dependent measures. Note that if there are only two dependent measures, then the test becomes identical to the univariate ANOVA performed on a single difference score.

Before shifting to the assumptions underlying multivariate analyses, it may be worth addressing a common source of confusion. Repeated measures can be arranged either in a univariate format (each data point in a separate row and identified by condition codes) or in a multivariate format (each subject's data points in the same row). The choice of data format is a separate issue from the choice of test statistic. Commercial statistics packages often use the multivariate format to compute the sums of squares using multivariate computations for reasons of efficiency, even when generating univariate statistics. For this reason, even univariate repeated measures statistics are often provided through the MANOVA functionality. However, if the test with repeated measures is an epsilon-corrected F test, it is not a MANOVA, no matter the label of the statistics module.

Multivariate ANOVA Assumptions

Similar to the univariate approach, multivariate normality and independence are assumptions (see previous discussion). Sphericity, by contrast, is not a requirement for multivariate analyses. Multivariate analyses account for differences in measure-to-measure covariances when computing test statistics. Although multisample sphericity is not required, the covariance matrices must be homogenous across levels of grouping factors.

An important limitation to multivariate tests is that they cannot be used when there are more variables than observations for mathematical reasons (the degrees of freedom of the denominator becomes zero or negative). This limitation refers not to the total number of scores per subject but rather the total number of levels for that one factor. Thus, for an electrode main effect, one would need more observations than electrodes. For testing interactions, the number of subjects needed is one less than the number of each of the levels, multiplied by each other (i.e., $[j-1][k-1][m-1]$). A dataset with only two-level factors would have no mathematical difficulties.

Applications to ERPs

Having completed the general review of repeated measures ANOVA, we can now address five special issues evoked when applying it to ERP datasets. The *Psychophysiology* editors have comprehensively addressed other more general considerations in ERP analysis (Picton et al., 2000).

Outliers   Although ANOVAs may be robust to deviations from normality, given equal numbers of subjects across levels of factors, they are quite sensitive to outliers. This is an issue for ERP data due to the occasional presence of artifacts or bad channels that escape detection. The following example shows this (from Stevens, 1990):

Gp1	Gp2	Gp3
15	17	6
18	22	9
12	15	12
12	12	11
9	20	11
10	14	8
12	15	13
20	20	30
	21	7

Upon examining the dataset, the value of 30 in group 3 appears to be an outlier. If the data point is included in the ANOVA, statistical significance is not attained at an alpha level of .05, $F(2, 25) = 2.61$, $p < .095$. However, with the outlier subject's data deleted, the results are statistically significant, $F(2, 24) = 11.18$, $p < .0004$. By omitting the outlier case, power of the test increases in two ways. First, the group mean for group 3 is reduced (11.89 with the case included, 9.65 when omitted), thus enhancing its distinction from the other two groups in this case. Secondly, the within variance of the cells is reduced and, thus, the pooled error term decreases.

Electrode × Condition Interactions   A second issue concerns interactions involving electrode factors (McCarthy & Wood, 1985). Consider a case where the P300 is measured at Cz, Pz, and Oz in response to Frequent and Rare stimuli. Following is the windowed mean amplitudes of the grandaveraged data.

	Cz	Pz	Oz
Frequent	1 μv	2 μv	1 μv
Rare	2 μv	4 μv	2 μv

In this experiment, we find that rare stimuli yield a P300 peak that is twice as large as frequent stimuli. Looking at the values for the three sites, we find that the readings have doubled at each site when rare stimuli were presented, compared to responses to frequent stimuli. The ANOVA results would be ideal if they stated whether there is: (1) a significant Stimulus effect, indicating that the frequency of stimuli makes a difference; (2) a significant Site effect, such that the center site detects a reading twice as large as the others; and (3) no interaction where the amplitude, but not the peak, is changing sites between the two conditions. Unfortunately, the ANOVA will not work this way. It will note that the rare effect is +1 for Cz and Oz but +2 for Pz. Because the effect of the frequency depends on the site, it will indicate there is an interaction. The problem is that an ANOVA looks for additive differences between groups, whereas in ERP data one tends to have multiplicative differences (in this example, a doubling). Thus, when one observes a site × frequency interaction, this does not necessarily mean that the centers of the ERP patterns are different in the two conditions.

McCarthy and Woods (1985) suggested that this complication could be addressed by following up with a test to confirm the electrode site effect. They described three methods for doing this, the second of which (vector scaling) they recommended and which has been adopted widely. In this procedure, the cells corresponding to each effect other than electrode are separately scaled by dividing the scores on the effect by the square root of their summed squares; in the present example, first the three Frequent values would be scaled, then the three Rare values. This procedure is intended to subtract the experimental effects, leaving only the electrode site differences, as can be seen below. If an ANOVA still produces a significant electrode interaction with the vector scaled data, the conclusion is that the interaction effect was in fact due to a topography change. Haig, Gordon, and Hook (1997) made a strong case that this vector scaling procedure should be applied "within-subject," applied separately to each subject's data rather than "between-subject" by pooling all the subject data and applying the same vector scaling to the aggregate data.

	Cz	Pz	Oz
Frequent	0.4 μv	0.8 μv	0.4 μv
Rare	0.4 μv	0.8 μv	0.4 μv

Some caveats are required to use this procedure appropriately. The first is that vector scaling is intended only to provide a test of the reliability of the interaction; the scaled numbers should not be directly interpreted as providing information about the scalp topography (Haig, Gordon, & Hook, 1997; Ruchkin, Johnson, & Friedman, 1999). When reporting results, one should indicate that the reliability of the interaction was confirmed with the procedure but nothing more need be reported.

A second caveat is that a significant interaction test can be caused by the presence of substantial levels of noise (Urbach & Kutas, 2002). The problem is that the scaling procedure estimates an amplitude measure for each set of electrode recordings. The background noise will affect the estimate of low-amplitude cells more than high-amplitude cells. This differential effect can result in an intact electrode interaction even in the absence of a true topography change. Although these authors argue that the vector scaling test is therefore invalid, we suggest instead a more moderate course. As long as it can rule out at least some interactions as not being reliable, the procedure still has utility. Given a significant interaction, authors should then graph the interacting cells to determine if the interaction is due to a topography change or due to insufficient correction for scaling. If the two graphs have the same relative distributions across the electrodes and differ only in the relative amplitude, then one can conclude that the significant interaction is instead due to insufficient correction by the vector scaling.

A third caveat is that activity in the baseline period can also produce artifactual significance in the vector scaling test (Urbach & Kutas, 2002). Because the baseline period is normally used to estimate the value of true zero in the EEG, activity in this period can result in misestimates of zero (Picton et al., 2000). The vector scaling test assumes that scalp topographies can only differ in shape (significant interaction) or in scaling (nonsignificant interaction). If, instead, the two scalp topographies differ in terms of their offset from "true" zero, then even identical scalp topographies may produce significant vector scaled interactions. Although this issue is a serious one, it is not grounds for discarding the test, as some advocate (Urbach & Kutas, 2002), because baseline effects are an issue for all ERP analyses. Taken to the extreme, one would have to abandon all ERP analyses by this logic.

One can also address this issue by mean-centering the data in each cell, prior to scaling them. The logic is the same as that used when standardizing data in statistical analyses. Even in the vector length framework McCarthy and Wood invoke, it is customary to correct for offsets from the origin. Mean-centering should be used judiciously because it can also eliminate genuine topographical differences. Haig, Gordon, & Hook (1997) provide an example of this scenario in a critique of McCarthy and Wood's other suggested approach, the normalization test, which has a similar issue. The researcher would have to make the case whether baseline correction or mean-centering provides a better approximation of zero. Standard vector scaling should be used if one can argue that baseline period activity is not present. Mean-centering should be used if one can argue that there is no danger of topographies differing by a fixed constant, as can happen if the electrode sites do not equally sample both sides of the dipolar field.

Reference Sites   A third issue to note is that ANOVA results are dependent on the reference scheme. A given dataset will produce different results when re-referenced. ANOVAs of ERP data are in effect contrasts between the recording sites and the reference site(s). Changing the reference site therefore changes the analysis results. The closer the reference site is to the tested electrode, the less likely significance will be detected. Dien (1998) offers a complete discussion.

Degrees of Freedom   A fourth issue is that using large numbers of individual electrode factors could inappropriately inflate the degrees of freedom (Robert Mauro, personal communication, 1994). The more observations entered into an ANOVA, the more reliable the results are assumed to be. This assumption is embodied in the decreasing levels of F-ratios necessary to meet significance thresholds with increasing degrees of freedom. However, in ERP data there are at least two relevant sources of error. The first is simple measurement imprecision. The second is subject variability, in the sense that individual differences exist in the nature of the signal due to differences in cognitive strategies and functional neuroanatomy. Increasing the number of electrode observations will help to attenuate the first source of error but not the second. The ANOVA procedure inappropriately treats both increases in number of subjects and number of electrodes as equivalent in regards to degrees of freedom. It seems quite evident to casual consideration that the quality of data provided by a hundred electrodes measured from two subjects is not equivalent to that provided by two electrodes from a hundred subjects for the purpose of making general conclusions about the population of all humans.

Electrode Factors   A final issue is that accounting for effects of important grouping factors in the presence of electrode factors requires careful thought. For example, if left hemisphere electrodes are likely to be systematically different from right hemisphere electrodes, then these effects should be separated by a hemisphere factor. Likewise, if dorsal locations are likely to vary systematically from ventral locations, one should include the dorsal-ventral factor. Taking such factors into consideration may reduce the error variance that includes the test for statistical significance, and add information about the conditions under which the other examined factors have effects.

A note of caution for adding factors is in order. If an additional factor does not represent a real source of variance, it may undermine the effects of other important factors in the analysis. Each additional term tested exacts a cost in the degrees of freedom for the MS_w, thus increasing the F-value necessary for statistical significance. If this cost in degrees of freedom is not offset by increased accuracy, as in the above examples, then the additional factor may be detrimental to the power of the test. Thus, researchers should avoid adding unnecessary factors. One should add grouping factors only if past evidence or theory-driven logic provides a rationale for doing so.

Another important consideration for an ERP researcher arises when matching variables on levels of a between-groups factor. Matched levels on a grouping factor must be comparable to be meaningful. Consider a case where the electrode locations are divided into two factors, a hemisphere factor and a location factor. The first factor divides the readings from the two sides of the head. The second factor consists of the locations ranging along the sides of the head, mirrored on the two sides. In this case, electrode pairs such as P3 and P4 will be matched on the hemisphere factor and will be treated as identical by the location factor test. The task of making sites comparable becomes even more complex when adding other factors such as anterior-posterior or dorsal-ventral to the analysis. Moreover, sites that do not have matching sites must be dropped from the analysis. For example, the sites along the midline must be dropped when hemisphere is used as the matching factor.

Suggested Data Analysis Procedure

Based on this review of univariate and multivariate repeated measures methodology, we will make two suggestions regarding how to optimize ERP data analysis: (1) employ multivariate statistical techniques; or (2) block electrode measures by region.

Use Multivariate Test Statistics

Both the epsilon-corrected univariate and the multivariate test statistics in repeated measures designs are considered to provide equivalent type I error control (rate of false positives that is equal or less than the nominal alpha); the question therefore is which provides more statistical power or ability to detect true differences (Stevens, 1999). Although the univariate approach is commonly regarded as more powerful, in actuality statisticians generally agree that it depends on the data being analyzed (Davidson, 1972).

The multivariate technique uses information about the interrelationships among dependent variables, whereas the univariate does not. When the population lacks sphericity, the multivariate approach is able to take those relationships into account; when sphericity is present, the univariate tests ignore any departures from it as random error. For example, at the $e = .49$ level the multivariate test can be roughly twice as powerful (Rasmussen, Heumann, & Botzum, 1989). Note that when the factor has only two levels, the univariate and multivariate approaches are literally the same, so no comparison is necessary. Other factors affecting relative power include the number of variables and the number of subjects (Davidson, 1972).

There is little consensus regarding when to use which type of statistic. Some statisticians advocate using the multivariate statistic unless the number of subjects n is less than $a + 20$ (Davidson, 1972) or $a + 10$ (Maxwell & Delaney, 1990), where a is the number of levels in the factor tested minus one. Others suggest using the multivariate test at low epsilons and the univariate at high epsilons (Rasmussen, Heumann, & Botzum, 1989). A recent simulation study suggests that all three parameters (number of subjects, number of levels, and epsilon value) need to be taken into account and provides some fairly complex guidelines (Algina & Keselman, 1997). Because predicting which will be more powerful is a complex endeavor, we echo the statisticians who have suggested the simpler procedure of using both epsilon-corrected univariate and multivariate tests in all cases, with the use of a .025 alpha to maintain the familywise type I error rate (Barcikowski & Robey, 1984; Looney & Stanley, 1989; Stevens, 1999). A recent evaluation of this strategy showed that it did not inflate the type I error rate but did not address its effect on power (Keselman, Keselman, & Lix, 1995). A possible exception is the case of an unbalanced design (between-subjects factors with unequal numbers of subjects per cell), for which the Welch-James test has been strongly recommended if the sample size is sufficiently large (Keselman, 1998). Because datasets from different labs will differ, it may be best to first evaluate the procedure against existing datasets before adopting this recommendation. Because the degrees of freedom of the interaction terms must be larger than the number of subjects to utilize the multivariate test statistics, we therefore make the second major recommendation of this review.

Regional Averaging

For exploratory statistical analysis of high-density montages, divide the electrodes into regions. Averaging the electrodes into regions has a number of advantages. It considerably improves ease of interpretation by organizing the factors and levels into descriptive units (e.g., posterior vs. anterior). It reduces the problem of magnitude changes showing up as significant interactions with location (cf. McCarthy & Wood, 1985). It provides a better fit to the ANOVA or MANOVA model by collapsing together electrodes that commonly covary, in much the same way that adding a factor will do, but without complicating the analysis by adding interaction terms. It helps control erratic locations by averaging them with other locations. The reduced number of variables allows the use of multivariate statistics. Finally, this method addresses the objection to the large, and probably illegitimate, degrees of freedom the multiple electrode readings afford.

A simple scheme would use three two-level regional factors: left vs. right hemisphere, anterior vs. posterior, and ventral vs. dorsal (lower vs. upper). The use of two-level factors for the regional averages facilitates the analysis. Two-level factors do not require epsilon correction factors for the univariate tests, as the levels are automatically spherical. Significant effects become easy to interpret, as there is no question where the differences lie. Only the task factor(s) may have multiple levels, simplifying matters. When computing the degrees of freedom needed for a multivariate interaction term, two-level factors are free in that they don't increase the number of necessary subjects. This scheme therefore makes it more feasible to use multivariate statistics. The primary objection to this regional approach is that it loses the fine resolution afforded by the high-density electrode net. One may address this objection by using follow-up descriptive analyses.

Example Data Analysis #1

For the following example, we have drawn data from an unpublished dataset. Thirty University of Oregon undergraduate students participated to help meet course requirements. For each of eight blocks of trials, subjects rated the same 45 five-letter stimulus words on a different adjective scale (e.g., good versus bad). Trials consisted of a one-second recording epoch followed by a subject response period. Each trial began with a 185-ms prestimulus baseline period. Words were then flashed on the screen for 810 ms; subjects were instructed to concentrate on emotionally judging the stimulus during this time. After an approximate 2-s pause, a rating scale appeared on the screen. The subject would then record his or her rating of the stimulus. A variable delay of 0–2 s ensued to minimize the contingent negative variation, followed by the next trial. Event-related potentials were measured from 65 electrodes, which were then average referenced. For the following analysis, the mean of the window from 284–334 ms. poststimulus was computed in the averaged data. The data are divided into three cells: words generally rated negative, neutral, and positive. The question is whether the emotional value of the words affected the ERP response.

Dataset Preparation

The variable names begin with a task condition identifier and end with the electrode number. The names contain a regional code to help identify their location:

A = Anterior
P = Posterior
L = Left
R = Right
D = Dorsal (upper)
V = Ventral (lower)

The electrodes are divided along three dimensions: anterior-posterior (AP), hemisphere (HEM), and dorsal-ventral (DV). Each of the eight regions thus formed have six or seven electrodes, for a total of 52 out of the full 65 measured sites. We have dropped electrodes located on region boundaries, such as the midline, or in outside positions, such as eye electrodes, from this example analysis.

As an initial screening, the data should be checked carefully for typographical errors and mislabeled variables. Then, compute means for each of these eight regions for each task. For example, combine and average electrodes 4, 7, 8, 11, 14, 15 and 19 for the task 1 condition to form TiALD. The new dataset includes 24 variables (8 regional factors × 3 tasks).

The next step is to screen the new dataset for violations of ANOVA assumptions. Problems may be detected by looking at descriptive statistics, such as the means, standard deviations, kurtosis, skewness, minimum values, and maximum values for the regional factors. Skewness and kurtosis within one or two units from the mean are acceptable, according to Glass (Glass, Peckham, & Sanders, 1972). To investigate the problem of skew, the z-score equivalents for the variables may be examined for outliers. Outliers may be specific data points, such as the result of an interruption or "glitch," or more general, such as if a subject's entire data set has been tainted by recording problems. In a normal distribution, about 99 percent of the observations should be within this three standard deviations of the mean; data with more extreme z-scores may be considered as possible outliers (Stevens, 1990). Because the decision to label extreme scores as outliers is often subjective, the best strategy for managing outliers is to verify the robustness of the properties of the dataset by examining the properties both with and without the outlier data.

In the present example, high kurtosis values are evident for variables T1PLD (4.70), T1PRD (6.36), T2ALD (8.54), T2PLD (3.06), T2PRD (8.54), T3PLD (3.03), and T3PRD (3.95). The z-scores indicate potential problems in the data that were collected from subjects 6 and 30. Both cases present at least four of 24 z-scores at magnitudes greater than 3.00. Due to the fact that several points within each case are problematic, we eliminated these subjects from the dataset.

Analysis of Variance

When looking at the output, consider significant interactions first and then, if none, interpret main effects if significant. In the presence of interactions the tests of the main effects are basically irrelevant, as discussed earlier. In the present example, one significant interaction emerged in both the multivariate and univariate tests. The multivariate results for this interaction are as follows:

	F-Value	df1	df2	Significance
Task × DV	6.86	2	26	$p = .004$

As discussed earlier, all four indexes for the multivariate F-value are the same, as the DV factor has only two levels. Thus, using the Pillai's Trace, Wilks' Lambda, Hotelling's Trace, or Roy's Largest Root will yield an F-value of 6.86 in this example.

The G-G and the H-F epsilon indexes provide information about sphericity. Recall that sphericity is a requirement for univariate repeated measures ANOVA. The general consensus in the empirical literature is that the more liberal H-F correction should only be used if there is reason to believe epsilon to be greater than .75. In this example, we estimated sphericity to be approximately 1.00 (.99 for G-G, 1.00 for H-F). Below are the univariate test results based on the G-G and H-F epsilon corrections, as well as the results based on a plausible assumption of sphericity among measures.

	Correction	F-Value	df1	df2	Significance
Task × DV	Sphericity assumed	6.97	2	54	$p = .002$
	G-G	6.97	1.98	53.37	$p = .002$
	H-F	6.97	2	54	$p = .002$

Due to compliance with the assumption of sphericity, the results are similar across the no correction, G-G correction, and H-F correction estimates.

Power estimates may be examined to investigate unexpected null results. For instance, power for the TASK × DV interaction is estimated to be 89 percent and 91 percent for the multivariate and univariate tests, respectively. Compare this to the power estimates for the nonsignificant TASK × HEM × DV interaction (16 percent for the multivariate and 24 percent for the univariate tests). These estimates suggest that, if the observed difference among the three task conditions is accurate and not due to error, then the test would only have a .16 chance of correctly reporting it as significant in the multivariate analysis (taking random error into account). This might indicate that not enough subjects were used to detect an effect of this size. Interpretation of power estimates requires reference to a measure of the effect sizes. In this case, the size is fairly small at an eta-squared value of .055 in the multivariate analysis. In the significant multivariate test of TASK × DV, the effect size was .345. Refer to earlier studies to determine the size of expected effects. If a previous study found a significant effect at the same effect size, the null effect might be the result of insufficient sample size or inflated error variance, both of which should be taken into consideration in replication studies.

Taken at face value, the significant TASK × DV interaction seems to suggest that the vertical distribution of the scalp topography differs between conditions. Application of vector scaling yields the following results:

	Test	F-Value	df1	df2	Significance
Vector scaled	Multivariate	3.12	2	27	$p = .089$
Task × DV	Univariate	3.12	2	54	$p = .052$

Strictly speaking, the nonsignificant results (with an alpha criterion of .025) indicate that there is not in fact a change in topography between task cells. This conclusion would have to be tempered by the near significance of the univariate test.

Post Hoc Examinations
When a significant effect is found, one may conduct post hoc tests to determine which levels of the factors are driving the observed effects. Because each of the eight regional factors have only two levels, such post hoc tests will only be necessary for the TASK factor with three levels. A suitable way of conducting these tests is with Hotelling t-tests. In effect, the analysis is rerun with only the two levels of TASK. The following is an example that forms a comparison between tasks 1 and 2. Looking at the TASK × DV interaction, we find that tasks 1 and 3 are significantly different.

	F-Value	df1	df2	Significance
Task 1 v. task 2	3.45	1	27	$p = .125$
Task 1 v. task 3	14.25	1	27	$p = .001$
Task 2 v. task 3	4.34	1	27	$p = .047$

When conducting post hoc tests for comparison among means, it is necessary to use a Bonferroni correction. One counts the total number of comparisons that could have been done (with k levels, there are $(k)!/2$ or in this case $(3 \times 2 \times 1)/2 = 3$ pairwise comparisons) and divides the criterion alpha level by that number. Thus, $.05/3 = .017$ is the criterion level for this test. The difference between task 2 and 3 initially would appear to be significant at the .05 level. However, due to the Bonferroni adjustment, this contrast would not be considered statistically significant ($p > .017$). See Keselman 1998 for an excellent review of multiple comparison procedures for repeated measures analysis.

Example Data Analysis #2

The following example illustrates that the proposed guidelines can make a difference to a real analysis and potentially mean the difference between being publishable or not. This dataset is a Novelty P3 dataset (Dien, Spencer, & Donchin, 2003). The data has been subjected to spatiotemporal principal components analysis (PCA) so the channels have been collapsed into factors representing scalp topographies described by the factor loadings. One factor of present interest is a frontal negativity factor, which has been localized to the orbital frontal cortex. The ANOVA has one stimulus factor (standard, target, novel).

	Test	F-Value	df1	df2	Significance
Stimulus	Multivariate	5.15	2	13	$p = .023$
	Univariate (G-G)	2.126	2	28	$p = .157$

Whereas the univariate test utterly misses significance, the multivariate test (all four are equivalent in this example) reveals significance even at the reduced alpha of .025, suggesting that the negativity is stronger for both novel and rare stimuli. As you can see, if only the univariate statistic had been reported, the effect would not even have merited mention of borderline significance.

Conclusion

Although the humble repeated measures ANOVA is often applied with little consideration, its principles can be quite complex. Misapplication of this technique can fatally flaw a study, whereas inefficient application can doom a study to nonsignificance. We hope that this review will help researchers apply this statistic to ERP datasets. Looking toward the future, note that researchers are developing new procedures that promise enhanced robustness to outliers and non-normality (Keselman, Wilcox, & Lix, 2003; Wilcox, 2001). Although ERP researchers have thus far been properly cautious about adopting these new techniques, the time may be approaching when more effective analyses may be widely available.

References

Algina, J., & Keselman, H. J. (1997). Detecting repeated measures effects with univariate and multivariate statistics. *Psychological Methods, 2*, 208–218.

Barcikowski, R. S., & Robey, R. (1984). Decisions in a single group repeated measures analysis: Statistical tests and three computer packages. *The American Statistician, 38*, 248–250.

Davidson, M. L. (1972). Univariate versus multivariate tests in repeated measures experiments. *Psychological Bulletin, 77*, 446–452.

Dien, J. (1998). Issues in the application of the average reference: Review, critiques, and recommendations. *Behavioral Research Methods, Instruments, and Computers, 30*, 34–43.

Dien, J., Spencer, K. M., & Donchin, E. (2003). Localization of the event-related potential novelty response as defined by principal components analysis. *Cognitive Brain Research, 17*, 637–650.

Glass, G. V., Peckham, P. D., & Sanders, J. R. (1972). Consequences of failure to meet assumptions underlying the fixed effects analyses of variance and covariance. *Review of Educational Research, 42*, 237–288.

Haig, A. R., Gordon, E., & Hook, S. (1997). To scale or not to scale: McCarthy and Wood revisited. *Electroencephalography and Clinical Neurophysiology, 103*, 323–325.

Hamm, J. P., Johnson, B. W., & Kirk, I. J. (2002). Comparison of the N300 and N400 ERPs to picture stimuli in congruent and incongruent contexts. *Clinical Neurophysiology, 113*, 1339–1350.

Huynh, H. (1978). Some approximate tests for repeated measurement designs. *Psychometrika, 43*, 161–175.

Jackson, J. E. (1991). *A user's guide to principal components*. New York: John Wiley & sons.

Keselman, H. J. (1998). Testing treatment effects in repeated measures designs: An update for psychophysiological researchers. *Psychophysiology, 35*, 470–478.

Keselman, H. J., Keselman, J. C., & Lix, L. M. (1995). The analysis of repeated measurements: Univariate tests, multivariate tests, or both? *British Journal of Mathematical and Statistical Psychology, 48*, 319–338.

Keselman, H. J., Keselman, J. C., & Shaffer, J. P. (1991). Multiple pairwise comparisons of repeated measures means under violation of multisample sphericity. *Psychological Bulletin, 110*, 162–170.

Keselman, H. J., Rogan, J. C., Mendoza, J. L., & Breen, L. J. (1980). Testing the validity conditions of repeated measures *F* tests. *Psychological Bulletin, 87*, 479–481.

Keselman, H. J., Wilcox, R. R., & Lix, L. M. (2003). A generally robust approach to hypothesis testing in independent and correlated groups designs. *Psychophysiology, 40*, 586–596.

Looney, S. W., & Stanley, W. B. (1989). Exploratory repeated measures analysis for two or more groups. *The American Statistician, 43*, 220–225.

Maxwell, S. E., & Arvey, R. D. (1982). Small sample profile analysis with many variables. *Psychological Bulletin, 92*, 778–785.

Maxwell, S. E., & Delaney, H. D. (1990). *Designing experiments and analyzing data*. Belmont, CA: Wadsworth Publishing Company.

McCarthy, G., & Wood, C. C. (1985). Scalp distribution of event-related potentials: An ambiguity associated with analysis of variance models. *Electroencephalography and Clinical Neurophysiology, 62*, 203–208.

Olson, C. L. (1976). On choosing a test statistic in multivariate analysis of variance. *Psychological Bulletin, 83*, 579–586.

Olson, C. L. (1979). Practical considerations in choosing a MANOVA test statistic: A rejoinder to Stevens. *Psychological Bulletin, 86*, 1350–1352.

Picton, T. W., Bentin, S., Berg, P., Donchin, E., Hillyard, S. A., Johnson, R., Miller, G. A., Ritter, W., Ruchkin, D. S., Rugg, M. D., & Taylor, M. J. (2000). Guidelines for using human event-related potentials to study cognition: Recording standards and publication criteria. *Psychophysiology, 37*, 127–152.

Rasmussen, J. L., Heumann, M. T., & Botzum, M. (1989). Univariate and multivariate groups by trials analysis under violation of variance-covariance and normality assumptions. *Multivariate Behavioral Research, 24*, 93–105.

Ruchkin, D. S., Johnson, R., Jr., & Friedman, D. (1999). Scaling is necessary when making comparisons between shapes of event-related potential topographies: A reply to Haig et al. *Psychophysiology, 36*, 832–834.

Scariano, S., & Davenport, J. (1987). The effects of violations of independence assumptions in the one-way ANOVA. *The American Statistician, 41*, 123–129.

Stevens, J. (1979). Comment on Olson: Choosing a test statistic in multivariate analysis of variance. *Psychological Bulletin, 86*, 355–360.

Stevens, J. (1990). *Intermediate statistics: A modern approach*. Hillsdale, NJ: Lawrence Erlbaum Associates.

Stevens, J. (1996). *Applied multivariate statistics for the social sciences*, 3rd ed. Mahwah, NJ: Lawrence Erlbaum Associates.

Stevens, J. (1999). *Intermediate statistics: A modern approach*, 2nd ed. Mahwah, NJ: Lawrence Erlbaum Associates.

Tabachnick, B. G., & Fidell, L. S. (1989). *Using multivariate statistics*. New York: Harper & Row, Publishers.

Urbach, T. P., & Kutas, M. (2002). The intractability of scaling scalp distributions to infer neuro-electric sources. *Psychophysiology, 39*, 791–808.

Vasey, M. W., & Thayer, J. F. (1987). The continuing problem of false positives in repeated measures ANOVA in psychophysiology: A multivariate solution. *Psychophysiology, 24*, 479–486.

Wilcox, R. R. (2001). *Fundamentals of modern statistical methods: Substantially improving power and accuracy*. New York: Springer.

II Data Analysis

5 Digital Filters in ERP Research

J. Christopher Edgar, Jennifer L. Stewart, and Gregory A. Miller

The processing of psychophysiological signals always includes some type of filtering. Although there are many different filtering techniques, all involve removing a portion of the recorded signal—either activity that is considered noise (e.g., 60-Hz activity), or some signal components to focus on others. Filtering is often conceptualized as removing particular sine wave frequencies from data that are treated as consisting solely of multiple sine waves, although the concept of filtering is entirely general, and real world signals rarely consist of invariant sine waves.

Filtering is routinely done by means of electronic circuits built into recording amplifiers or electrically interposed between the amplifier and the recording device, such as an analog-to-digital (A/D) converter. Such electronic (or *analog*) filters applied to a continuous (usually varying) voltage contrast with *digital* filters that are applied to a discrete, numeric representation of the numerically recorded signal. (For an introduction aimed at psychophysiologists, see Cook & Miller, 1992; for an extensive overview of digital filtering methods for the advanced psychophysiologist reader, see Ruchkin, 1988.) Digital filtering has several clear advantages over analog filtering (see Picton et al., 2000). First, the original data can be retained for evaluation using alternative filter settings. Second, one can construct digital filters so that they do not alter the phase (see box 5.1) of frequencies in the waveform. Third, digital filtering can more easily adapt its settings than filtering that depends on hardware components. It is generally appropriate to restrict analog filtering to what is required to prevent aliasing (due to signal frequencies too high to be represented accurately at a given sampling rate; see box 5.2) or blocking of the A/D converter (due to signal amplitude exceeding its input range) and to use digital filtering for subsequent signal analysis.

Reliance on digital filters is increasing, thanks to the pervasiveness of powerful desktop computers, along with growing interest in psychophysiological research, leading individuals, labs, and companies to create publicly available software (e.g., Wellcome Department of Cognitive Neurology [SPM], Richard Coppola [EEGSYS], Oxford Image Analysis Group [FSL], Medical Numerics [MEDx], NeuroScan [SCAN and CURRY], James Long Company [EEG Analysis System], Michael Scherg [BESA], Edwin Cook

[FWTGEN], Electrical Geodesics [Analysis Tools], Scott Makeig [EEGLAB], CorTech Labs [FreeSurfer], Neuromag [Neuromag], Brain Innovation B.V. [BrainVoyager], Brain Products Vision Analyzer) that allow investigators to manipulate and analyze psycho-physiological signals, relieving the investigator of the need to write custom digital filtering programs. However, one should use the available software only with a full appreciation for the algorithms and options it provides.

As others have explained characteristics of analog filters and differences between analog and digital filters (e.g., Coles et al., 1986; Cook & Miller, 1992; Nitschke, Miller, & Cook, 1998; Picton et al., 2000), the present discussion focuses on digital filtering techniques, emphasizing practical information of use to psychophysiologists, rather than formal mathematical treatments available in engineering and signal processing texts. This overview concludes with a discussion of filtering features in some popular software aimed at the ERP research community, with a particular focus on the variability across and within programs. We present a method to determine the gain function of a given filter, so that users of publicly available software can evaluate the behavior of the filters used.

Analog and Digital Filtering: Concepts and Terms

The most commonly considered electronic filters used in psychophysiology are *high-pass* and *low-pass*, which selectively attenuate low-frequency and high-frequency components, respectively. (More ambiguously, the term "high cutoff" can refer to the high-pass setting or the low-pass setting, and similarly for the term "low cutoff." "High-pass" and "low-pass" are unambiguous and preferable.) Deployed in series, a combination of a high-pass and a low-pass filter constitutes a *bandpass* filter, which passes frequencies within a single range. Another hybrid, the *bandstop* filter, selectively attenuates frequency components within a specified range. Typically, band-stop filters, often referred to as *notch filters*, attenuate a narrow range of frequencies in the vicinity of power line noise (50 or 60 Hz). The range of frequencies that a filter will pass without substantial attenuation is its *pass band*. The range of frequencies in which little energy is passed is the *stop band*, and the range of frequencies in which gain is intermediate is the *transition band*. In an ideal filter, there might be no transition band, or the boundary between the transition band and the pass or stop band would be discrete. In realistic filters, such boundaries cannot be so sharp; descriptions of such boundaries must be understood as approximate. In principle, one could construct a filter with any combination of pass and stop bands. One can also subject the same set of data to several filters in parallel, producing alternative sets of filtered output (e.g., for different EEG bands). Whether analog or digital, more complex filters can achieve narrower transition bands, which may be required in situations where the signal of interest and the noise or artifact to be rejected contain similar frequency components.

Box 5.1

Phase

In the context of ongoing sine waves, *phase* (or *phase angle*) refers to where in the cycle a given sinusoidal waveform is at a particular time. A sine wave starts at time t_0 and continues indefinitely, changing moment to moment; but at any given moment one can ask what the phase is of that sine wave. That is, at what point in its cycle is it? Specifying its amplitude, frequency, and phase at t_0 allows projection of its value at any future moment. If the wave starts at 0 v at time t_0, ranges from $+10$ to -10 v, and oscillates at 10 Hz (completing a cycle every 100 ms), it will return to 0 v every 50 ms. It will reach $+10$ v at 25 ms and again at 125 ms. At every multiple of 100 ms, it will be back at 0 v, headed positive. After 1000 ms, it will have completed 10 cycles and be back at 0 v.

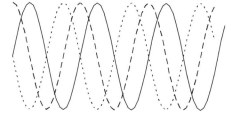

——— 0 degrees = 0 radians = 360 degrees = 2 pi radians
– – 90 degrees = pi/2 radians (= cosine at 0 degrees)
· · · 180 degrees = pi radians

There are two common conventions for quantifying the phase of a sine wave: degrees and radians. One complete cycle of a sine wave can be characterized as taking 360 degrees or as taking $2 * \text{pi}$ radians, because of the relationship of the sine function to proportions of a circle. At the beginning of a cycle, the sine wave is at 0 degrees or at 0 radians. Halfway through a cycle, a sine wave is at 180 degrees or at pi radians. After one full cycle, it is at 360 degrees or at $2 * \text{pi}$ radians, which is the same as 0 degrees or 0 radians. In the figure, the solid line is a sine wave that starts at 0 degrees and completes three cycles. The dashed line shows the same sine wave, except that the sine wave starts at its maximum positive voltage rather than at 0 v. Thus, only its phase differs from the solid line. Because 10 v is one-quarter of the full cycle of the solid line, the dashed line is said to be at a phase of 90 degrees or pi/2 radians. One can also say that the solid and dashed lines differ by 90 degrees or pi/2 radians. Finally, the dotted line is perfectly "out of phase" with the solid line, meaning that it is a mirror image, although otherwise identical. Formally, the dotted line begins at a phase (phase angle) of 180 degrees or pi radians.

Box 5.2

The Nyquist Rule and Aliasing

In order for a time series to represent a continuous waveform adequately, the *sampling rate* (f_s in samples per second, the inverse of the sampling period in seconds per sample) must be more than twice the fastest frequency present in the original waveform. (More strictly, one must sample more than twice the bandwidth, but in most applications this includes 0 Hz.) Similarly, if the sampling is of the scalp surface (via ERP electrode density), rather than time, the spatial frequency of sampling must be more than twice the spatial frequency of topographic change on the head surface (see Srinivasan, Tucker, & Murias, 1998, for more discussion of this issue). The same spatial sampling density issue arises in fMRI research. This requirement follows from the fact that only if samples are obtained at least twice per cycle can a discrete time series accurately represent the frequency of a sine wave. This axiom is referred to as *Nyquist's rule*; one-half the sampling frequency is referred to as the *Nyquist frequency*. If the rule is violated, the resulting digitized waveform may contain low-frequency components not present in the original data. This phenomenon is known as *aliasing*, because a signal component appears at a frequency in the sampled data different from its frequency in the original signal.

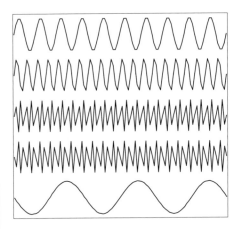

The figure illustrates the effect of aliasing. The *x* axis is 1000 ms, and the five signals are digitized at 100 Hz, thus providing a Nyquist frequency of 50 Hz. The five signals begin at 0 degrees phase and have identical amplitudes but differ in frequency, top to bottom: 10, 20, 40, 60, and 97 Hz. For the 10-Hz signal, the 100-Hz A/D rate does a good job of representing the original continuous waveform, seeming to lose just a bit at the peaks of the cycles. The 20-Hz signal is very recognizable, though the tracing is a bit choppy. Inspection verifies that 20 cycles are completed. To the eye, the 40-Hz signal looks very choppy and perhaps composed of several frequencies. But because it is below the Nyquist frequency it is still

Box 5.2
(continued)

accurately represented: there are 40 downward peaks. This illustrates that sampling at more than twice the frequency in the signal does not ensure an attractive representation. Importantly, the 60-Hz signal is misrepresented. It appears to be identical to the 40-Hz signal except for a 180-degree phase reversal. Frequency analysis would unambiguously (though incorrectly) show that it is composed of a single, pure 40-Hz component. The 60-Hz signal has been aliased down to 40 Hz, because 60 and 40 are equidistant from the Nyquist frequency of 50 Hz. Finally, the bottom tracing shows an extreme and intriguing example of aliasing. Even though the 97-Hz signal is below the 100-Hz sampling rate, the signal is very badly distorted. The signal appears to be a perfect 3-Hz signal, because 97 and three are equidistant from the Nyquist frequency. This example is particularly impressive because the time series looks deceptively clean.

We can offer several caveats regarding aliasing. First, Nyquist's rule requires sampling at twice the fastest frequency present in the original waveform—not merely twice the fastest frequency in which the investigator is interested. Second, treatment of the aliasing problem generally assumes that real-world phenomena are well represented by sinusoidal components. To the extent the raw data are not perfectly sinusoidal (and physiological data generally are not), a higher sampling frequency is necessary. Third, strict conformance to the Nyquist rule is not necessarily sufficient to provide a digitized signal that will illustrate the raw data well. Even a pure sine wave sampled at fewer than five samples per cycle may look very choppy, and signals composed of multiple components may require a much higher sample rate in order to provide good visual fidelity. The Nyquist rule only addresses the aliasing issue about whether frequencies will be systematically misrepresented. A raw signal composed of sine waves and sampled at more than twice the frequency of the highest component will not be aliased and can be treated numerically with confidence, but the vector of samples may not be very presentable graphically. Fourth, sampling density is not an issue when a single observation is of interest. For example, if the research question is focused on activity at the Cz recording site rather than on topography or source localization, the spatial density of other electrode placements is not an issue. Similarly, if one cares only about activity 400 ms after stimulus onset, one need only digitize a single value at that latency, without concern about aliasing.

Some analog filters are occasionally called *anti-aliasing filters*. This term can be confusing, as it actually refers to the use to which the filter is put rather than to any property of the filter. One can avoid aliasing by employing a low-pass analog filter prior to digitizing a signal. One would need an additional, anti-aliasing filter only if the amplifier does not provide a suitable setting relative to the frequency characteristics of the signal and the sample rate, in terms of either f_c or roll-off. Typically, anti-aliasing filters have very steep roll-offs, perhaps 45 dB/octave.

Because of possible errors in estimating the highest frequencies in real-world data, noise introduced by amplifiers and A/D converters, and the nonsinusoidal nature of many phys-

Box 5.2
(continued)

iological signals, many have suggested (e.g., Attinger, Anne, & McDonald, 1966; Coles et al., 1986) that the sample rate be as much as 5–10 times higher than the Nyquist rule suggests. On the other hand, when the noise power introduced at high frequencies is minimal, less intensive sampling may suffice and the resulting (trivially small) aliased noise ignored. A second situation in which it is sometimes possible to violate the Nyquist rule is where all high-frequency noise sources are a harmonic of a single frequency. With the right sampling period, the sampling will occur at the same phase of the noise cycle with every sample (e.g., power-line noise at 50 or 60 Hz). However, the obtained samples may include a DC offset that can vary by as much as the full peak-to-peak range of the noise, which may or may not be problematic in a given context. For example, in a long-interval CNV study, Simons, Öhman, and Lang (1979) sampled the EEG at 30 Hz, which is largely impervious to 60-Hz noise. Because they deviated epochs of interest from a prestimulus baseline, their data were not vulnerable to the DC offset problem. Aliasing is important in selecting parameters for digital data acquisition and filtering. A more rigorous treatment of aliasing, based on power spectrum analysis, appears in appendix A of Cook and Miller 1992.

For simplicity, we will largely restrict the present discussion to simple high-pass and low-pass filters, although we will note other types. Also, the present discussion will focus on filters characterized in terms of their response to sine wave input. That is how psychophysiology, including the literature on event-related brain potentials (ERPs), usually characterizes filter performance, although other approaches are possible.

In common use, the term *gain* indicates an increase in magnitude, but more generally it refers to any ratio of output to input. Gain may be greater than, equal to, or less than 1.0. In discussions of electrical circuits, one generally considers segments of the circuit designed to boost signal magnitude (gain > 1.0), regardless of frequency (amplifiers), separately from segments designed to reduce magnitude (gain < 1.0) selectively as a function of frequency (filters). Thus, filters normally have a frequency-dependent gain ranging from 0.0 to 1.0. (In some cases gain may even be negative, meaning that the polarity of the signal is inverted.) The relationship between frequency and gain is typically plotted as the *gain function* for a particular filter, with frequency on the *x* axis and signal magnitude on the *y* axis represented in amplitude (voltage) or power (roughly the square of voltage; box 5.3 discusses their relationship). Figure 5.1 illustrates the gain function for a low-pass filter. The upper left shows the ripple that some types of filters introduce in the pass-band and/or stop-band. When the gain goes below zero (or is negative), the effect is an inversion of the signal.

Filters are sometimes characterized in terms of the approximate boundaries of the transition band. Alternatively, a specific frequency within the transition band may be

Box 5.3
Power, Amplitude, and Cutoff Frequency

For expository purposes, one can often use power and amplitude interchangeably to convey the magnitude of a signal or a component of a signal. However, quantitatively, power and amplitude are not the same concepts. As a first approximation, power is the square of amplitude, so that power is never negative. More precisely, voltage = current $*$ resistance (Ohm's law), and power (in watts) = voltage $*$ current. As a result of these relationships, power = voltage $*$ voltage/resistance. Thus, power is proportional to the square of voltage. Commonly in treatments of these relationships, resistance is implicitly set to 1.0, so that power is the square of voltage.

This distinction is important in describing the characteristics of digital filters. Filters are often described in terms of the frequency at which the output of the filter is half that input. Sometimes authors put this explicitly in terms of half amplitude or half power, but often neither is specified. The frequency at which the output amplitude is half the input amplitude is not, in general, the frequency at which the output power is half the input power. This follows readily from the observation that $.707^2 = .5$. With power the square of amplitude, the frequency at which power is reduced by 50 percent is the frequency at which amplitude is reduced by 29.3 percent. Conversely, given $.5^2 = .25$, the frequency at which amplitude is reduced by 50 percent is the frequency at which power is reduced by 75 percent. Depending on the gain function of a filter, the half-amplitude and half-power frequencies may be quite different. It is important that authors (and publicly available software) make clear whether their frequency cutoffs are specified in terms of power or amplitude. In the present chapter, f_c always refers to cutoff frequency in the strict sense of the half-power frequency, following its usual definition in the electrical engineering literature. We use *cutoff frequency* more generically, referring to either half power or half amplitude. These are its common uses, but in some contexts cutoff frequency refers to some other threshold on the gain function (see Cook & Miller, 1992, for some examples).

cited as the "cutoff" or "corner" frequency, f_c. The definition of f_c varies across authors and even across amplifier manufacturers. In the electrical engineering literature, f_c is defined fairly consistently as the half-*power* frequency—that frequency within the transition band where the gain (ratio of output power to input power) is .5. Some standard sources in the psychophysiology literature also define f_c as the half-power frequency. However, other sources treat f_c as the half-*amplitude* frequency, which is not the half-*power* frequency. In addition, two other ways of reporting filter cutoffs involve the time constant and decibels (see box 5.4 and box 5.5).

Another feature of transition bands sometimes reported is the "roll-off," usually expressed in dB per unit change in frequency, usually octave (a doubling or halving of frequency) and sometimes decade (a tenfold change in frequency). Thus, a 6-dB/octave filter has a much narrower transition band (steeper roll-off) than a 6-dB/decade filter,

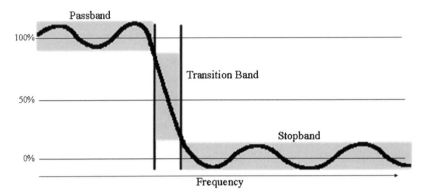

Figure 5.1
The gain function of a filter is divided into the pass band, transition band, and stop band. The gain function shown is for a low-pass filter, without magnitude as a percentage of input magnitude.

though one could describe both (ambiguously) as having a "6-dB roll-off." Note that analog and digital filters can be designed with gain functions different from those for a simple RC filter, including cascading several RC circuits in series. As a consequence, the slope or roll-off within the transition band can be more or less steep. Thus, a filter might be characterized as having a 24-dB/octave slope.

Literatures more remote from the electrical engineering tradition may use an altogether different means of characterizing filters. For example, it is common in current functional magnetic resonance literature to apply (spatial) smoothing characterized in terms of its *FWHM*, or full-width/half-maximum value. Typically, this refers to a (normally) symmetrical weighting function, and the acronym FWHM is the width (in mm) of the function at half its maximum value.

This variety of methods of characterizing filters reflects the variety of disciplines from which psychophysiology draws, but inconsistencies in reporting such characteristics can be problematic. Ideally, authors would routinely include a figure showing the gain function of their filters. Minimally, authors should report filter characteristics unambiguously. For example, one should not report a cutoff frequency without making clear whether this refers to half power, half amplitude, the start of the transition band, or some other reference point.

This discussion of analog and digital filters is equally applicable to signals sampled over time and signals sampled over space. From the standpoint of a numeric operation on a vector of values, it is irrelevant whether the values represent a phenomenon unfolding over time or over space. For practical reasons, analog filters are generally confined to time-domain applications, but digital filters are equally applicable to time and space contexts.

Box 5.4
RC Circuits, Time Constants, and Phase Delay

The time constant is a property of certain types of simple analog electrical circuits. For present purposes, a resistor (R) and a capacitor (C) in series will suffice. A constant voltage applied across this circuit (such as from a battery) will, in effect, cause charge to flow through the resistor and accumulate on the capacitor. As the charge accumulates, the capacitor begins to resist the flow of additional charge. Thus, over time, voltage builds up across the capacitor, while current through the resistor declines. The circuit reaches a steady state when the voltage across the capacitor matches the voltage applied to the circuit, at which time current is zero. The voltage build-up and current decline are mirror images, each asymptotic functions of time. The eventual voltage across the capacitor depends entirely on the voltage applied to the circuit, not on the R or C values. However, the time taken to reach asymptote does not depend at all on the applied voltage. It depends solely on the R and C values. Thus, the circuit behaves consistently over time regardless of the amplitude of the voltage input. For a given RC combination, the time constant (TC) is defined at the time in seconds to reach approximately 63 percent of the asymptotic state, and it happens that $TC = R * C$. The cutoff frequency f_c can be defined in terms of R and C: $R * C = TC = 1/(2\pi f_c)$.

This account extends readily to the case of varying voltage input that is typical of psychophysiological signals. Inversion of the polarity of the voltage source will cause current to reverse direction and charge to empty from the capacitor. The rate at which that happens is again governed by the time constant of that RC combination. Some amplifier settings are labeled in time constant units (seconds) rather than frequency units (cycles per second). Reference in the literature to the time constant of a circuit has sometimes meant the high-pass f_c. Thus, a filter might be characterized by a time constant and a low-pass f_c. However, formally this is ambiguous, as any given RC circuit can serve as either a high-pass or low-pass filter, depending on whether the voltage across the resistor or the capacitor is taken as the output of the filter. In fact, a single RC circuit can serve both functions simultaneously, such as in the crossover circuit in a multispeaker audio system, separating treble and bass frequencies for different speakers.

The role of the capacitor in RC filters accounts for the phase distortion that such filters create. It takes time for charge on the capacitor to accrue and empty, more time for lower input frequencies. Thus, the output of the circuit is a delayed representation of the input (already a distortion), and that delay varies with frequency (a further distortion). To further appreciate the phase delay inherent in a real or simulated analog filter, consider a simple RC circuit employed as a high-pass filter typically found in an amplifier. Essentially, lower frequency components of the signal are removed as their charge builds up slowly and dissipates slowly on the capacitor. Each moment's input voltage is blurred with recent moments' voltages. The filter thus has some memory. A sudden (high-frequency) change to a new input level is reflected immediately in the output until the new level has been sustained long enough to build up charge across the capacitor. There will be no noticeable

Box 5.4

(continued)

build-up if the frequency of the new input has a sufficiently high frequency. But if the new input level is sustained (low frequency or even 0 Hz—a true level change), the capacitor charge will gradually build up. Thus, the output level will reflect the input level only after some delay—a phase distortion, the degree of which depends on the frequency of the input. This is the basis of the familiar rising and falling curve associated with an RC circuit's time constant.

The amount of this phase distortion is a function of frequency. An RC filter will distort not only the latency but also the shape of the input waveform. Phase shift is of particular concern in psychophysiological research when the timing of an event (e.g., a peak of an ERP component) is the focus of investigation. Analog low-pass filters will generally increase the apparent latencies of such events, with the amount of this increase depending on the frequency components of the event and specific characteristics of the filter design—the lower the cutoff frequency (equivalently, the longer the time constant), the greater the distortion. This phase shift may be a desirable feature when the researcher seeks to replicate and extend previous research conducted with analog filters (e.g., Cook et al., 1991). Some software provides a backward filter (see Zero Phase Shift and Simulated Analog Settings section, p. 106) that allows one to compensate for the phase shift caused by the analog filters.

Issues in Understanding Digital Filters

Having reviewed some general principles and issues in filtering, we now address digital filtering more specifically. We can use the term "digital filter" for a wide range of techniques that may only have in common the fact that they are mathematical procedures that are applied to discrete numeric representations of discrete or continuous waveforms in order to selectively augment or more commonly to attenuate certain frequencies. Psychophysiologists using a wide range of physiological measures routinely work with such representations. Any parameter that can be recorded repeatedly over time or space can be treated as a vector of observations of the form:

$$X_t, X_{t+d}, X_{t+2d}, X_{t+3d}, \ldots, X_{t+nd}$$

If these values are recorded over time, the data are sometimes called a *time series*. The subscripts refer to the time at which the variable X is observed, with t the time at which recording began and d the *sampling period* (the time or distance between adjacent samples, a constant in most applications, and assumed constant in the present discussion). Event series (where time between events, in ms, differs from event to event) such as heart periods can be converted to time series with a constant sampling period (Cheung & Porges, 1977; Graham, 1978; Miller, 1986).

Box 5.5
Decibels

Characterization of the cutoff frequency of a filter in terms of decibels (dB) involves a log function of the gain, with different but equivalent equations for power and amplitude and with negative values meaning a gain less than 1.0. In dB, a gain of $(P_{out}/P_{in}) = .5$ power is $10 \log_{10}(P_{out}/P_{in}) = 10 \log_{10}(.5) = -3$ dB. A gain of $(V_{out}/V_{in}) = .5$ amplitude is $20 \log_{10}(V_{out}/V_{in}) = 20 \log_{10}(.5) = -6$ dB. As noted in box 3, voltage = current * resistance (Ohm's law), and power (in watts) = voltage * current. Therefore, power = voltage * voltage/resistance. Thus, power is proportional to the square of voltage. Commonly in treatments of these relationships, resistance is implicitly set to 1.0, and power is said to be the square of voltage. The half-power frequency f_c is often referred to as the frequency at which the gain is "3 dB down." At the half-amplitude frequency, output is 6 dB down. It must be appreciated that the half-power frequency and the half-amplitude frequency are not the same frequency, because power and amplitude are different values. That is, the frequency at which the filter will reduce the power by half is not the frequency at which it will reduce the amplitude by half. This is a common source of confusion in the ERP literature. Generally, the half-amplitude frequency will be further from the center of the passband than is the half-power frequency. A characterization of a filter in terms of the frequency at which output is cut in half is ambiguous unless it is made clear whether this is half of the power or half of the amplitude.

Representing Waveforms in the Frequency Domain

A time series that indicates voltage or some other parameter as a function of time is considered a representation "in the time domain." An alternative representation of the same information is based on the principle that any stationary waveform (i.e., from which long-term trends or changes in level have been removed and in which the frequency components do not change in amplitude or phase over time) may be represented as the sum of a set of sinusoidal waveforms, each of a different frequency and having an associated amplitude (or power) and phase. This principle (the Fourier theorem) is the basis of *Fourier analysis*, which determines the amplitudes and phases of the constituent sinusoids as a function of frequency. This representation of a signal is "in the frequency domain." A *direct Fourier transform* converts a digitally represented signal from the time domain to the frequency domain; an *inverse Fourier transform* does the converse (see box 5.6). No information is lost in either transform— each is simply a way to represent the original vector of data. Figure 5.2 provides two examples of how a set of sine waves can combine to form an apparently nonsinusoidal time series.

The interchangeability of time-domain and frequency-domain representations of a given waveform bears emphasis. Consider a set of j sine waves. Given the stationarity assumption, the frequency, amplitude, and phase of each sine wave are constant throughout the analyzed epoch. At any particular time during the epoch, the different sine waves may be at different points in their cycles. Summing across the set of sine waves produces a single composite waveform in which the constituents may be difficult to identify. One could digitize the composite waveform, describing it as a single vector of values arranged in time. Alternatively, one could describe it with amplitude and phase vectors (known as the amplitude and phase spectra) arranged in order by frequency. Either description—in the time domain or in the frequency domain—completely specifies all of the information contained in the digitized composite waveform. One description may be more tractable for a given set of analyses or more intuitively appealing for a given question, but the same information is available in the two representations. Although more familiar in analyses of ongoing EEG, one can use Fourier analysis in conventional ERP paradigms (e.g., Pfurtscheller & Lopes da Silva, 1999). The inverse Fourier transform is also used in the conversion of raw

Box 5.6
The Fourier Theorem, Stationarity, and Epoch Length

The Fourier approach to analyzing a finite time series of length T (in seconds) is built around a sine wave of frequency $1/T$ (in cycles per second) and its harmonics. Fourier modeling of the time series will work properly only when the slowest frequency in the data, other than overall level (0 Hz), is exactly $1/T$. In other words, Fourier assumes that there is a frequency contributing to the activity in epoch T that has a cycle length exactly equal to T. Furthermore, all other (faster) frequencies in the data are assumed to be limited to the harmonics $2/T$, $3/T$, etc. In the output of the forward Fourier transform (FFT), each such frequency is sometimes called a frequency *bin*. The longer the epoch T is, the finer the frequency resolution of the Fourier transform.

Some confusion can come from the terminology of the Fourier transform. In reality, the data are not "transformed." The original data remain, but new vectors are created that describe a set of sine waves. There is a power or amplitude vector, with one value for each harmonic, and a phase vector, again with one value for each harmonic. Just as multiple regression as a computational procedure determines the best-fitting line by computing weights for the available predictors, the FFT as a computational procedure figures out a set of sine wave characteristics that describe a vector of data.

It may seem counterintuitive that increasing the sample rate does not improve the frequency resolution. What increasing the sample rate does is extend the number of harmonics, or bins, in the spectrum that the Fourier Transform computes (see box 5.2 on the Nyquist rule and aliasing). Thus, to represent a broader range of frequencies, one should increase the sampling rate. To improve the frequency resolution, one should increase the epoch length.

Box 5.6
(continued)

The Fourier transform can be applied in reverse, creating a time series from a set of sine waves. Thus, the transformation goes in both directions, with no loss of information in either direction.

The impact of the assumption that a time series can be modeled as the sum of a specific set of sine waves is often underappreciated. Brigham (1974, chapter 6) and Glaser and Ruchkin (1976, chapter 3) provide graphical illustrations of the misallocation of frequency information, called leakage, that occurs when nonharmonic frequencies are present. Fourier analysis is best when the Fourier transform is applied to a time series of infinite length, because this leakage into inappropriate frequency bins will not occur. This point can readily be understood as follows: as T approaches infinity, $1/T$ approaches 0.0. As a result, the width of each bin approaches zero, and the frequency resolution becomes extremely high, so that virtually any activity is close to a harmonic. Very long analysis epochs are thus much less vulnerable to leakage of nonharmonic activity.

On the other hand, long analysis epochs are vulnerable to violation of the stationarity assumption of no changes in the constituent frequencies over time. The Fourier transform from the time to the frequency domain produces a set of amplitude and phase values, one amplitude and one phase value for each harmonic. Because the entire time series will be described by a (static) set of frequencies of specified amplitude and phase, this approach cannot deal correctly with any change in the amplitude or phase of a given frequency during the T epoch. In that sense, the data must be stationary during the epoch analyzed.

One way to deal with the stationarity assumption is to divide a long time series into shorter epochs, on the assumption that data will be more stable over shorter periods. Thus, for example, a 60-s time series might be analyzed as 60 1-s epochs, rather than as a single 60-s epoch.

Real-world psychophysiological data routinely violate the Fourier method's requirement of stationarity, meaning that the time series to be analyzed is composed of invariant sine waves. Rather than viewing stationarity as a requirement of Fourier analysis, it is better to think of it as an assumption. In other words, Fourier analysis characterizes any arbitrary time series as a set of sine waves. If in fact that time series is anything other than a set of sine waves, the characterization will be off the mark. How far off the mark and how problematic that is are judgment calls the investigator must make.

As noted elsewhere in this chapter, whether the original data vector contains values arrayed in time or values arrayed in space, virtually all comments here apply to both. Thus, for example, one can model a one-dimensional spatial (rather than temporal) vector as the sum of a series of sine waves, where the frequencies are in terms of cycles per unit distance (rather than per unit time). This is common in magnetic resonance imaging, for example. It can also be done with a set of electrodes—most simply, those arrayed in a single plane, equally spaced. Issues of epoch length and stationarity apply equally to distance and to time.

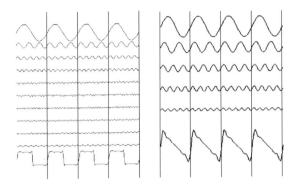

Figure 5.2

Two illustrations of the summation of pure sine waves to approximate apparently nonsinusoidal times series. In the left panel, 10 sine waves (all odd harmonics) sum to an approximation of a square wave. In the right panel, five sine waves (all even harmonics) sum to an approximation of a sawtooth wave. In either case, adding additional sine waves of the appropriate frequency, amplitude, and phase would improve the approximation.

magnetic resonance imaging data to images. Appendix A of Cook and Miller (1992) details the computational steps for the direct and inverse Fourier transforms; that is, for shuttling between time and frequency domain representations.

Note that the fidelity of a Fourier analysis is limited by the extent to which modeling the data as a sum of invariant sinusoids is appropriate to the raw data. Because Fourier-transformed data in the frequency domain contain exactly the information in the original time-domain waveform, the Fourier transform, in either direction, does not introduce distortion into the data. However, characterization of the data via a set of sine waves does not ensure that the original physiological phenomena were indeed sinusoidal or that scoring in terms of sine waves are high-fidelity representations of those phenomena.

Implementing Digital Filters

We noted earlier that a wide range of mathematical procedures applied to time series may be considered digital filters (for an extended and intuitively appealing presentation of this perspective, see Donchin & Heffley, 1978). If one simply requires that the procedure selectively attenuate certain frequencies, then digital filters are pervasive in psychophysiology. For example, the calculation of the mean of a time series may be construed as a digital filter that attenuates all frequencies except 0 Hz (DC). Computation of the variance of the time series is the complementary operation, removing the DC component while retaining (and combining) all other frequencies. The present discussion focuses on procedures that yield a time series (one from which certain frequencies have been removed) rather than a single value such as the mean.

In a common type of digital filter, each filtered output point is defined as a weighted or unweighted average of some number of input data points. Let vector W consist of $2j + 1$ weights (subscripted $-j$ to $+j$) that will be used to compute output vector Y from input vector X. Typically, X and Y are the same length (Y may be a bit shorter, as some filters are not applicable near the ends of the time series), and W is much shorter. The sample period (distance in time or space between the points in X), the number of weights, and the values of those weights affect the gain function of the filter. $2j + 1$ input data points (a portion of vector X) will be included in the computation of each filtered output point (to be stored in vector Y). Each value in Y is computed by *convolving* the $2j + 1$ weights in W with $2j + 1$ values in X. Convolution is the sum of the cross-products of the weights and corresponding X values:

$$Y_t = \sum_{i=-j}^{j} W_i \times X_{t+i} \tag{5.1}$$

The number and magnitude of the weights in W clearly affect the gain function of such a filter. Note that the convolution of two vectors is similar to the correlation between them, but in correlation the means are removed from each vector, and each is divided by its standard deviation—that is, correlation normalizes the two vectors.

Another factor that affects the gain function is the temporal relationship between the points in X convolved with W and the point in Y in which the summed cross-product is stored. In equation 5.1, the $2j + 1$ weights are applied symmetrically around the point in X being filtered. Typically in such a case, the set of weights is symmetric about the unpaired center weight W_0 (i.e., $W_j = W_{-j}$). An alternative approach employs just points in X up to and including the point corresponding to the Y value that the filter will output, with j weights:

$$Y_t = \sum_{i=0}^{j} W_i \times X_{t-i} \tag{5.2}$$

This aligns W with j points in X, the last of which is the time point corresponding to the value being computed for Y. When the values in X are digitized in time, this approach has the advantage of not needing points collected later than a given Y value in order to filter X into Y. This allows application of filtering in real time. A disadvantage is that this tactic introduces a phase shift into Y: Y_t reflects concurrent and previous but not subsequent values in X. In effect, a portion of the variance in X is shifted later in Y. The approach in equation 5.1 does not introduce this phase shift, as long as the weights are symmetrical about the unpaired center weight.

Equations 5.1 and 5.2 only employ values in X in computing values in Y. Yet another factor that affects filter performance is the option to employ previously filtered points in computing the filtered value for Y. This uses portions of the Y vector to compute a given value in Y. The general form of such a filter with j weights is:

$$Y_t = X_t + \sum_{i=1}^{j} W_i \times Y_{t-i} \tag{5.3}$$

One can understand the effect that this re-use of filtered points has in terms of the *impulse response* of the filter. Filters that define output points solely on the basis of input points have a *finite impulse response* (FIR), because the effect of a single aberrant input point (an "impulse") disappears after a finite amount of time, after the last filtered point that includes the aberrant unfiltered point in its computation. For example, in equation 5.1, the impact of the value in X_t extends only from X_{t-j} to X_{t+j}. In contrast, filters that define each filtered point at least in part based on filtered points have an *infinite impulse response* (IIR), because the effect of a single X_t will propagate to all subsequent points: X_t will affect Y_t, Y_t will affect Y_{t+1}, Y_{t+1} will affect Y_{t+2}, and so on. *Nonrecursive* and *recursive* are synonyms for FIR and IIR filters, respectively.

Infinite impulse response digital filters represent something of a hybrid between analog filters and FIR digital filters, sharing characteristics of both. A thorough discussion of IIR filters is beyond the scope of the present paper (see Ackroyd, 1973; and Cook & Miller, 1992, for a comparison of analog and digital filters). We will restrict the following presentation to FIR filters.

FIR Filters in ERP Research

The ERP literature has described a variety of explicit and implicit FIR filters, particularly for smoothing (removing high frequency components from) time series. Researchers often accomplish smoothing time series data by redefining each point in the original time series as the average of itself and a symmetric number of additional points before and after it, per equation 5.1. Such a filter is frequently referred to as a *moving-average filter*, reflecting the fact that computation of the average around each unfiltered point X_t is repeated to define each filtered point Y_t. This type of filter is also sometimes called a *boxcar* filter, reflecting the shape of the weights ($1/n$) plotted as a function of lag relative to the output point. Moving-average filters vary only in the number of data points averaged together. The gain function this produces is a function of the number of data points and the temporal or spatial sample rate. Ruchkin and Glaser (1978; Glaser & Ruchkin, 1976; Ruchkin, 1988) discuss equal-weight filters in detail and provide an equation for their gain. Nitschke, Miller, and Cook (1998) explore the effect of sample rate (and thus the temporal or spatial distance between weights) on the gain function.

A particular advantage of moving-average filters is the rapidity with which each filtered point can be computed. In general for FIR filters with j weights, convolution of each filtered point requires j multiplications and $j - 1$ additions. But if the weights are equal, one can instead do $j - 1$ additions and then a single division by j.

Although moving-average filters with both equal and unequal weights are frequently used in data reduction, their gain functions are not generally reported and may not be generally recognized. Using frequency-domain methods summarized in the next section and presented more formally in appendix B of Cook and Miller (1992), one can compute the gain function for filters having any set of symmetric weights.

In addition to the explicit filtering and smoothing applications described above, a wide range of other procedures common in the ERP literature and elsewhere can be understood within an FIR framework. Particularly relevant are FIR filtering methods used in template-matching algorithms. The "template" can be seen simply as a set of W_j weights with a particular configuration of values, and the weights may not be symmetric. The basis for selecting weights may differ greatly across applications, but in general it will reflect a specific notion the investigator has about the signal being sought. For example, if the template is simply a 10-Hz sine wave, then convolution of that template with raw EEG will constitute an alpha-band band-pass filter. One might search EOG or EEG for an eye blink by establishing a filter template whose weights outline a blink. The Woody (1967) filter technique used for latency correction of ERPs uses as its template a portion of the pre-correction average waveform for a given subject. Thus, one can customize the template for each subject and channel. A simpler variation on the Woody technique employs a sine wave half cycle or a triangular wave half cycle as the template (e.g., Ford et al., 1994). In all of these examples, one slides the template along the data, convolves, and notes the latency of maximum cross-product as the most likely latency of the signal one is filtering. These examples represent additional ways psychophysiology already uses digital filters.

Design and Evaluation of Digital Filters in the Frequency Domain

All of the FIR filters described above involve convolving a time series with a (usually symmetric) weight series (itself a time series), yielding a filtered time series. As noted above, any time series can be represented in the frequency domain rather than the time domain. A common approach to design and evaluation of digital filters relies on representing both the original time series X and the weight series W in the frequency domain. The amplitude spectrum of a filtered time series is equal to the amplitude spectrum of the original time series, multiplied frequency-by-frequency by the cosine component of the amplitude spectrum of the weight series (see appendix A of Cook & Miller, 1992). Moreover, the power spectrum of the resulting time series is equal to the power spectrum of the original time series, multiplied frequency-by-frequency by the squared cosine component of the weight series. These properties are fundamental to the construction of FIR filters using Fourier transform methods.

Gold and Rader (1969) describe the specific steps for constructing such filters (see also Ackroyd, 1973; Cook & Miller, 1992; Oppenheim & Schafer, 1975; Ruchkin, 1988), and software implementing the steps is available for easy creation and evaluation of a custom set of W weights (e.g., Cook, 1981). The technique involves four steps: (1) Specify the filter's ideal gain function. (2) Apply the inverse Fourier transform to the gain function in order to obtain the initial set of weights. This is a simple transformation from the frequency domain to the time domain; the gain function in the former becomes the set of weights in the latter. (3) It is typically desirable to reduce the number of weights and to taper the weights in order to balance requirements related to transition bandwidth, computational limits, maximum filter width, and "ripple" (the degree to which the gain function varies around 1.0 in the pass band and around 0.0 in the stop band). (4) Evaluate the reduced filter and repeat the process until obtaining an acceptable filter. Appendix B of Cook and Miller 1992 describes these steps in detail.

A complementary approach is also based on frequency-domain representation. This approach requires three steps: (1) Use a direct Fourier transform to transform the original time series into the frequency domain. (2) Set those elements of the transform that correspond to frequencies to be eliminated to zero. (3) Use an inverse Fourier transform to recreate the original time series, minus those frequencies for which the direct transform was set to zero.

Application Notes

A comparison of several EEG data sets illustrates some of the issues in digital filter design. In a standard ERP study, one often wants to identify components that are roughly half-sinusoids and quantify their peak amplitude and the latency of that peak. The filter should have either a narrow transition band or f_c well above the frequencies of the component(s) of interest. In data digitized at 125 Hz, Giese-Davis, Miller, and Knight (1993) expected the main ERP components of interest to be below 5 Hz and wished to remove alpha band information (around 10 Hz) prior to scoring. A low-pass filter with a half-amplitude cutoff of 5 Hz would require a moderately narrow transition band, in order to pass low frequencies and still remove alpha. A 31-weight filter proved adequate, with an amplitude gain of 96 percent at 0 Hz, 87 percent at 2 Hz, and 2 percent at 10 Hz.

In contrast, in order to look at baseline EEG (Etienne et al., 1990), a 31-weight filter constructed to pass just alpha (8–13 Hz half-amplitude cutoffs) was less effective. The gain was only 61 percent at 10 Hz, then down to 25 percent at 6 and 16 Hz and to 2 percent at 3 and 18 Hz. The high attenuation at 10 Hz was due to that frequency being relatively close to both of the cutoff frequencies; very narrow transition bands, requiring many weights, are necessary in such a case. A 91-weight version would have been very effective: 99 percent at 10 Hz, 1 percent at 6 and 15 Hz.

A quite different case is the measurement of very slow phenomenon underlying fast EEG activity. For contingent negative variation (CNV) data in a paradigm with a relatively long warning interval, Yee and Miller (1988) employed a moving-average filter to remove conventional EEG, averaging together the last 250 ms of EEG to score the CNV (sometimes called an "area" measure, although such measures are more properly characterized as "average amplitude"; a true area measure would have units of milliseconds-microvolts). Such a case where signal and noise are presumed to be far apart in frequency permits a wide transition band, and one can benefit from the simplicity and speed of the moving-average method.

We can make some general comments with respect to the design of digital filters. A filter with a narrow transition band is usually preferable to one with a wide transition band. This is because the former will pass more (signal) on the pass band side of the cutoff frequency and attenuate more (noise) on the stop band side of the cutoff frequency. Thus, a narrower transition band allows the separation of closer frequencies. In principle, it is possible to construct a digital filter with transition band(s) that approach zero width. However, for a given type of filter, a narrower transition band requires more weights. Thus, there is a trade-off between resolution in the frequency domain (narrowness of the transition band) and resolution in the time domain; more on this below.

When not otherwise indicated, one should construct digital filters with symmetrical weights. Because bioelectric signals generally contain multiple frequency components, a traditional RC analog filter and an FIR digital filter with asymmetric weights will distort not only the latency but also the shape of the input waveform by introducing a phase shift and doing so differentially as a function of frequency. No phase shift occurs if the FIR filter has symmetrical weights.

The frequency domain method described in appendix B of Cook and Miller (1992) provides a general method for designing complex, unequal-weight filters to meet a variety of specifications of pass band, transition band, and ripple. The reader can consult the engineering literature for other approaches to digital filter design. Requirements of replication might lead an investigator to choose one type of filter over other similar filters. Practical issues, including computation time when the filter is to be implemented on-line, may also constrain the choice of filter. Researchers will continue to develop new methods of digital filtering (e.g., Mallat, 1999).

Digital Filtering in Marketed ERP Analysis Software

Increased interest in psychophysiological research as well as inexpensive computing power has fostered the development of marketed analysis software, both commercial and freeware. These products often include features such as artifact rejection, selective averaging, and baseline removal. Typically, software also provides limited digital filtering capabilities that are not thoroughly documented. We intend the present discussion to help users of marketed programs understand the features of the digital filter provided in their package, so they can optimally use and accurately report this information. We also describe a procedure below that allows one to determine the gain function of a filter.

Marketed programs typically provide a single type of filter. For example, BESA 2000 (BESA Manual, Version 2000) and NeuroScan (Neurosoft Inc., Version 4.1) use a Butterworth filter, which optimizes the flatness of the pass band at the expense of a relatively broad transition band. Other filters have different characteristics. For example, the Chebyshev filter has a relatively narrow transition band at the expense of passband ripple. Other programs provide preset filters but may also provide a means by which the user can insert filters with any possible gain function. Despite differences in the type of filter used, terminology, and the user interface, there are three basic features shared by most filtering software surveyed for this chapter: setting the low- and high-pass frequencies, selecting a zero-phase-shift method or a simulated analog method that provides a phase shift, and adjusting the steepness of the gain function in the transition band, each of which we discuss below.

Low- and High-Pass Filter Settings

All programs surveyed for this chapter (James Long Company EEG Analysis System EEGCONV Version 7.589, BESA 2000, EEGLAB Version 4.03, NeuroScan Version 4.1, Instep Version 4.2, Neuromag Plotter Version 4.6.2, EGI Net Station) allow the user to specify low- and high-pass filter settings. Programs typically also allow the user to specify bandpass and bandstop (notch) filters. Where a bandpass filter option is not available, enabling both the low- and high-pass filter options constitutes a bandpass filter. Virtually none of the products allows more than one instance of each type of filter, such as multiple pass bands (desirable to eliminate both EEG alpha and 50- or 60-Hz power-line noise), although several programs allow one to set multiple notch/bandstop filters. Apparently only one commercial product (James Long Company) allows users to import custom weights and apply any convolution vector to the dataset, allowing the user to employ many types of filters.

Importantly, there is variability across programs in whether "cutoff frequency" means the half-*power* frequency (in accordance with much of the electrical engineering literature) or the half-*amplitude* frequency (common in laboratory practice in the ERP literature). As noted above, this corresponds to the frequency at which the gain has decreased by either 3 dB (50 percent power) or 6 dB (50 percent amplitude). In some cases, it is not made explicit whether amplitude or power values are used. For example, in BESA 2000, a plot showing the filter gain function graphs f_c as the 50 percent cutoff frequency but does not state whether the y axis reflects amplitude or power. (Michael Scherg, personal communication, 04/18/2003, clarified that BESA plots amplitude.)

Across products, there is also variability in the way low- and high-pass filters are set. The more common method is when one sets separate low- and/or high-pass filter settings via specifying the 50 percent amplitude or power point explicitly. The second method is often used to set a notch filter or a band-pass filter (each of which has both high- and low-pass points). In this case, one explicitly specifies the desired midpoint of the stop band or pass band, and then sets the cutoff frequencies indirectly by explicitly adjusting the width of the stop or pass band. For example, when creating a filter to pass only EEG alpha (8–12 Hz), one might set the midpoint at 10 Hz and the width at 4 Hz. If software (e.g., BESA 2000) interprets the width setting as the half-point frequencies for the high- and low-pass cutoffs, this would place the high-pass at 8 and the low-pass cutoff at 12 Hz. The effect of such settings is to remove 50 percent of the signal at both 8 and 12 Hz, retaining more activity at intermediate frequencies. In addition, given that the filter is not perfect, it passes some amount of theta (4–8 Hz) and beta (13–20 Hz) activity. Increasing the width parameter includes more alpha band activity at the expense of also including more theta and beta (figure 5.3). In other programs (e.g., Neuromag), when defining stop band parameters, one sets a midpoint and the width defines where the gain returns to unity instead of the 50 percent cutoff point. In general, the exact gain function at frequencies below and above f_c are unknown, although as shown below, one can easily compute these values. Note that this example is ambiguous as to what 50 percent of the signal means. Given that products vary in whether their use of f_c refers to half power, half amplitude, or possibly something else and that this is not always made clear, the example must be vague in order to be general.

Aside from the variability in the way one sets cutoff frequencies, there is considerable variability in terminology, both within and across software. For example, the Neuromag "filter shaping" display provides a convenient set of slider bars for setting the low-pass, high-pass, and notch filters. For each filter, one adjusts a "Center frequency" and a "Width" slider bar. The setting labeled "Center frequency" can be confusing, in that for setting the notch filter it refers to the center of the notch (the center of its stop band), whereas for setting the low-pass or high-pass filter it refers to the center of the transition band. The manual states (p. 16) that in setting the "Center frequency" point, the user sets the −3 dB point. However, it is the −6 dB frequency that the user actually specifies directly, rather than the −3 dB frequency. Neuromag confirmed that it is the half-amplitude frequency that the software intends and that the manual should say −6 dB rather than −3 dB in order to be consistent with the table on the same page (Matti Kajola, personal communication, 6/11/03).

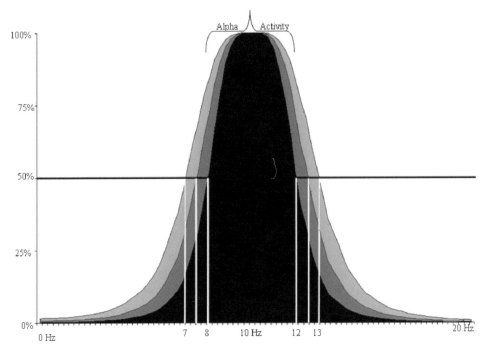

Figure 5.3
The gain function (amplitude) of a passband filter with a midpoint at 10 Hz and width settings of 4, 5, and 6 Hz. Increasing the width parameter includes more alpha-band activity, at the expense of also including more theta and beta.

Zero Phase Shift and Simulated Analog Settings

Along with deciding on low- and/or high-pass settings, some software provides a choice of a zero-phase-shift filter or a simulated-analog filter. (If not specified explicitly, it is likely, but should not be assumed, that the default is zero phase shift.) A number of different conventions are used to input the settings for simulated analog filters. For example, Neuroscan 4.1 provides a button labeled "Analog Simulation," and the Neuroscan 4.1 manual (p. 156) notes that an analog simulation filter is a one-pass (forward) Butterworth filter, which is 3 dB down at the cutoff frequency (we describe characteristics of the Butterworth Filter below when discussing zero-phase settings). BESA 2000 provides the same option and additionally allows the user to specify the analog simulation by selection of time constants of 1, 0.3, or 0.1 s (see box 5.4). These capabilities allow investigators to replicate the high-pass analog filter built into most amplifiers. However, aside from this purpose, the use of simulated analog filters is not recommended, due to the frequency-dependent phase distortion it introduces.

Applying a filter that induces identical phase distortion when applied in both the forward and backward directions cancels the distortion and thus allows one to maintain the temporal shape of the waveform. This is how some software implements the zero-phase-shift setting. For example, in BESA 2000 and NeuroScan 4.1, zero-phase-shift filtering involves a Butterworth filter applied twice, once in the forward direction and once in the reverse direction.

It is important to note that, with each application of the Butterworth filter (either a forward or backward pass), the -3 dB and -6 dB frequencies shift, and thus the net cutoff frequency and transition band slope change. For example, whereas a single pass of the Butterworth Filter with an 8-Hz high-pass setting places f_c (-3 dB) at 8 Hz (slope 6 dB/octave), two passes of the filter result in a two-fold increase in the attenuation at 8 Hz (-6 dB; slope 12 dB/octave). Now 8 Hz is the half-amplitude frequency and is no longer f_c, the half-power frequency. Four passes (two backward and two forward) create a filter that is -12 dB at 8 Hz (slope $=24$ dB/octave). This characteristic of filter settings is frequently not noted, nor is it always clear in available software whether the filter parameters the user enters directly specify the characteristics of the single-pass filter or the net effect of a multipass filter. Figure 5.4 illustrates the gain function of a filter provided by BESA 2000 with 8–12 Hz half-amplitude bandpass. Three different low-pass slopes (24 dB/octave, 48 dB/octave, 96 dB/octave) are implemented by different numbers of passes of a Butterworth filter. Because the half-amplitude frequency does not change as a function of slope (and thus as a function of the number of passes), it is apparent that the BESA user interface interprets the user's specifications in terms of the net cutoff desired rather than in terms of the (single-pass) Butterworth filter itself. Investigators should report the net effect of the filter on the gain function. Reporting characteristics of an individual pass in a multipass filter method is of little interest and can actually be misleading.

Adjusting the Slope of Filter Roll-Off

The number of times the filter is applied is closely related to the filter's roll-off. Just as software differs in the way cutoff frequencies are set, there are also differences in the way roll-off settings are expressed. In general, the differences depend upon whether the input value reflects the roll-off value due to a single pass of the filter or the net effect of multiple passes. One can understand these differences by first considering the slope set in an analog filter and then considering slope settings in a digital filter. In effect, analog filters are applied once in the forward direction. Because the filter is only applied once, it is termed a first-order filter. A Butterworth filter applied once has a cutoff frequency at -3 dB and a slope of 6 dB/octave. Off-line, the same filter can be applied multiple times, in forward and reverse directions, to create higher order filters that will have zero phase shift if applied an even number of times. Aside from maintaining phase information, each application of the filter increases the steepness of the roll-off. For

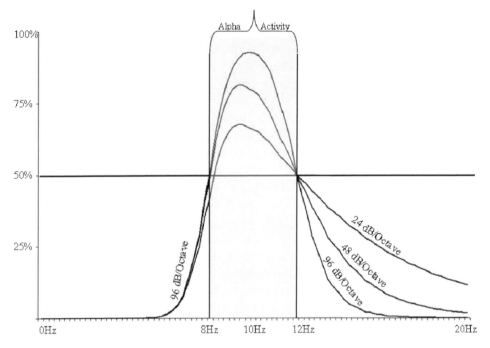

Figure 5.4
Illustration of the effect of overlap of low-pass and high-pass transition bands as a function of slope settings for the low-pass filter.

example, a Butterworth filter that is applied once in each direction is a second order filter with a final slope of 12 dB/octave (6 dB/octave for each pass). Overall, in order to narrow the width of the transition band one simply needs to run the data through the filter multiple times.

As noted above, some of the variability across software packages in the way they define roll-off values is a function of whether the input settings reflect the single pass roll-off value or the net effect of multiple passes of the filter. Versions of Neuroscan prior to 4.1 reported roll-off values in terms of that for a single forward or backward pass, although both forward and backward passes were completed, so that the net effect was twice what the user specified: a single-pass roll-off value was set (e.g., 12 dB/octave), with the filtered data actually characterized by a roll-off twice this value (24 dB/octave). Some other programs select the net roll-off value. In BESA 2000, this depends on whether one enables the zero-phase-shift option. The roll-off value the user enters characterizes the single-pass filter, but additionally selecting the zero-phase-shift option doubles the net effect, due to the two passes made with that filter. The manual spells this out, but it is not apparent in the user dialog box (confirmed by Patrick Berg, personal communication, 4/18/03). Users should understand the method employed.

When allowing the user to set the cutoff frequency explicitly, programs generally provide a way to adjust the width of the transition between the pass band and the stop band. However, in programs where a midpoint frequency and width value are selected (e.g., stop band and pass band settings), and where it is not possible to also simultaneously vary the steepness of the roll-off, one is forced to rely on the default roll-off settings.

When high- and low-pass settings are nearby or the transition band is broad, a combination of high- and low-pass settings determine the gain function in the low- and high-pass transition bands. For example, as figure 5.4 shows, with cutoff frequencies at 8 and 12 Hz and with relatively steep roll-offs (96 dB/octave), there is little overlap between the two transition bands. Although the 8- and 12-Hz cutoffs are quite close to each other, such a filter passes virtually all of the 10-Hz activity. However, if the low-pass transition band is widened via a 48-dB/octave slope, the two transition bands begin to overlap, so that both low- and high-pass filters remove a portion of frequencies in the center of the pass band. A very significant distortion in the high-pass transition band is observed with a 24 dB/octave low-pass slope. In designing a filter, it is not necessary to have the same roll-off for high- and low-pass filters. However, roll-off is particularly important when the high and low cutoffs are close, such that their transition bands may overlap, cutting into the pass band more than the investigator foresees. The overall gain function a filter procedure produces is influenced by multiple factors, and when implementing filters in software it is often difficult to determine in advance the final gain function. The next section details a method to determine gain values at all frequencies.

Determining Exact Gain Values at Each Frequency

Unfortunately, software often provides exact gain values at only a few frequencies. In particular, exact gain values may only be stated at f_c (50 percent power, 70.7 percent amplitude) or at 50 percent amplitude. Some products provide an on-screen plot of the entire gain function, which is very valuable in selecting one's filters but may be imprecise for determining and reporting filter behavior at a specific frequency.

Although the full gain function is rarely made available, often one can easily obtain this empirically, using a variant of the methods described above and in appendixes A and B of Cook and Miller (1992). In general, what is needed is the ability to calculate a Fourier transform (converting the data from the time to the frequency domain) on both the original unfiltered data and the filtered data, and the ability to output the resulting power or amplitude spectrum of both time series. Marketed analysis programs often include the ability to calculate a Fourier transform. If not included, widely available, general-purpose software such as MATLAB or Excel has built-in Fourier transform functions, although a small amount of additional computation may be needed to obtain the power or amplitude spectrum from the output of such functions (see Cook & Miller, 1992, appendix A).

The power or amplitude spectrum will be a new vector, with values for a series of sine waves. When T is the real-time size of the epoch submitted to the Fourier transform, each value in the spectrum provides the power or amplitude for a frequency that is a harmonic of the frequency given by $1/T$, as box 5.6 explains.

In a time series collected at 250 Hz, an epoch that contains 512 points (2^9) spans $T = 2.048$ seconds of data. The size of the step between adjacent frequencies in the power or amplitude spectrum is $1/2.048 = 0.488$ Hz. The first bin or entry in the vector will contain $0/T = 0$ Hz (DC) power, the second bin $1/T = 0.488$ Hz, the third $2/T = 0.977$ Hz, and so on up to $256/T = 125$ Hz. Software allows one to set the epoch length T (sometimes with number of points constrained to a power of 2). Once both the unfiltered and filtered datasets have been created and the bin size determined, one can calculate the filtered/unfiltered ratio for each frequency bin to obtain the filter's gain function.

As an illustration, figure 5.5 plots the gain function (amplitude) with data digitized at 250 Hz and epoch lengths of .512 seconds (128 points), 1.024 seconds (256 points), 2.048 seconds (512 points), and 4.096 seconds (1024 points). Each case employed a band-pass filter with the midpoint set at 10 Hz and a width of 4, setting the half-amplitude points at 8 and 12 Hz. The graphs show that, as epoch length increases, frequency resolution also increases. For short epoch lengths one can only very generally approximate the desired frequency boundaries. For example, to compute a measure of total alpha activity, with an epoch size of .512 seconds, at the low end of the alpha band one must choose between 7.81 and 9.77 Hz and at the high end between 11.71 and 13.67 Hz. Exact values of 8 and 12 Hz are not available, because the spectrum contains only harmonics of $1/T$. That is, the researcher's choice of T dictates that the activity in the epoch will be modeled as the sum of just $1/T$ and its harmonics—no other frequency can be represented accurately. As figure 5.5 shows, increasing the epoch length to 4.096 s decreases the step size to $1/T = 1/4.096 = .244$ Hz. Although increased frequency resolution is desirable, it necessarily comes at the expense of decreased temporal resolution.

Conclusion

Digital filters are pervasive in the ERP literature and in related disciplines, and reliance on them will surely increase. Publicly available software collectively provides a wide array of choices, but these vary across programs, are often not well documented, and are rarely described adequately in research publications that rely on them.

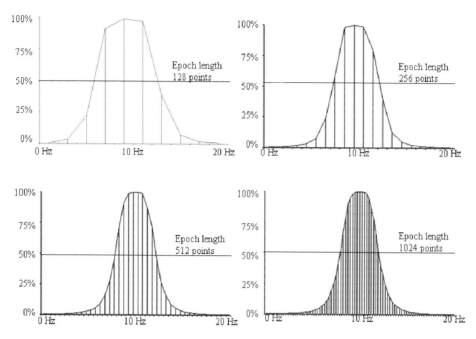

Figure 5.5
Each panel plots the gain function of a bandpass filter, identical except for the real-time length of the data epoch being filtered. The panels illustrate that the longer the epoch (and thus the poorer the temporal resolution), the better the frequency resolution.

The present discussion touches on a number of fundamental and practical issues in understanding and selecting appropriate digital filters. A major strength of digital filtering is its flexibility; however, that flexibility means that the researcher must make many choices (knowingly or not). With each choice come trade-offs that the researcher needs to weigh. Marketed software can save the researcher considerable time, but it often undercharacterizes its algorithms and options. Despite the apparent convenience of point-and-click interfaces, researchers should not exercise those options without understanding them, especially the assumptions and limitations they entail. Faithful replication relies on authors providing adequate description of their filters.

Acknowledgments

This research was supported by grants from the National Institute of Drug Abuse (R21 DA14111) and the National Institute of Mental Health (RO1 MH65304, T32 MH19554). Address reprint requests to: Gregory A. Miller, Director, Biomedical

Imaging Center, University of Illinois, Urbana, IL 61801, USA. Tel: (217)-244-0600, email: gamiller@uiuc.edu.

The authors use none of the commercial software cited here except Neuromag and BESA 2000, have no financial interest in any of the cited companies, and received no financial or other consideration for the informal evaluations done for this chapter. There are numerous other freeware and commercial packages available, and users should evaluate them as thoroughly as possible before and after selecting a product.

References

Ackroyd, M. H. (1973). *Digital filters*. London: Butterworth.

Cheung, M. N., & Porges, S. W. (1977). Respiratory influences on cardiac responses during attention. *Physiological Psychology, 5*, 53–57.

Coles, M. G. H., Gratton, G., Kramer, A., & Miller, G. A. (1986). Principles of signal acquisition. In M. G. H. Coles, E. Donchin, & S. W. Porges (Eds.), *Psychophysiology: Systems, processes, and applications—A handbook* (pp. 183–221). New York: Guilford Press.

Cook, E. W. (1981). FWTGEN—An interactive FORTRAN II/IV program for calculating weights for a non-recursive digital filter. *Psychophysiology, 18*, 489–490.

Cook, E. W., & Miller, G. A. (1992). Digital filtering: Background and tutorial for psychophysiologists. *Psychophysiology, 29*, 350–367.

Donchin, E., & Heffley III, E. F. (1978). Multivariate analysis of event-related potential data: A tutorial review. In D. A. Otto (Ed.), *Multidisciplinary perspectives in event-related brain potential research* (pp. 555–572). Washington, D.C.: Environmental Protection Agency.

Etienne, M. A., Deldin, P. J., Giese-Davis, J., & Miller, G. A. (1990). *Differences in EEG distinguish populations at risk for psychopathology*. Paper presented at the annual meeting of the Society for Psychophysiological Research, Boston.

Ford, J. M., White, P., Lim, K. O., & Pfefferbaum, A. (1994). Schizophrenics have fewer and smaller P300s: A single-trial analysis. *Biological Psychiatry, 35*, 96–103.

Giese-Davis, J., Miller, G. A., & Knight, R. (1993). Evidence for a memory deficit in subjects at risk for psychosis. *Psychophysiology, 30*, 646–656.

Glaser, E. M., & Ruchkin, D. S. (1976). *Principles of neurobiological signal analysis*. New York: Academic.

Gold, B. & Rader, C. M. (1969). *Digital processing of signals*. New York: McGraw-Hill.

Graham, F. K. (1978). Constraints on measuring heart rate and period sequentially through real and cardiac time. *Psychophysiology, 15*, 492–495.

Mallat, S. (1999). *A wavelet tour of signal processing*, (2d ed.). Chestnut Hill, MA: Academic Press.

Miller, G. A. (1986). Automated beat-by-beat heart rate editing. *Psychophysiology, 23*, 121–122.

Nitschke, J. B., Miller, G. A., & Cook, E. W. (1998). Time- and frequency-domain digital signal processing in EEG/ERP analysis: Some technical and empirical comparisons. *Behavior Research Methods, Instruments, and Computers, 30*, 54–67.

Oppenheim, A. V., & Schafer, R. W. (1975). *Digital signal processing.* Englewood Cliffs, NJ: Prentice-Hall.

Pfurtscheller, G., & Lopes da Silva, F. H. (1999). Event-related EEG/MEG synchronization and desynchronization: basic principles. *Clinical Neurophysiology, 110*, 1842–1857.

Picton, T. W., Bentin, S., Berg, P., Donchin, E., Hillyard, S. A., Johnson, Jr., R., Miller, G. A., Ritter, W., Ruchkin, D. S., Rugg, M. D., & Taylor, M. J. (2000). Guidelines for using human event-related potentials to study cognition: Recording standards and publication criteria. *Psychophysiology, 37*, 127–152.

Ruchkin, D. S. (1988). Measurement of event-related potentials: Signal extraction. In T. W. Picton (Ed.), *Handbook of electroencephalography and clinical neurophysiology*, vol. 3, revised series (pp. 7–43). Amsterdam: Elsevier.

Ruchkin, D. S., & Glaser, E. M. (1978). Some simple digital filters for examination of CNV and P300 waveforms on a single trial basis. In D. Otto (Ed.), *Multidisciplinary perspectives in event-related brain potential (ERP) research* (pp. 579–581). Washington, D.C.: U.S. Government Printing Office, EPA-600/9-77-043.

Simons, R. F., Ohman, A., & Lang, P. J. (1979). Anticipation and response set: Cortical, cardiac, and electrodermal correlates. *Psychophysiology, 16*, 222–233.

Srinivasan, R., Tucker, D. M., & Murias, M. (1998). Estimating the spatial Nyquist of the human EEG. *Behavior Research Methods, Instruments, & Computers, 30*, 8–19.

Woody, C. D. (1967). Characterization of an adaptive filter for the analysis of variable latency neuroelectric signals. *Medical and Biological Engineering, 5*, 539–553.

Yee, C. M., & Miller, G. A. (1988). Emotional information processing: Modulation of fear in normal and dysthymic subjects. *Journal of Abnormal Psychology, 97*, 54–63.

6   Methods for the Estimation and Removal of Artifacts and Overlap in ERP Waveforms

Durk Talsma and Marty G. Woldorff

In an ideal world, one would have no need for artifact detection mechanisms at all. Event-related potentials (ERPs) are calculated using the approach of averaging the recorded EEG activity of many repetitions of the same stimulus condition (often referred to as "trials"), which assumes that for any given repetition, the recorded EEG consists of a signal part (ERP) and a noise part (background EEG). The noise part is assumed to be uncorrelated with the signal, and therefore, given an infinite number of trials, the noise part should cancel out and the remaining ERP would be a reflection only of the event-related brain activity.

Unfortunately, such an ideal world does not exist. In reality, various recording artifacts do tend to correlate with the signal; some artifacts are always of the same polarity (and thus do not cancel out during signal averaging), subjects may blink their eyes or make movements at consistent times relative to the onset of a visual stimulus (causing large time-locked amplitude deflections on the frontal EEG channels), and it is never possible to record an infinite number of trials to lose these artifacts completely. Moreover, as we will see later in this chapter, the very nature of the experimental design required for specific scientific questions, namely that of ERP components from adjacent trials that are overlapping onto the current one, may introduce a more subtle type of distortion (Woldorff, 1993). As we will discuss later, overlap can be a specific problem when stimulus presentation rates are high.

Above we distinguished three different elements contributing to any given single trial: signal (ERP), noise (background EEG), and artifacts. Although not explicitly mentioned, it follows intuitively from this description that whereas cerebral activity generates the signal and the background EEG noise, artifacts are typically generated by external sources, such as eyes, muscles, or recording equipment. We therefore propose the following working definition of an artifact:

Artifacts are occurrences of any given electrical activity that can be recorded by EEG equipment, which is not originating from cerebral sources, and either clearly distinguishable from the recorded background EEG or substantially large enough to modify the observed ERP waveform from its true waveform.

According to this definition, overlap is not a true artifact, because brain activity generates the overlapping ERP components. However, this activity is unwanted, because it is activity that is not the result of processing the current trial type, but of processing the preceding or succeeding trial.

Because artifacts can distort the observed ERP waveform, it is necessary to find some way to estimate and remove these artifacts from the EEG signal. One method is based on the principle of detecting artifacts and excluding trials on which they are detected. In general, this method is effective; however, one should keep in mind that when using very strict criteria, the rejection method may result in a large number of false alarms because naturally occurring high-amplitude EEG waves may trigger the artifact detection algorithm, therefore excluding a large number of trials and, hence, yield again a very poor signal-to-noise ratio. For this reason, artifact removal based on the exclusion of artifact-contaminated trials should strive for a careful balance between the severity of the artifacts rejected and the number of trials included in the final average. The spike, drift, and eyeblink detection algorithms we discuss below are good examples of this group of methods.

Other methods are based on the principle of not only detecting the presence of artifacts, but also on estimating the relative size of the artifact and correcting (i.e., removing) it. One obvious advantage of these methods is that correcting artifacts leaves more trials available for averaging, and thus makes it possible to obtain a better signal-to-noise ratio of the observed ERP. A disadvantage of this method, however, is that if the estimations of the artifact are poor, the errors induced by subtracting these can be large enough to substantially distort the observed ERP. This group of methods includes the eyeblink correction and overlap removal methods.

This chapter discusses three different types of artifacts and presents methods to remove them. In order of increasing complexity, we will discuss the following types of artifacts: (1) instrumentation artifacts, (2) eye movement artifacts, and (3) overlap from adjacent trials.

Instrumentation Artifacts

A number of sources can generate instrumentation artifacts. Instrumentation artifacts consist, among others, of high-frequency transient activity or high-frequency background noise; or low-frequency drifts that can be caused by slow polarization of electrodes, cephalic skin potentials (e.g., Picton & Hillyard, 1972), or badly placed electrodes. In many cases, these artifacts are in the frequency range that is outside that of interest in ERP research (which is typically from about 0.1 to about 20 Hz). When this is the case, applying an off-line digital bandpass filter (i.e., applied after the fact) might be sufficient to reduce the noise contributed by the artifact to acceptable levels (see chapter 5 of this volume). When this is not the case, there are other methods to eliminate—or at least greatly attenuate—these types of artifacts from the ERPs.

Transient Activities

Fisch (1991) identifies a number of different artifacts that, although marked by differences in amplitude, frequency of occurrence, and scalp distribution, share one useful common characteristic for automatized detection of these artifacts. In particular, they mostly consist of high-amplitude spikes that are easily detectable using a peak-to-peak amplitude test. These artifacts are caused by muscle activity, movement, electrocardiographic (ECG) activity, blood-flow pulse waves, and electrode or equipment problems. We base the description of each artifact in the following section mainly on Fisch 1991, chapter 6.

Muscle Activity   Muscles can cause transient high-amplitude spikes, which are mainly generated by scalp and face muscles in frontal and temporal regions; however, they may be recorded by electrodes nearly anywhere on the scalp surface. This type of artifact can often be reduced, or even completely eliminated, by asking the subjects to relax, drop the jaw or open their mouth slightly, or change their position. When this type of artifact occurs on a single electrode, pushing on or reapplying the electrode can sometimes stop it.

Movement   Head and body movements or movement of electrode wires can cause artifacts even when all electrodes make good mechanical and electrical contact. These types of artifacts are often erratic and not repetitive, unless the movement is rhythmical. This type of artifact can result from tremor, chewing or sucking, breathing, or head movements.

Electrocardiographic Activity   ECG activity can be picked up in the EEG mainly in recordings with wide interelectrode distances, especially in linkages across the head and to the left ear. The artifact may appear in all channels if a common reference is used and it is being picked up at that reference, or it can be in just a few channels. Small artifacts may reflect the R-wave of the ECG, whereas larger artifacts can reflect additional ECG components. The R-wave usually appears maximally over the left posterior scalp regions, because the main cardiac dipole producing the R wave is positive and directed diagonally from right to left and from anterior to posterior.

Pulse-Wave Artifacts   Periodic waves of smooth or triangular shape may be picked up by an electrode on or near a scalp artery as the result of blood pulse waves producing slight changes of the electrical contact between electrode and scalp. Fisch (1991) reports that this is more likely to happen with electrodes in the frontal or temporal areas than with electrodes in the posterior scalp regions.

Electrode- or Equipment-Related Artifacts   Most artifacts in this category are distinguished from cortical activity in that they seem to be superimposed on cortical recordings and/or appear only in channels connected to one electrode. Although some of these have characteristic shapes, others might resemble cerebral activity. A common artifact in this category is "electrode popping," which is due to a sudden change of electrode contact, causing large amplitude changes that rise and fall abruptly. Other electrode artifacts drift more slowly and may resemble cerebral slow waves (see below). Because this type of artifact is mainly due to faulty electrodes or equipment, the first step in avoiding these types of artifacts is to check all the connections: the electrode may be detached or loose, the lead wire may be broken, or the conductive paste may have dried. Next, check the electrode impedance. In addition, check that all connections between electrodes and amplifier are sufficiently dry. We have experienced that a residual amount of moistness in the connectors linking the electrocaps to the switchboard (as a result of washing the caps after a previous recording session) can cause substantial drifts on a number of channels. Finally, carefully consider using disposable sponge disks (to redistribute the pressure of cap-mounted electrodes on the subject's head), as we have experienced that these can lift the electrodes from the scalp and cause frontal channels to drift.

Spike Detection   When the number of trials containing spikes is low, relative to the number of clean trials, and the onset of the artifact is random with respect to the onset of the event of interest, selective averaging will by itself largely reduce the distortion of the ERP waves due to spike occurrence. For example, if a typical ERP consists of averaging together 100 trials and a spike has an average amplitude of 50 μV, then after averaging, the contribution of each single spike to the final average is reduced to 0.5 μV, assuming that these spikes do not overlap in time. Although this example shows that selective averaging can seriously reduce amplitude deflections from spike artifacts in EEG data, even averaging a full 100 trials will reduce the effect of spike artifacts to an amplitude difference that is of the same magnitude of amplitude as a typical ERP effect.

   To illustrate this, we present data from a single subject originally collected for a study on non-spatial intermodal attention (Talsma & Kok, 2001). Figure 6.1 shows this subject's ERP response to a visual stimulus. In this particular recording, some of the trials were contaminated by large-amplitude spike artifacts, but they were very low in number. More specifically, on 4 out of 105 trials, spikes with amplitude changes of up to 160 μV between two consecutive samples (4 ms) were detected, due to a popping reference electrode. These spikes were detected using a relatively simple peak-to-peak amplitude detection algorithm (see appendix II) configured to detect amplitude

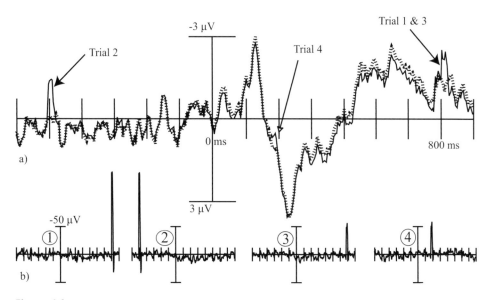

Figure 6.1
Example of the effectiveness of excluding trials containing spike artifacts on ERP averages. (*a*) Comparison of an ERP waveform with spike trials included (solid) and excluded (dotted line). Including trials containing spike artifacts in this example can lead to distortions of about 1–2 μV in the final averages. (*b*) examples of four individual trials containing spikes. Panel (*a*) indicates the distortion caused by each of these spike-trials. Notice that trials 1 and 2 actually contain the same spike, but shifted in time, due to the relatively high stimulus presentation rate.

deflections of more than 50 μV per 4 ms. As figure 6.1 shows, including spike trials in the average results in spike-related distortions of about 1 μV in the averaged ERP wave.

It is best to reject trials when spikes with high amplitudes are present (i.e., more than 150 μV). It is difficult to give an exact criterion for spike rejection, because the relative distortion of the averaged ERP waveforms depends on both frequency and amplitude of spike occurrence. In general, excluding a few trials with high-amplitude spikes will help improve the quality of the ERP waveform, but excluding many trials with low-amplitude artifacts will generally not help improve this quality further—it may even cause the quality of the ERP waveform to decrease because of an unacceptably high number of rejected trials. Because of this, sometimes an alternative method is useful, determining the spike rejection criteria on the basis of the statistical properties of the signal. An example of such a method excludes trials from further analysis on which electrical activity exceeds that of two or more standard deviations of the mean voltage. Although this method appears to work reasonably well, it is still susceptible to false rejections of trials when low background activity in the recorded EEG causes this method to use low rejection criteria.

As an alternative, when the duration of the artifact is short—not more than a few milliseconds—one could also consider correcting the artifact by interpolating around the occurrence of the artifact. In general, the estimated interpolation error will be small, compared to the error caused by the artifact. Therefore the signal-to-noise ratio of ERPs composed of artifact-interpolated trials will be larger than that of ERP averages composed of either all the trials (with no correction or rejection), or than that of ERP averages composed of only the artifact-free trials (i.e., after rejection of the trials with artifacts).

Periodic Noise

The next type of basic recording artifacts we cover consists of periodic noise. We subdivide this group of artifacts into two different categories. The first consists of exogenous artifacts, mainly caused by sources of interference outside the subject (i.e., from the recording equipment or the electrical environment). The second source of periodic "artifact" is endogenous to the subject and consists primarily of unwanted rhythmic brain activity with a disproportionately large amplitude.

Interference   The most common artifact due to interference comes from power lines and equipment. This interference has a frequency of 60 Hz in North America, and of 50 Hz in most other countries. This artifact is most typically picked by electrodes with poor connections, that is, by electrodes with high impedances, which causes the wires running from these electrodes to function as antennae, picking up environmental electrostatic noise. Although faulty or high-impedance electrodes may pick up this artifact, and they may appear in one or a few channels, inordinately strong interference can cause artifacts even with good recording electrodes and equipment; these artifacts are then likely to appear in all channels of all recordings made in this particular setting. Interference artifacts may be introduced either electrostatically by unshielded power cables and regardless of current flow, or electromagnetically by strong currents flowing through cables and equipment such as transformers or electromotors. Shielding the offending power cables and using a shielded room for the recording can reduce electromagnetic interference by proper wiring of the power cables. An effective method of removing line noise is by applying a low-pass moving average (see figure 6.2). Figure 6.2b shows the frequency response of a number of moving average filters with lengths of 4, 9, and 27 points. We can compute the frequency response of such a moving average filter using the following equation

$$H[f] = \frac{\sin(\pi f M)}{M \sin(\pi f)}$$

where H is the frequency response function and M is the length of the moving average filter. The frequency f runs between 0 and 0.5 times the sample frequency. For $f = 0$,

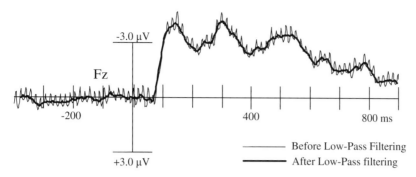

a) The effect of line noise removal on ERPs

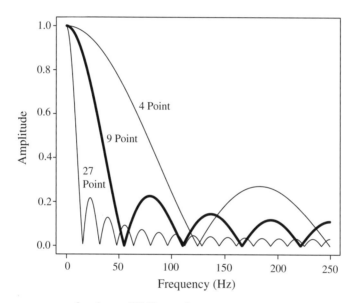

b) Frequency-response functions at 500 Hz sample rate

Figure 6.2

Effectiveness of line-noise removal. (*a*) Shown here is a grand average ERP, which was obtained by averaging 19 single-subject ERPs. Each single-subject ERP was composed of approximately 100 single trials. In the unfiltered data (thin line), a high-frequency noise component is clearly present, even in the grand average waveform, because stimulus presentation was time locked to the 60-Hz refresh cycle of the computer screen. Low-pass filtering, using a 9-point moving average filter, effectively removed this high-frequency noise component. (*b*) Frequency response curves for 4-, 9-, and 27-point moving average filters, for a digital signal sampled at 500 Hz. A 9-point moving average fully attenuates frequencies at 56 Hz and strongly attenuates frequencies around 60 Hz.

use $H[f] = 1$. As figure 6.2b shows, using a 9-point moving average will fully attenuate frequencies at 56 Hz and strongly reduce frequencies in the band around 60 Hz, effectively removing line-noise artifacts.

Rhythmic Activity   Although technically not an artifact according to our working definition, rhythmic EEG activity can pose a number of problems to an experimenter that are similar in nature to real artifacts. Therefore, we conclude this section on periodic noise with a brief discussion of these EEG waves and the specific problems they pose in ERP research.

One of the most common brain rhythms consists of sinusoidal waveforms in the frequency band between 8 and 12 Hz, known as the alpha band, and which peaks at 10 Hz. These alpha waves are observed mostly over parietal and occipital recording sites and more so when subjects have their eyes closed or are drowsy. Thus, they can be an indication of a subject's fatigued state. Alpha activity takes many trials to average out, because it is of high amplitude and because of the tendency of alpha waves to sometimes synchronize with stimulus presentation. The presence of alpha waves differs strongly from subject to subject, and when a subject is producing a particularly large amount of alpha activity, it may be necessary to discard him or her from inclusion in the analysis.

Large alpha waves might be a particular problem when ERPs are composed of limited numbers of trials. For example, in many attention studies, subjects are required to respond to an infrequent number of so-called target stimuli. Because targets are infrequent, ERPs to these targets are therefore composed of only a low number of trials. Therefore, these ERPs are generally more difficult to interpret, because of the lower signal-to-noise ratio.[1] This is particularly a problem when large alpha waves are found, because the residual alpha wave activity in the targets will be substantially larger than the alpha activity still present in more frequent non-target ERPs (see figure 6.3).

Residual alpha activity in ERP averages can be reduced by jittering the stimulus presentation, in ranges of 100 ms, or multiples of 100 ms. By jittering the stimulus presentation from trial to trial, the onset of the ERP response will be random with respect to the phase of the alpha wave in the background of the ERP. Because the dominant frequency in the alpha band is around 10 Hz, one cycle of the alpha wave will take about 100 ms to complete. Therefore, randomly jittering the stimulus presentation over such a 100 ms range will, on average, have the stimulus presentation occur equally on each phase of the alpha wave, causing the background alpha activity to cancel out during averaging.

Slow Drifts and Amplifier Saturations
Slow-wave activity such as those related to anticipatory processes ([CNV]; Walter et al., 1964), directing of attention (Hopf & Mangun, 2000), or working memory processes

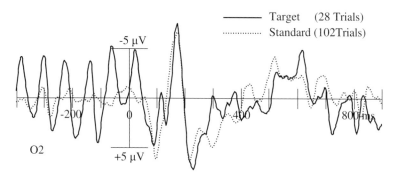

Figure 6.3

Illustration of excessive rhythmic brain activity (large alpha waves). Plotted here are the ERP waveforms to a visual target stimulus composed of 28 artifact free trials, vs. a similar attended standard, consisting of 102 artifact free trials. Notice that because the target ERP is composed of only one-third of the trials as the standard ERP, the signal-to-noise ratio is significantly reduced and the contribution of background activity is still present, obfuscating the true ERP components such as the P1 or the N1.

(Klaver et al., 1999) typically has the same frequency content as slow drifts caused by skin potentials or incorrectly placed electrodes. Slow drifts are mainly a problem when EEG recordings are made in DC mode, that is, when no high-pass filter is applied during data acquisition. This type of recording is typically made when slow wave activity, such as described above, is of interest. Therefore, if such is the case, it is necessary to detect large linear drifts in these recordings and reject those trials in which any given channel yields a linear trend that exceeds a previously established threshold. Trend detection can be done through linear regression by minimizing the following equation, to determine a and b

$$\chi^2(a,b) = \sum_{i=1}^{N} \left(\frac{y_i - a - bx_i}{\sigma_i} \right)^2 \tag{6.1}$$

in which x represents the observed time series, b any linear trend present in the observed time series x, and a an intercept (DC value) at x_0. After minimizing equation 6.1, the value of b can be compared to a preset threshold and if this threshold is exceeded, this trial can be rejected.

Figure 6.4 shows ERP data from a single subject that was originally recorded for a study on spatial intermodal attention (Talsma & Kok, 2002). In this particular recording a substantial amount of drifting channels were observed, because of a loosely connected reference electrode. Figure 6.4 shows an auditory ERP generated by averaging 182 trials, including trials containing drifting channels. This full ERP is compared to

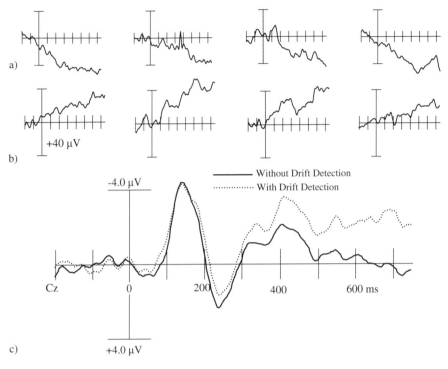

Figure 6.4
Effectiveness of drift removal using linear trend detection on ERP waveforms. (*a*) Example of four
individual trials containing a large positive-going drift; (*b*) example of four similar trials, but now
drifting negatively; (*c*) difference in the resulting single-subject ERP, resulting from excluding trials
with large drifts.

the same ERP response, where 77 trials with either a positive or negative linear trend of
more than 10 $\mu V/s$ were excluded from the average, thus leaving 105 drift-free trials.

This example illustrates two important aspects of drift detection: (1) Despite the fact
that slow channel drift was exceptionally high in this particular recording, and also
despite the fact that the degree of drift on affected trials was high, the difference in
observed ERP between including and excluding drifting trials is relatively small. The
reason for this is that in this example the direction of drift (positive or negative) was
random with respect to stimulus presentation and therefore positive and negative
drifts largely cancelled out. (2) Even though the difference in ERP signal resulting from
excluding drifting channels is relatively small in our example, it is still somewhere
in the order of 1 to 2 μV, which is in the same order of magnitude as a typical experimental ERP effect, and therefore there would be an advantage of rejecting or correcting
for drifting channels. When using a drift detection mechanism as described above, one

should make sure to use a substantially long time window (preferably 1 or 2 s) to calculate the drift, because otherwise the drift detection algorithm is susceptible to local amplitude changes. Instead of rejecting trials containing large drifts, one could also choose to correct these trials by subtracting the estimated linear trend from the observed data.

One should take a number of issues into consideration when detecting drifting channels. First, in some cases, channels can show a rapid drift into one direction, which is then followed by a much slower drift into the opposite polarity. When detecting drifting channels, the experimenter should make sure to detect both the negative and positive drifts. Otherwise the "drift free" ERPs will generally be distorted by a net drift that could be even worse, because negative- and positive-going drifts do not cancel out anymore. We will give an illustration of this below, when we discuss the consequences of not correctly detecting the post blink-return drift in the vertical EOG channel (see figure 6.5).

Another problem related to drifting channels is amplifier or digitization saturation. Saturation occurs when a continuously increasing (or decreasing) EEG signal reaches the edge of the amplification or digitization range, at which point the true signal is clipped off at the maximum (or minimum) digitization value and will appear as a flat line. Again, this problem is most frequently encountered when data is recorded in DC mode (i.e., without the use of a hardware high-pass filter). Amplifier saturation artifacts can be detected by scanning the digitized output signal for repeated occurrences of the same digitization unit. However, line noise can cause small fluctuations in the digital output, making the strict versions of the above-described test fail. Therefore, it is better to scan for flat lines using a blocking/flat line algorithm that allows for the very small variations in signal that may occur even during blocking, such as the one appendix III describes. The main difference between the peak detection algorithm from appendix II and the flat line detection algorithm is that the latter reports a positive identification when the peak-to-peak amplitude is smaller than the threshold, whereas the former reports a positive identification when the observed peak-to-peak amplitude is larger than this threshold. Obviously, one should use this function to check whether the recorded signal stays within a very small amplitude range, such as 1 μV, for a substantial period of time (e.g., 500 ms).

Eye Movements and Eyeblinks

Two distinctly different processes generate ocular artifacts originating from eyeblinks and saccades. The eyeball is polarized, with the cornea being positive with respect to the retina. Saccade potentials are caused by rotation of this corneoretinal dipole, whereas blink potentials are caused by the eyelid sliding down over the positively charged cornea, permitting current to flow up toward the forehead region (Lins et al.,

1993b; Matsuo, Peters, & Reilly, 1975). The potentials both of these processes generate are typically large, and therefore these eye movements and blink related activities should always be recorded in an electro-oculogram (EOG) using electrodes near the eyes (Picton et al., 2000). Typical EOG recordings consist of the recording of a vertical EOG (vEOG), expressed as a differential recording between two electrodes placed at locations directly above and below the eyes, and a horizontal EOG (hEOG), which is the difference of two electrodes placed at the outer canthi of the left and right eye. In some cases, a radial EOG (rEOG) is obtained, which is the average amplitude of the two vertical EOG electrodes, referenced against a distant electrode location, such as Pz or Oz. The rEOG is generally not employed in EOG correction (e.g., Croft & Barry, 2002), but some think it is necessary to account for eye movement in the plane perpendicular to both horizontal and vertical planes (Elbert et al., 1985) and others use it to account for the eyelid component of blinks (Croft, 2000). Although ocular artifacts most strongly affect frontal electrodes, diminishing in amplitude as one moves posteriorly back over the scalp, they can still be observed on electrodes located as far away from the eyes as O1 or O2.

Because ocular artifacts are of such large amplitude, one should inform subjects about the effect of artifacts on EEG recordings. In many EEG studies, therefore, subjects are instructed to fixate their eyes on a central point throughout length of a block of trials and to try to minimize blinking during a trial as much as possible. When subjects comply with this, the number of ocular artifacts on any given run is typically low (on the order of 10 percent of all trials). Trials that do contain EOG artifacts can then be handled in a number of different ways, as described below.

Approaches to Handling EOG Artifacts

Rejection of Contaminated Trials   A common procedure in dealing with ocular artifacts is to reject trials in which the electrical activity at the EOG or other frontal channel exceeds a certain criterion level. When subjects have complied with the instructions described in the previous section, the number of EOG-contaminated trials is relatively low, and these trials can be rejected from further analysis. In many cases, there are good reasons for excluding trials containing ocular artifacts; in experiments studying visual processes, one wants to be sure that on each trial subjects were actually perceiving the stimuli from the correct location, that is, that they fixated at the designated location, and also that they perceived the stimulus correctly (i.e., that their eyes were actually open during stimulus presentation). Therefore, one should reject trials in which subjects did not properly fix their eyes, or closed their eyes during visual stimulus presentation. Such trials may not reflect the brain processes the experimenter intended to measure (Simons, Russo, & Hoffman, 1988).

The rejection method is relatively straightforward, but there are also some inherent problems in this method. Although it is relatively easy to refrain from blinking for a short period of time, it is generally impossible not to blink for the entire length of a block of trials. In addition to instructing subjects that they should not blink, the experimenter should also emphasize that subjects should not make blink-control a secondary task that takes up so many resources that it impairs the subject's behavior on the primary task or reduces ERP waveforms in amplitude (see, e.g., Weerts & Lang, 1973). Especially fast-rate ERP designs have trials that overlap in time (see also below). It is therefore unavoidable that a number of trials will contain ocular artifacts and have to be rejected from further analysis. Although this problem is in general relatively small with healthy young adults, the problem of recording artifact-free ERPs in other age groups, such as small children or seniors, or in patient groups such as attentional deficit/hyperactivity disorder (ADHD) or autistic children, can be considerably more problematic.

Researchers have reported a number of additional problems with the EOG rejection method. First, the ocular artifacts can show a considerable variation in amplitude, and the smaller blinks and saccades are generally difficult to detect (see, e.g., Talsma et al., 2001). Croft and Barry (2002) argue that in order to achieve the same accuracy as obtained with common EOG correction methods, the rejection criteria for EOG artifacts would have to be set to values as impractically low as 2.6 μV. That is, at frontal EEG channels, any vertical EOG activity exceeding 2.6 μV would already cause an ERP estimation error equal to or larger than the error induced by EOG artifact correction methods. Along similar lines, Verleger (1993) argues that it is impossible to determine whether or not a given trial is contaminated by blink or eye-movement artifacts.

Finally, incorrectly rejecting eyeblink trials may lead to ERP waves that are much more distorted than not rejecting any eyeblink trials at all. Figure 6.5 shows an example of this. Eyeblink EOGs are typically characterized by a relatively large initial voltage change, as the eyelid moves across the cornea. This initial amplitude change is then followed by a much slower blink-return drift of the EOG signal to the baseline recording level. In this example we show a grand-average auditory ERP (data from Talsma 2001). We performed eyeblink detection by scanning for peak-to-peak amplitude changes that exceeded 50 μV in a moving time window of 100 ms (see appendix II). The left column of figure 6.5 compares the results from correctly rejecting blink trials with the results obtained by averaging all the trials (i.e., including the eyeblink trials). Here we started detecting eyeblinks on every trial in a moving window starting about 500 ms before stimulus onset. The center and right two columns of figure 6.5 illustrate the reason for starting blink detection a few hundred milliseconds before stimulus onset. Here, blink detection started at stimulus onset, and although this enabled the detection of any blinks following stimulus onset, the procedure failed in detecting

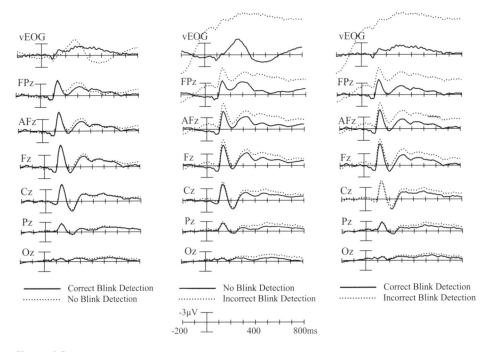

Figure 6.5
Example of eyeblink artifacts on ERPs. Shown here are the results of correct and incorrect eyeblink detection on the vertical EOG channel and the effect of eyeblink activity on the midline ERPs from anterior to posterior electrode positions. (*Left*) The effect of correctly rejecting eyeblink contaminated trials. When eyeblink trials were included (dashed line) EOG activity was larger than when these trials were excluded (solid line). Consequently, the ERPs are distorted by this ocular artifact. (*Center*) Effect of incorrectly conducted eyeblink detection. When blink detection started at stimulus onset (dashed line), the blink detection algorithm failed to catch the post blink return drift in the signal, resulting in a large negative drift in the signal around stimulus onset, which led to a distortion of the ERP wave that was much larger than the distortion caused by not rejecting any blink-contaminated trial (solid line). (*Right*) Comparison of correctly and incorrectly rejected eyeblinks.

blinks that had occurred right before stimulation. Because the peak-to-peak amplitude test was not sensitive enough to detect the post-blink return drift, the selective exclusion of only those trials where blinks occurred directly after stimulation resulted in ERP averages that were much more distorted than either ERPs excluding no blink activity from the average (center column), or ERPs excluding all blink activity (right column).

To avoid problems such as these, researchers have proposed a number of correction methods (see, for example, Brunia et al., 1989, for a comparison among different methods). The most widely used method for removing ocular artifacts from EEG recordings subtract part of the monitored EOG signal from each EEG signal. This approach is based on the assumption that the EEG recorded on the scalp consists of the true EEG plus a linearly scaled fraction of the EOG. This fraction (or propagation factor) represents how much of the EOG signal spreads to the EEG recording electrode.

For effective artifact correction, one must solve two problems: computing the propagation factors for each electrode site, and performing the correction. To compute the propagation factors accurately it is important to have enough variance in the eye activity. Blinks produce consistently large potentials and are usually frequent enough to compute propagation factors using the recorded data. Because the scalp distribution of eyeblink artifacts is distinctly different from the scalp distribution of artifacts related to saccades, one should calculate separate propagation factors for eye movements and blinks. Although eye movements in recorded data may be small but consistent enough to affect ERP averages, they may nevertheless be too small to allow an accurate estimation of propagation factors. If this is the case, it is best to estimate these propagation factors using separate calibration recordings in which consistent saccades of the order of about 15 degrees are generated in left, right, up, and down directions.

There are a number of approaches to estimating the propagation factors and subtracting the EOG activity from EEG recordings. These approaches include time or frequency domain based regression, dipole source modeling, and independent component analysis (ICA). In the following sections we discuss advantages and disadvantages of each of these methods.

Regression Methods   Linear regression is a technique to describe the relation between two sets of variables. One can use linear regression to predict the distortion of EEG recordings by estimating the linear relation between EEG and EOG recordings (see appendix I for a mathematical description of the use of linear regression in ocular artifact correction). It is one of the earliest developed methods for removing ocular artifacts from EEG recordings. Regression can correct EEG recordings for ocular artifacts in both time domain (Gratton, Coles, & Donchin, 1983; Verleger, Gasser, & Möcks, 1982) and the frequency domain (Gasser, Sroka, & Möcks, 1985; Woestenburg, Verbaten, & Slangen, 1983).[2] Although both methods are based on the same underlying regression model, differences in implementation can lead to small but consistent differences between the various methods.

Time Domain Regression   Simple time domain linear regression is the basis of a number of correction methods that have been successfully applied in ERP research (e.g., Gasser, Sroka, & Möcks, 1986; Verleger, Gasser, & Möcks, 1982). A problem with this basic method, however, is that correlations between EEG and EOG that are not due to ocular artifacts may bias the estimation of the propagation factors. For example, one may observe similar event-related activity on both EEG and EOG channels, which will bias the estimation phase of the propagation factors. For this reason, Gratton, Coles, and Donchin (1983) developed an improved method that is based on the simple regression method, but differs in that it subtracts any event-related activity from both EEG and EOG recordings and uses only event-unrelated EEG and EOG activity to estimate the regression coefficients.

Frequency Domain Regression   One limitation of the simple regression model is that it cannot account for frequency-dependent and delayed (phase-shifted) transfer from EOG to EEG (Brillinger, 1975; Kenemans et al., 1991). In contrast, a multiple-lag time domain (multiple) regression model describes both transfer characteristics. Researchers have used such models in many multiple lag time domain EOG correction algorithms (Kenemans, Molenaar, & Verbaten, 1991; Kenemans et al., 1991). The mathematical operation used to correct EEG signals in the multiple regression method, known as convolution, is equivalent to a multiplication in the frequency domain. Generally, the convolutions involved in time domain multiple-lag regression require considerably more computation time than the equivalent multiplications in the frequency domain (fast Fourier transformations included; see Beauchamp & Yuen, 1979). Although computation time is currently much less a consideration as it was more than twenty years ago, it still follows that multiple-lag ocular artifact correction is best performed in the frequency domain.

Figure 6.6 (see color plate 1) illustrates the frequency domain regression method. Shown here is an ERP waveform of one senior participant of an aging study described by Talsma (2001, chapter 8). Although still an active society member at the age of 79, this person had severe problems controlling his eyeblink. Using the rejection method would have resulted in the exclusion of all trials. Figure 6.6 shows an auditory ERP. The vertical eye channels contain a considerable amount of electrical activity, which is transferred onto the EEG recordings, specifically channels FP1, FPz, and FP2. After correction, the undistorted auditory ERP remains intact, whereas the distortion due to eyeblinks has been removed. The method used in this example is based on a description by Kenemans et al. (1991).

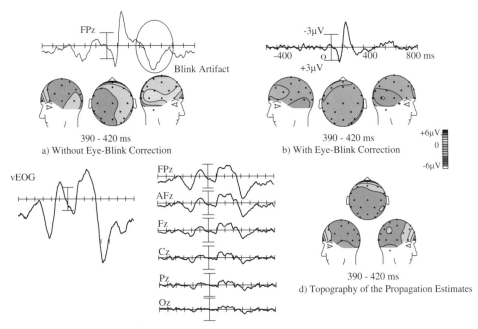

c) Estimated Propagation of EOG Activity From FPz to Oz EEG Channels

Figure 6.6
Example of ocular artifacts on ERPs with and without correction, using the frequency domain regression method. (See plate 1 for color version.)

Dipole Source Modeling Scherg and Berg (1995) and Berg and Scherg (1991) argue that the traditional regression methods can distort the spatial distribution of EEG recordings so much that frontal sources (including the auditory areas) can no longer be modeled adequately. There are two reasons for this argument: (1) according to Scherg and Berg (1995), the EOG reflects only part of the true oculo-electric activity; and (2) EEG activity also transfers to the EOG channels (Iacono & Lykken, 1981). Therefore, the regression methods may remove not only ocular activity but also part of the EEG activity at frontal channels. As an alternative to regression they therefore propose a dipole modeling solution, which estimates the eye activity independent of the frontal EEG. Instead of considering propagation factors between EOG and EEG, source components or "characteristic topographies" are computed for each type of eye activity. These source components are then combined with a dipole model (Berg & Scherg, 1994; Lins et al., 1993a) or principal components analysis (PCA)-based topographic description (Ille, Berg, & Scherg, 1997) of the brain activity to produce an operator that is applied to the data matrix to generate waveforms that are estimates of the overlapping eye and brain activity. The estimated eye activity is then subtracted from all EEG (and EOG) channels using the propagation factors defined by the source components.

According to the authors of the BESA dipole localization program, this method has a number of advantages over the traditional regression approach. First, they claim that it generates a better estimate of ocular activity than that provided by EOG channels. Second, it allows them to use the EOG channels for their EEG information. Third, if separate source components are generated for different types of ocular artifacts, their estimated waveforms provide an estimate of these different types of ocular artifacts independently.

Disadvantages of this method are, however, that it relies heavily on the use of dipole localization software and involves a labor-intensive construction of an adequate dipole model for estimating and separating the underlying ERP and EOG activities. The method also requires using a considerable number of periocular electrodes for estimating ocular activity, which cannot be used for recording brain activity at other locations. This may especially be a problem when recording with a limited number of electrodes (e.g., 32 or fewer).

Independent Component Analysis Independent components analysis (ICA) is a new, data-driven method for extracting individual signals from mixtures of signals (see e.g., Stone, 2002, for a good introduction of the ICA technique). More specifically, ICA can separate mixtures of signals recorded from N channels into a maximum of N separate components. Although ICA is still a fairly new technique, it has been used in analyzing a wide variety of problems (e.g., Jung et al., 2000, 2001), including separating eye movement activity from EEG recordings (Jung et al., 2000). ICA is similar to the spatial PCA approach (Ille, Berg, & Scherg, 1997) in that both ICA and PCA find spatial components representing ocular artifacts. Corrected EEG can than be obtained by removing these components through inverse computation. ICA differs from PCA in that it can detect components that are statistically independent, but not necessarily uncorrelated, whereas PCA components are by definition always uncorrelated. For this and other reasons, PCA cannot completely separate artifacts from cerebral activity, especially when both have comparable amplitudes (Lagerlund, Scharbrough, & Busacker, 1997), whereas ICA would be theoretically capable of doing so.

A limitation of ICA, however, is that the algorithm assigns ocular artifacts arbitrarily to one of the detected independent components. Therefore ICA requires the visual inspection of each solution to determine which component represents the estimated ocular artifact that is to be removed. In addition, ICA is a very novel technique that still needs to be validated and compared to some of the more established methods.

Overlapping ERP Components

Electromagnetical event-related brain activity typically consists of components that can last up to 1 or more seconds. Of these components, the P300 can be of particularly high amplitude and is usually followed by a negative slow wave returning to baseline, which can last for up to one or more seconds. Many experiments present stimuli at a relatively slow rate (i.e., less than one stimulus per second), to prevent ERP waves from adjacent trials overlapping. At higher presentation rates, ERPs elicited by successive stimuli can overlap in time, which can result in distortion of the ERP averages (Woldorff, 1993).

There are many experimental situations, however, that require a high rate of stimulus presentation (reviewed in Woldorff, 1995). In studies of selective attention, for example, a relatively low rate of stimulus presentation makes it very difficult to selectively focus on one relevant stimulus type and ignore others. High stimulus presentation rates, on the other hand, seem to enable a more selective focusing of attention. This view is also strongly supported by empirical data indicating that the early differentiation of processing of attended and unattended stimuli is enhanced by, or even requires a faster rate of stimulus presentation (Hansen & Hillyard, 1984; Hillyard et al., 1973; Parasuraman, 1978; Schwent, Hillyard, & Galambos, 1976; Woldorff, Hansen, & Hillyard, 1987; Woldorff, Hackley, & Hillyard, 1991; Woldorff & Hillyard, 1991; Woldorff et al., 1993; Woldorff et al., 1998).

At high rates of stimulus presentation, however, there exists the potential for waveform distortion that needs to be dealt with. In this section we describe a number of approaches one can take to minimize or remove the distortions resulting from overlapping ERPs. More specifically, we will describe the ADJAR iterative post-experimental deconvolution method and the "no-stim" subtraction method in detail. Additional overlap correction methods use Fourier transforms (Hansen, 1983), or the General Linear Model (Brillinger, 1981) to model the distortion due to overlap from adjacent trials.

Approaches to Estimate Overlap

To date, researchers have taken various approaches to resolve the problem of overlapping ERP responses. One approach has been to increase the high-pass cutoff of the filter settings, which effectively attenuates the longer latency, lower frequency portion of the ERPs. This technique artificially "forces" the response to be finished, or at least to appear to be finished, by the time the next stimulus is presented. Such high-pass filtering may achieve a reasonable solution when only the early high-frequency waves of the ERP are of interest, but may be of limited value when the longer latency waves are of interest, or when these waves contain significant power in the higher frequencies. Therefore, if studying these longer latency waves, one needs to apply one or more techniques to actually estimate the overlap from adjacent responses and subtract the estimated overlap from each waveform. In this section we will discuss two basic methods for estimating and removing overlap. We should emphasize that the use of either of these methods should be taken into consideration while designing the experiment, because a number of criteria will have to be met in order to successfully estimate the overlap from adjacent trials.

In general, one can considerably reduce the problem of overlap by fully randomizing and first-order counterbalancing the stimulus sequence. This procedure ensures that each trial type will contain approximately the same overlap as each other trial type. Therefore, contrasting two trial types that are each distorted with exactly the same overlap with each other will reveal the true difference between these two trial types. There are, however, some caveats in this method: (1) Woldorff (1993, 103–105) discovered that under certain circumstances stimulus randomization does not control for differential overlap. More specifically, when the experimental condition varies between runs (e.g., attend left vs. attend right), thereby changing the responses to the adjacent trial types, the observed overlap may not necessarily be the same for all trial types, even if the stimulus presentation sequence was fully randomized. (2) Sometimes, ERPs from two separate stimuli will be combined (e.g., one auditory [A] and visual [V] stimulus) and compared to ERPs elicited by the simultaneous presentation of a multi-object stimulus (e.g., one audiovisual multisensory object). One can combine ERPs when the ERP waves of interest represent independently evoked perceptual processing of these stimuli only (e.g., Giard & Perronet, 1999; Molholm et al., 2002; Teder-Sälejärvi et al., 2002; Talsma & Woldorff, in revision). When this assumption is valid, the combined waveform can be compared to a similar multi-object response. When overlap distorts these ERP waveforms, however, the assumption of sensory processing only is violated and the summated waveforms will contain twice the overlap distortion as the multi-object ERPs waveforms and therefore obfuscate the effects of interest. (3) Although randomization can enable the extraction of the differential response between two trials, the raw ERPs of both types will still be distorted by overlap.

Interstimulus Interval Jittering At stimulus rates where successive ERP waveforms overlap, every response included in the average (except the first and the last in the sequence) will have superimposed upon it portions of the ERP response to the preceding stimulus and portions of the response to the succeeding stimulus. Randomly varying or jittering the ISIs around a mean value can partially cancel or "smear out" these overlapping responses, thereby mitigating the distortion of the final average. An empirical rule of thumb is that the effective jitter range needs to be larger than the period of the slowest dominant waves in the overlapping responses (Woldorff, 1993). Given a few assumptions, the effect of ISI jitter on the overlap from adjacent responses can be approximated as a low-pass filtering operation on the adjacent response with either a negative or positive time shift (see Woldorff, 1993, for a full discussion).

Postexperimental Deconvolution (ADJAR)   As described above, jittering the ISI be-tween successive trials acts as a low-pass filter, which mitigates the distortion caused by overlapping ERP components. However, as with a high-pass filtering method described earlier, this approach still leaves a residual amount of overlap in the ERP waveforms. One mathematical framework of methods estimating this residual distortion makes use of the distribution of ISIs between successive stimuli. This framework, known as the adjacent response (ADJAR) technique (Woldorff, 1993), estimates overlapping ERP waveforms by convolving preceding and succeeding ERP responses with their respec-tive ISI adjacent event distributions (figure 6.7, plate 2).

Advantages of the ADJAR technique are that it allows for postexperimental decon-volution, which makes it suitable to apply to a large number of experimental designs. In addition, ADJAR requires a relatively minor number of changes to existing experi-mental designs. In general, to successfully correct ERP data using ADJAR, one should ensure that ISIs are reasonably well jittered. It also helps to have the stimulus sequence reasonably well randomized, but this is not critical (see below). In addition, the ADJAR technique is suitable for deconvolving various subranges of the ISI event distribu-tions, which allows the analysis of extremely rapid stimulus sequences. Because ADJAR makes use of the actual event distribution of the trial sequences that estimate the overlap, instead of a theoretical distribution, ADJAR will work when unequal num-bers of trials are present in different conditions. Finally ADJAR also works when event-distributions are skewed, or when stimulus sequences are not fully randomized. For example, in "S1/S2" paradigms, a stimulus of one type (i.e., a cue) is always followed by a stimulus of another type (i.e., an imperative stimulus), but two stimuli of the same type (i.e., two cues) never follow each other.

ADJAR has proven relatively difficult to implement. In addition, the time domain deconvolution process is computationally intensive and therefore a time-consuming process (although theoretically the time domain convolutions could be replaced by a frequency domain multiplication). Finally, because of the low-pass filter characteristics of jittering ISIs and the convergence of the iterative approach, ADJAR does not handle the removal of overlap from low-frequency responses, such as CNVs, or negative slow waves.

Inclusion of "No-Stim" Trials   As an alternative to the ADJAR post-experimental deconvolution, one can choose to estimate the distortion on ERP waves by including a substantially large enough proportion of "no-stim" trials in the experimental design.

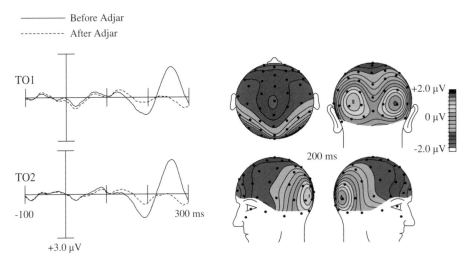

a) The effect of removing an overlapping   b) The scalp topography of the overlapping visual
   visual stimulus on ERP waveforms   ERP as estimated and removed by ADJAR

Figure 6.7
Illustration of the use of the ADJAR overlap correction technique in a multisensory experiment.
Auditory and visual stimuli were presented in close temporal proximity. (*a*) Shown here is the ERP
response to an auditory stimulus that was followed in time by a visual stimulus (between about 75–
125 ms). The delayed visual response can clearly be seen in the uncorrected ERP waveform (solid
line). After ADJAR correction, the contribution of the visual stimulus has been removed (dashed
line). (*b*) The scalp topography of the difference between corrected and uncorrected ERP waveforms.
This scalp topography is typical of a visual ERP waveform, showing that ADJAR was successful in
removing the visual ERP, but maintaining the auditory ERP. (See plate 2 for color version.)

This approach borrows from the functional imaging (fMRI) literature, where no-stim
trials were first introduced to provide a way to estimate the overlap from the slow,
event-related, hemodynamic response signals (blood oxygen dependent, or BOLD signals) used in functional MRI (Buckner et al., 1998; Dale & Buckner, 1997; Burock et al.,
1998). No-stims can best be thought of as points in time that are randomly inserted
into the stimulus stream, and which have the same randomization as the regular
stimuli, but without the actual occurrence of a stimulus. In such a case, the time-locked
averages to no-stim trials will contain on average the same response overlap from adjacent trials as any other trial type will contain. When the proportion of no-stims and
the jitter rate of the ISI between trial types satisfy the conditions Busse and Woldorff
specify (2003), one can assume that the no-stim events do not evoke a response
themselves. Therefore, selectively averaging the no-stim events will only reflect the

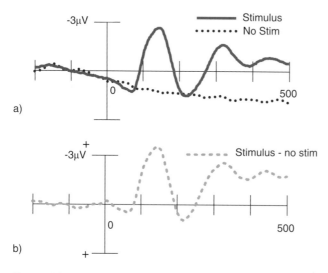

Figure 6.8

Illustration of the effectiveness of subtracting time-locked averages "no-stim" trials from the time-locked averaged ERPs elicited by real stimuli. In this example, ERPs were collapsed across all trial types in one condition of a multisensory integration condition. Panel (*a*) shows superimposed the time-locked averaged ERP waveforms to the real stimulus trials and to the no-stim trials. Panel (*b*) shows the same ERP waveform after subtracting the response to the no-stim trials. Notice that the slanted baseline, which is equally present for the both stimulus trials and for the no-stim trials in panel (*a*), has disappeared in panel (*b*).

summated response overlap from adjacent trials. Thus, subtracting the average no-stims ERP from the observed ERP averages from the other trial types will subtract out the response overlap, revealing the true ERP waveform to these other trial types.

As an example, we present data from a study on the interaction between multisensory integration and attention (Talsma & Woldorff, in revision). To test the effectiveness of estimating overlap using the no-stim method, visual-only, auditory-only, and multisensory ERPs were collapsed (to obtain a very high signal to noise ratio) for one attention condition (attend left); no-stim ERPs from the same attention condition were subtracted from this waveform. Figure 6.8a clearly shows that baseline activity (resulting from overlapping responses) is equally present in both ERPs evoked by stimulus trials as well as ERPs evoked by no-stim trials. Subtracting the no-stim ERPs from the stimulus ERPs therefore eliminates any baseline activity from the stimulus ERPs.

The no-stim approach can have several advantages over ADJAR. First of all, subtracting out no-stim ERP responses is a mathematically simple procedure, which is also easy to implement in existing ERP software. However, the use of this method needs to be carefully planned in the design stage of the experiment. Because no-stims pick up any overlapping ERPs in exactly the same way as normal ERPs would, the no-stim method is also able to correct for overlap from all types of low-frequency activity, including late negative slow waves, or stimulus preceding, anticipatory negativities.

There are, however, also a number of limitations to the no-stim method. First, it is necessary to include a relativly high number of no-stim trials in the design to get a clean estimate of the overlap. There are two reasons for this. First, as with regular ERPs, the signal-to-noise ratio of no-stim ERPs is directly proportional to the square root of the number of trials. Therefore, one needs to have at least the same number of no-stim trials as there are regular trials in one condition, to obtain an estimate of the overlap that has the same signal-to-noise ratio of the ERP waves. Second, as Busse and Woldorff (2003) show, the total number of no-stim trials should be a considerable proportion of the total number of trials, to avoid the no-stim trials from evoking an omitted stimulus response. These authors showed that this is even more true at rates of one stimulus per second or faster, as the omitted stimulus response is even more likely to be elicited at such rates. For these reasons, it is not advisable to use no-stims in long experiments, because the inclusion of a substantial number of no-stims would make an already long experiment even longer.

For reasons given above, the no-stim method works best in fully randomized and counterbalanced designs. When experimental designs are not fully counterbalanced, the assumption that all stimulus types are equally distorted by overlap is violated, and therefore, subtracting no-stim ERPs from real stimulus ERPs will not accurately remove the adjacent-response overlap and reveal the true ERPs. In such circumstances, ADJAR or other deconvolution approaches would be more advisable.

Comparison of ADJAR versus No-Stims

From the description of the two main overlap removal techniques it follows that each technique has its own strengths and weaknesses. Whereas ADJAR is flexible and adaptable, it is relatively hard to configure or implement correctly. The no-stim subtraction method, by contrast, is more limited to specific types of experiments and has certain requirements, but is easy to use. It also may be better at estimating overlap caused by very slow potentials. There are many situations where either method is applicable, and there is no principal requirement to limit oneself to one method.

Conclusion

This chapter has discussed a number artifacts and methodological problems that are commonly dealt with in ERP research. More specifically, we have discussed recording artifacts, such as spikes, drifts, and noise from power lines, ocular artifacts, including blinks and saccades, and finally, we have discussed a number of problems that might arise as the stimuli are presented more rapidly and the ERPs elicited by adjacent trials in the sequence overlap in time and distort the averages.

Common recording artifacts, such as spikes and drifting channels, can be detected through mathematically easy procedures that are generally fairly successful at excluding from the average any trials containing these artifacts. We have argued, however, that in certain cases it is possible to correct trials containing such artifacts. We have further illustrated that the amplitude of artifacts on single trials might be considerable. After averaging, the amplitude of spike and drift artifacts are substantially reduced. However, the amplitudes of these artifacts are still large enough to be falsely identified as experimental effects. Therefore, one should carefully determine the parameters used in artifact exclusion or artifact correction procedures.

Similarly, ocular artifacts are commonly dealt with by removing any trials on which they are detected. There are, however, a number of useful alternatives to the trial removal approach. The first of these methods consists of computing the propagation of electro-ocular activity into the EEG through linear regression. There are a number of different algorithms based on this technique. Simple regression assumes instantaneous and frequency independent transfer between EOG and EEG. Multiple regression, on the other hand, is able to handle delayed and frequency dependent transfer from EOG to EEG. These two techniques both operate in the time domain. Frequency domain regression techniques are mathematically equivalent to the time domain multiple lag regression method, but are computationally more efficient than the time domain method.

An alternative to the regression technique is to model both cortical and ocular activity by using a dipole model. The ocular activity can then be estimated through a spatial dipolar pattern, which can be subtracted from the spatial pattern that is explained by the cortical dipoles. Similarly, one can use independent component analysis to estimate a statistically independent spatial pattern that can be subtracted from the EEG channels.

Finally, at fast rates of stimulus presentation, the ERPs to successive stimuli in the sequence can overlap, thereby distorting the ERP averages. We discussed two methods to estimate and remove such overlap. The ADJAR approach is an iterative deconvolution technique that subtracts better and better estimates of the adjacent-response overlap from the ERPs. The second method relies on including no-stim trials in the randomized sequence that do not evoke ERPs themselves, but whose time-locked averages reflect the same overlap from adjacent trials as do the other stimulus types. Both of these methods has its specific strengths: ADJAR is a more general approach, but not so easy to implement and slow to converge for removing very slow wave overlap. The no-stim method imposes certain design restrictions (e.g., inclusion of a number of additional trials of null events) and assumptions (no elicitation of omitted stimulus responses), but it can be very useful under certain circumstances, such as removing slow wave overlap.

Appendix I: Ocular Artifact Removal Using Linear Regression

In its most elementary form, time domain regression methods perform a simple linear regression between signal and artifact. Consider for example the following equation,

$$y_t = hx_t + e_t \tag{6.2}$$

which represents the linear relation between two signals x (EOG) and y (EEG), which vary as a function of time. Time is indexed by t, ranging from 0 to $T - 1$ (T being the number of samples) and e_t represents the error made when predicting y_t from x_t. Minimizing the mean square of e_t (across t), we find a least square estimate for h in equation 6.2:

$$h = \frac{w_{xy}}{w_{xx}} \tag{6.3}$$

where w_{xy} is the covariance between x and y, and w_{xx} denotes the variance of x. Using the value of h from equation 6.3 the EOG artifact in signal y can now be corrected by subtracting hx_t from y_t.

Equation 6.2 can be extended and turned into a multiple regression model by including as predictors past and future values of x:

$$y_t = \sum_{u=-T}^{T} h_u x_{(t-u)} + e_i \tag{6.4}$$

where u indexes the lag for prediction. Equation 6.4 represents a general model for multiple lag regression. As for equation 6.2, we can solve equation 6.4 using a least square estimate:

$$H = W_{xx}^{-1} W_{xy} \tag{6.5}$$

where H is a vector containing the h_u, for u ranging from $-U$ to U. W_{xx} is a symmetrical $(2U + 1) \times (2U + 1)$ matrix, containing the covariances between x_t and x_{t-u}, $u = -U, \dots, U$—i.e., the autocovariance function of x. W_{xy} is a vector containing the covariances between x_t and $y_{(t-u)}$, $u = -U, \dots, U$, i.e. the cross-covariance function of x and y. After obtaining H from equation 6.5, the observed EEG signal can be corrected for ocular artifacts by convolving the observed EOG signal with the regressors H and subtracting the estimated artifact from the observed EEG signal, e.g.:

$$EEG_{t,corr} = EEG_{t,obs} - \sum_{u=-T}^{T} h_u EOG_{(t-u)} \tag{6.6}$$

Appendix II: Sample C++ Code for Spike Detection

Excessive amplitude fluctuations in EEG signals can be detected using a relatively straightforward moving peak-to-peak amplitude test. The following C++ code can be used to perform such a test. This function scans if the EEG signal fluctuates more than the value of `maxAmpDiff` within a moving time window of length duration. If the detected amplitude fluctuation exceeds the maximally allowed amplitude fluctuation, the function stores the observed maximum amplitude variation in the variable `*amplitude` while also returning the first sample number at which this violation occurred. Otherwise, the function returns 0 to indicate that the EEG signal in this epoch has passed the test.

```
01 int detectSpikes (double *data,
02                   double maxAmpDiff,
03                   int duration,
04                   int start,
05                   int end,
06                   double *amplitude)
07 {
08      double ampDiff;
09      int index;
10
11      for (int j = start; j < (end-duration); j++)
12      {
13          for (index = 0; index <= duration; index++)
14          {
15              ampDiff = fabs (data [j] - data[j + index]);
16              if (fabs (ampDiff >= maxAmpDiff))
17              {
18                  *amplitude = ampDiff;
19                  return j;
20              }
21          }
22      }
23      *amplitude = 0;
24      return 0;
25 }
```

This function can scan for artifacts of different amplitude and duration by modifying one of the following arguments:

```
double *data: A vector containing EEG data.
double maxAmpDiff: The maximum peak-to-peak amplitude fluctuation
        allowed within the envelope.
```

```
int duration: The length of the time window used for the peak-to-
              peak amplitude test.
int start: The first EEG data point that is tested.
int end: The last EEG datapoint that is tested.
```

Appendix III: Sample C++ Code for Flat Line Detection

Extended periods of little or no EEG activity (e.g., indicating amplifier saturations or blocking) can be detected using a modified version of the peak-to-peak amplitude test described in appendix II. The following C++ code can be used to perform such a test. This function is similar to the spike detection algorithm; however, it scans the EEG signal to see if it fluctuates less than the value of minAmpDiff within a moving time window of length duration. If the detected maximum amplitude fluctuation stays within the minimally allowed amplitude fluctuation for the entire window, the function stores the recorded maximum amplitude variation in the variable *amplitude while also returing the first sample number at which the violation occurred. Otherwise, the function returns 0 to indicate that the EEG signal in this epoch passed the test. The advantage of a method such as this over scanning for the occurrence of repeated series of identical digitization units is that this method will allow for small fluctuations due to line noise.

```
01 int detectFlatline (double *data
02                     double minAmpDiff,
03                     int duration,
04                     int start,
05                     int end,
06                     double *amplitude)
07 {
08      double ampDiff;
09      double localMax = 0;
10      int index;
11      for (int j = start; j < (end-duration); j++)
12      {
13          for (index = 0; index <= duration; index++)
14          {
15              ampDiff = fabs (data[j] - data[j + index]);
16              if (fabs(ampDiff) > localMax)
17                  localMax = fabs(ampDiff);
18          }
19          if (fabs (localMax <= minAmpDiff))
20          {
21              *amplitude = ampDiff;
```

```
22                    return j;
23            }
24        }
25        *amplitude = 0;
26        return 0;
27 }
```

This function can scan for artifacts of different amplitude and duration by modifying one of the following arguments:

```
double *data: A vector containing EEG data.
double minAmpDiff: The minimum peak-to-peak amplitude fluctuation
               required within the time window.
int duration: The length of the time window used for the peak-to-
               peak amplitude test.
int start: The first EEG data point that is tested.
int end: The last EEG datapoint that is tested.
```

Acknowledgments

We wish to thank Chad Hazlett, Tineke Grent-'t Jong, Wayne Khoe, and Roy Strowd for their helpful comments on earlier drafts of this chapter and/or other assistance. Durk Talsma also wishes to thank various colleagues in Amsterdam and Utrecht for assistance in implementing some of the algorithms discussed in this chapter.

Notes

1. There are additional interpretation difficulties related to target stimuli, such confounds caused by motor response related ERP components. These problems are, however, beyond the scope of this chapter.

2. Time domain refers to the most common method of representing EEG or ERP waveforms. In the time domain, electrical voltages are represented as a function of time, known as a time series. Any time series X_t (where $t = 0, \ldots, t = N$) can be decomposed into a series of sine and cosine wave frequencies F_f (where $f = 0, \ldots, f = N/2$). The representation of a signal as a series of frequencies is known as the frequency domain representation of a signal. The conversion between time domain and frequency representation can be done through a computational technique known as the discrete Fourier transform.

References

Beauchamp, K. G., & Yuen, C. K. (1979). *Digital methods for signal analysis*. London: George Allen & Unwin.

Berg, P., & Scherg, M. (1991). Dipole models of eye movements and blinks. *Electroencephalography and Clinical Neurophysiology, 79*, 36–44.

Berg, P., & Scherg, M. (1994). A multiple source approach to the correction of eye artifacts. *Electroencephalography and Clinical Neurophysiology, 90*, 229–241.

Brillinger, D. R. (1975). *Time series: Data analysis and theory.* New York: Holt, Rhinehart & Winston.

Brillinger, D. R. (1981). The general linear model in the design and analysis of Evoked Response Experiments. *Journal of Theoretical Neurobiology, 1*, 105–119.

Brunia, C. H. M., Möcks, J., van den Berg-Lenssen, M., Coelho, M., Coles, M. G. H., Elbert, T., Glaser, T., Gratton, G., Ifeachor, E. C., Jervis, B. W., Lutzenberger, W., Sroka, L., van Blokland-Vogelesang, A. W., van Driel, G., Woestenburg, J. C., Berg, P., McCallum, W. C., Tuan, P. H. D., Porock, P. V., & Roth, W. T. (1989). Correcting ocular artifacts: A comparison of several methods. *Journal of Psychophysiology, 3*, 1–50.

Buckner, R. L., Goodman, J., Burock, M., Rotte, M., Koutstaal, W., Schacter, D., Rosen, B., & Dale, A. M. (1998). Functional-anatomic correlates of object priming in humans revealed by rapid presentation event-related fMRI. *Neuron, 20*, 285–296.

Burock, M. A., Buckner, R. L., Woldorff, M. G., Rosen, B. R., & Dale, A. M. (1998). Randomized event-related experimental designs allow for extremely rapid presentation rates using functional MRI. *Neuroreport, 9*(16), 3735–3739.

Busse, L., & Woldorff, M. G. (2003). The ERP omitted stimulus response to "no-stim" events and its implications for fast-rate fMRI. *Neuroimage, 18*, 856–864.

Croft, R. J. (2000). The differential correction of eyelid-movement and globe rotation artefact from the EEG (reply to Verleger). *Journal of Psychophysiology, 14*, 207–209.

Croft, R. J., & Barry, R. J. (2002). Issues relating to the subtraction phase on EOG artefact correction of the EEG. *International Journal of Psychophysiology, 44*, 187–195.

Dale, A., & Buckner, R. M. (1997). Selective averaging of rapidly presented individual trials using fMRI. *Human Brain Mapping, 5*, 329–340.

Elbert, T., Lutzenberger, W., Rockstroh, B., & Bierbaumer, N. (1985). Removal of ocular artifacts from the EEG: A biophysical approach to the EOG. *Electroencephalography and Clinical Neurophysiology, 60*, 455–463.

Fisch, B. J. (1991). *Spehlmann's EEG primer*, 2d ed. Amsterdam: Elsevier.

Gasser, T., Sroka, L., & Möcks, J. (1985). The transfer of EOG into the EEG for eyes open and eyes closed. *Electroencephalography and Clinical Neurophysiology, 61*, 181–193.

Gasser, T., Sroka, L., & Möcks, J. (1986). The correction of EOG artifacts by frequency dependent and frequency independent methods. *Psychophysiology, 23*, 404–712.

Giard, M.-H., & Perronet, F. (1999). Auditory-visual integration during multimodal object recognition in humans: A behavioral and electrophysiological study. *Journal of Cognitive Neuroscience, 11*, 473–490.

Gratton, G., Coles, M. G. H., & Donchin, E. (1983). A new method for off-line removal of ocular artifacts. *Electroencephalography and Clinical Neurophysiology, 55*, 468–484.

Hansen, J. C. (1983). Separation of overlapping waveforms having known temporal distributions. *Journal of Neuroscience Methods, 9*, 127–139.

Hansen, J. C., & Hillyard, S. A. (1984). Effects of stimulation rate and attribute cueing on event-related potentials during selective auditory attention. *Psychophysiology, 21*, 394–405.

Hillyard, S. A., Hink, R. F., Schwent, V. L., & Picton, T. W. (1973). Electrical signs of selective attention in the human brain. *Science, 182*, 177–180.

Hopf, J. M., & Mangun, G. R. (2000). Shifting attention in space: An electrophysiological analysis using high spatial resolution mapping. *Clinical Neurophysiology, 111*, 1241–1257.

Iacono, W. G., & Lykken, D. T. (1981). Two-year retest stability of eye-tracking performance and a comparison of electrooculographic and infrared recording techniques: Evidence of EEG in the electro-oculogram. *Psychophysiology, 18*, 49–55.

Ille, N., Berg, P., & Scherg, M. (1997). A spatial components method for continous artifact correction in EEG and MEG. *Biomedical Techniques and Biomedical Engineering, 42(Suppl 1)*, 80–83.

Jung, T.-P., Makeig, S., Humphries, C., Lee, T.-W., McKeown, M. J., Iragui, V., & Sejnowski, T. J. (2000). Removing electroencephalographic artifacts by blind source seperation. *Psychophysiologoy, 37*, 163–178.

Jung, T.-P., Makeig, S., McKeown, M. J., Bell, A. J., Lee, T.-W., & Sejnowski, T. J. (2001). Imaging brain dynamics using independent component analysis. *Proceedings of the IEEE, 89*, 1107–1122.

Jung, T.-P., Makeig, S., Westerfeld, M., Townsend, J., Courchesne, E., & Sejnowski, T. J. (2001). Analysis and visualization of single-trial event-related potentials. *Human Brain Mapping, 14*, 166–185.

Jung, T.-P., Makeig, S., Westerfield, M., Courchesne, J. T. E., & Sejnowski, T. J. (2000). Removal of eye activity artifacts from visual event-related potentials in normal and clinical subjects. *Clinical Neurophysiology, 111*, 1745–1758.

Kenemans, J. L., Molenaar, P. C. M., Verbaten, M. M., & Slangen, J. L. (1991). Removal of ocular artifact from the EEG: A comparison of time and frequency domain methods with simulated and real data. *Psychophysiology, 28*(1), 114–121.

Kenemans, J. L., Molenaar, P. C. M., & Verbaten, M. N. (1991). Models for estimation and removal of artifacts in biological signals. In R. Weitkunat (Ed.), *Digital biosignal processing*. New York: Elsevier.

Klaver, P., Talsma, D., Wijers, A. A., Heinze, H.-J., & Mulder, G. (1999). An event-related potential correlate of visual short-term memory. *Neuroreport, 10,* 2001–2005.

Lagerlund, T. D., Scharbrough, F. W., & Busacker, N. E. (1997). Spatial filtering of multichannel electroencephalographic recordings through pricipal component analysis by singular value decomposition. *Journal of Clinical Neurophysiology, 14,* 73–84.

Lins, O. G., Picton, T. W., Berg, P., & Scherg, M. (1993a). Ocular artifacts in EEG and event-related potential. II. Source dipoles and source components. *Brain Topography, 6,* 65–78.

Lins, O. G., Picton, T. W., Berg, P., & Scherg, M. (1993b). Ocular artifacts in EEG and event-related potentials. I. Scalp topography. *Brain Topography, 6,* 51–63.

Matsuo, F., Peters, J. F., & Reilly, E. L. (1975). Electrical phenomena associated with movements of the eye-lid. *Electroencephalography and Clinical Neurophysiology, 38,* 507–511.

Molholm, S., Ritter, W., Murray, M. M., Javitt, D. C., Schroeder, C. E., & Foxe, J. J. (2002). Multisensory auditory-visual interactions during early sensory processing in humans: A high-density electrical mapping study. *Cognitive Brain Research, 14,* 115–128.

Parasuraman, R. (1978). Auditory evoked potentials and divided attention. *Psychophysiology, 15,* 460–465.

Picton, T. W., Bentin, S., Berg, P., Donchin, E., Hillyard, S. A., Johnson Jr., R., Miller, G. A., Ritter, W., Ruchkin, D. S., Rugg, M. D., & Taylor, M. J. (2000). Guidelines for using human event-related potentials to study cognition: Recording standards and publication criteria. *Psychophysiology, 37,* 127–152.

Picton, T. W., & Hillyard, S. A. (1972). Cephalic skin potentials in electroencephalography. *Electroencephalography and Clinical Neurophysiology, 33,* 419–424.

Scherg, M., & Berg, P. (1995). *BESA Brain Electric Source Analysis. User Manual.* Version 2.1. Munich.

Schwent, V. L., Hillyard, S. A., & Galambos, R. (1976). Selective attention and the auditory vertex potential. I. Effects of stimulus delivery rate. *Electroencephalography and Clinical Neurophysiology, 36,* 191–200.

Simons, R. F., Russo, K. R., & Hoffman, J. E. (1988). Event-related potential and eye-movement relationships during psychophysical judgements: The biasing effect of rejected trials. *Journal of Psychophysiology, 2,* 27–37.

Stone, J. V. (2002). Independent component analysis: An introduction. *Trends in Cognitive Science, 6,* 59–64.

Talsma, D. (2001). *Selective attention and its role in sensory processing, working memory, and cognitive aging: Event-related potential studies of potentially related events.* Doctoral dissertation, Universiteit van Amsterdam.

Talsma, D., & Kok, A. (2001). Non-spatial intermodal selective attention is meditated by sensory brain areas: Evidence from event related potentials. *Psychophysiology, 38,* 736–751.

Talsma, D., & Kok, A. (2002). Intermodal spatial attention differs between vision and audition: An event-related potential analysis. *Psychophysiology, 39*, 689–706.

Talsma, D., Wijers, A. A., Klaver, P., & Mulder, G. (2001). Working memory processes show different degrees of lateralization: Evidence from event related potentials. *Psychophysiology, 38*, 425–438.

Talsma, D., & Woldorff, M. G. (in revision). Selective attention and multisensory integration: Four phases of effects on the evoked brain activity. Submitted to *Journal of Cognitive Neuroscience*.

Teder-Sälejärvi, W. A., McDonald, J. J., Di Russo, F., & Hillyard, S. A. (2002). An analysis of audio-visual crossmodal integration by means of event-related potential (ERP) recordings. *Cognitive Brain Research, 14*, 106–114.

Verleger, R. (1993). Valid identification of blink artifacts: Are they larger than 50 µV in EEG records? *Electroencephalography and Clinical Neurophysiology, 87*, 395–404.

Verleger, R., Gasser, T., & Möcks, J. (1982). Correction of EOG artifacts in event-related potentials of the EEG: Aspects of reliability and validity. *Psychophysiology, 23*, 472–480.

Walter, W. G., Cooper, R., Aldridge, V. J., McCallum, W. C., & Winter, C. V. (1964). Contigent negative variation: An electric sign of sensorimotor association and expectancy in the human brain. *Nature, 203*, 380–384.

Weerts, T. C., & Lang, P. J. (1973). The effects of eye fixation and stimulus response location on the Contingent Negative Variation (CNV). *Biological Psychology, 1*, 1–19.

Woestenburg, J. C., Verbaten, M. N., & Slangen, J. L. (1983). The removal of eye-movement artifacts from the EEG by regression analysis in the frequency domain. *Biological Psychology, 16*, 127–147.

Woldorff, M. G. (1993). Distortion of ERP averages due to overlap from temporally adjacent ERPs: Analysis and correction. *Psychophysiology, 30*, 98–119.

Woldorff, M. G. (1995). Selective listening at fast stimulus rates: So much to hear, so little time. In Karmos et al. (Eds.), *Perspectives of Event-Related Potentials Research (EEG Suppl. 44)*, pp. 32–51. Amsterdam: Elsevier.

Woldorff, M. G., Gallen, C. C., Hampson, S. A., Hillyard, S. A., Pantev, C., Sobel, D., & Bloom, F. E. (1993). Modulation of early sensory processing in human auditory cortex during auditory selective attention. *Proceedings of the National Academy of Science of the USA, 90*, 8722–8726.

Woldorff, M. G., Hackley, S. A., & Hillyard, S. A. (1991). The effects of channel-selective attention on the mismatch negativity wave elicited by deviant tones. *Psychophysiology, 28*, 30–42.

Woldorff, M. G., Hansen, J. C., & Hillyard, S. A. (1987). Evidence for effects of selective attention in the mid-latency range of the human auditory event-related brain potential. In R. Johnson Jr., J. W. Rorhbough, & R. Parasuraman (Eds.), *Current trends in event-related potential research (EEG suppl. 40)* (pp. 146–154). Amsterdam: Elsevier.

Woldorff, M. G., & Hillyard, S. A. (1991). Modulation of early auditory processing during selective listening to rapidly presented tones. *Electroencephalography and Clinical Neurophysiology, 79,* 170–191.

Woldorff, M. G., Hillyard, S. A., Gallen, C. C., Hamson, S. R., & Bloom, F. E. (1998). Magneto-encephalographic recordings demonstrate attentional modulation of mismatch-related neural activity in human auditory cortex. *Psychophysiology, 35,* 283–292.

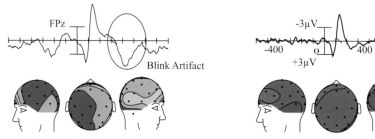

Blink Artifact

390 - 420 ms
a) Without Eye-Blink Correction

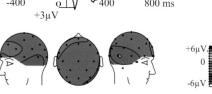

390 - 420 ms
b) With Eye-Blink Correction

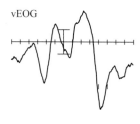

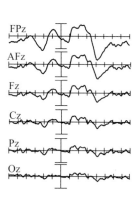

c) Estimated Propagation of EOG Activity From FPz to Oz EEG Channels

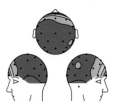

390 - 420 ms
d) Topography of the Propagation Estimates

Plate 1

Example of ocular artifacts on ERPs with and without correction, using the frequency domain regression method. See chapter 6.

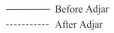

—— Before Adjar

------ After Adjar

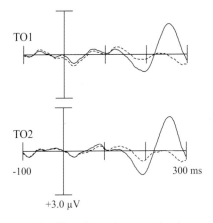

TO1

TO2

-100   300 ms

+3.0 µV

a) The effect of removing an overlapping
visual stimulus on ERP waveforms

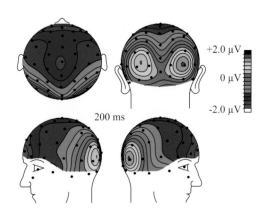

+2.0 µV

0 µV

-2.0 µV

200 ms

b) The scalp topography of the overlapping visual
ERP as estimated and removed by ADJAR

Plate 2
Illustration of the use of the ADJAR overlap correction technique in a multisensory experiment. Auditory and visual stimuli were presented in close temporal proximity. *(a)* Shown
here is the ERP response to an auditory stimulus that was followed in time by a visual stimulus (between about 75–125 ms). The delayed visual response can clearly be seen in the
uncorrected ERP waveform (solid line). After ADJAR correction, the contribution of the
visual stimulus has been removed (dashed line). *(b)* The scalp topography of the difference
between corrected and uncorrected ERP waveforms. This scalp topography is typical of a
visual ERP waveform, showing that ADJAR was successful in removing the visual ERP, but
maintaining the auditory ERP. See chapter 6.

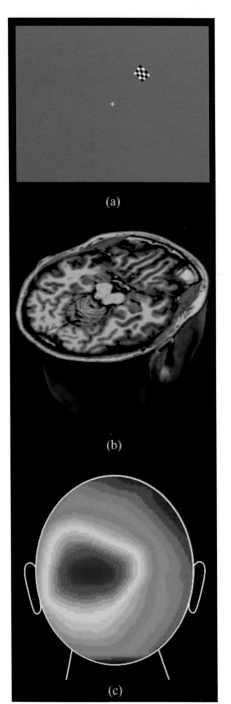

(a)

(b)

(c)

Plate 3

(a) Stimulus display with fixation cross at center and checkerboard probe at 4° visual angle in the upper right visual field, measuring 1° along each edge. (b) High-resolution anatomic MRI, with reconstructed skin surface. Only elements below a selected axial slice are shown. The head volume is rotated clockwise and the view is from posterior and above. The cortical activity in left ventral visual area V1 elicited by the stimulus is shown in yellow with a red outline, as assessed using functional MRI (fMRI). (c) Posterior view of scalp voltage topography elicited 100 ms following probe onset. Red, yellow, cyan, and blue indicate progressively decreasing voltage amplitudes, respectively. The left posterior voltage maximum is due to the underlying left ventral V1 activity. See chapter 7.

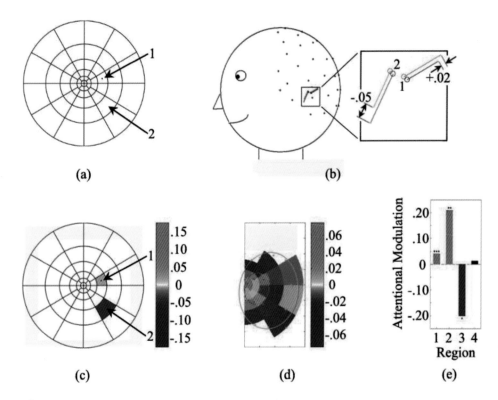

(a)   (b)

(c)   (d)   (e)

Plate 4

(a) Outline of checkerboard stimulus identical to that shown in figure 7.4a, except using an outer diameter of 15.6° visual angle was used. While maintaining central fixation, participants attended to a small color reversing circle, indicated by the black dot, located 2.6° in eccentricity. Probe 1, at the attended location, and probe 2 were selected to illustrate the procedure used to quantify attentional modulation. The response to these probes during attention to the left visual field served as baseline. (b) Left: profile of a head model with electrodes and best-fit dipoles corresponding to probe 1 and probe 2 in the attend right and attend left conditions, shown in red and black, respectively. Right: the dipole magnitude corresponding to probe 1 is larger in the attend right than the attend left condition; this difference of magnitude is a measure of attentional modulation. A positive difference of magnitude indicates attentional facilitation while a negative difference of magnitude indicates attentional inhibition, as with probe 2. (c) The difference of dipole magnitude values corresponding to probe 1 and probe 2 were projected onto the stimulus display using the color bar. Red indicates attentional facilitation and blue attentional inhibition. (d) Mean difference of magnitude values across all participants. Magenta asterisks demarcate the outer boundary of the contiguous facilitatory region and cyan asterisks demarcate the outer boundary of the contiguous inhibitory region. These boundaries were fit with elliptical models that defined a facilitatory region and inhibitory region. (e) Statistical significance of attentional modulation within region 1, the attended probe; region 2, probes within the facilitatory region; region 3, probes within the inhibitory region (excluding probes from regions 1 and 2); and region 4, probes outside of the inhibitory region. ***p < 0.001, **p < 0.01, *p < 0.05. See chapter 7.

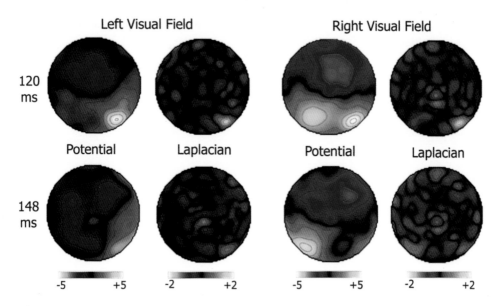

Plate 5

Topographic maps of potential and Laplacian of the ERP at two time points following the presentation of the target stimulus, 1000 ms after the offset of the cueing stimulus. Times shown on the figure are after the target stimulus arrives. Potentials are in units of microvolts. Laplacians are in units of microvolts per squared centimeter. See chapter 8.

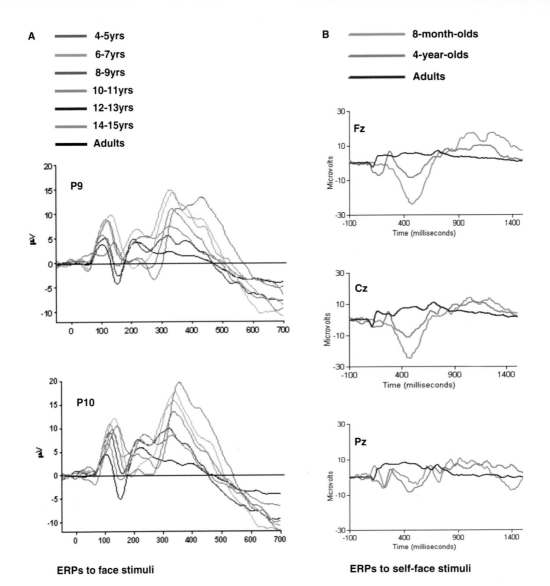

ERPs to face stimuli

ERPs to self-face stimuli

Plate 6

(A) Grand averaged ERPs from posterior, inferior temporal electrodes P9 (left parietal lobe) and P10 (right parietal lobe) in response to face stimuli for seven age groups. *(B)* Grand averaged ERPs from midline electrodes taken from a pilot study in which 8-month-olds, 4-year-olds, and adults passively viewed images of their own face in the context of a face recognition task. *(A* courtesy of Dr. Margot Taylor, Centre National Cervau et Cognition, Toulouse, France; *B* courtesy of Lisa S. Scott, Institute of Child Development, University of Minnesota.) See chapter 12.

FRONTALS

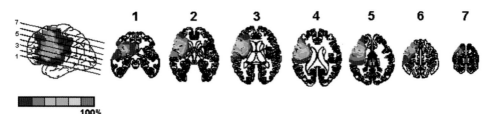

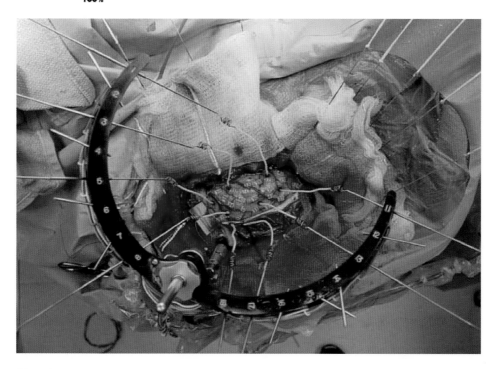

Plate 7
Averaged lesion reconstructions for the group of 11 frontal patients illustrate dorsolateral PFC damage with variable extent into ventrolateral prefrontal cortex, the anterior temporal tip, and insular cortex. Lesions were estimated from CT or MRI scans and transcribed onto sequential axial templates. All lesions are projected onto the left hemisphere. The scale indicates the percentage of patients with damage in the corresponding areas. Lines through the lateral view show the level of the axial cuts from ventral (1) to dorsal (7). (Adapted from figure 2 of Swick & Knight, 1999.) See chapter 13.

Plate 8
The picture depicts a typical electrode mounting apparatus, the horseshoe-shaped cortical crown. The carbon ball electrodes can be seen at the end of the white wires connected to the crown. The numbers tag the locations of cortical stimulation during language or motor mapping. See chapter 14.

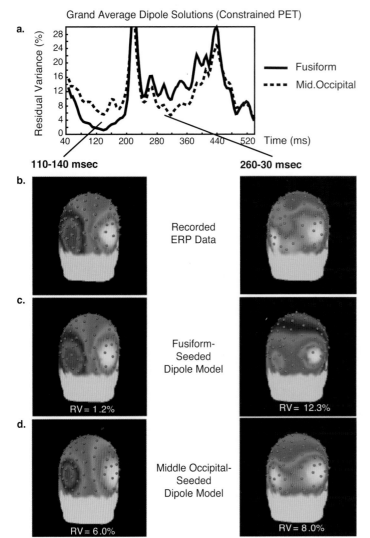

a. Grand Average Dipole Solutions (Constrained PET)

Residual Variance (%)

— Fusiform
---- Mid.Occipital

Time (ms)

110-140 msec

260-30 msec

b. Recorded ERP Data

c. Fusiform-Seeded Dipole Model

RV = 1.2%   RV = 12.3%

d. Middle Occipital-Seeded Dipole Model

RV = 6.0%   RV = 8.0%

Plate 9

(a) Graph depicting the percentage of scalp voltage variance not accounted for ("residual variance") when measuring the goodness of fit between dipole models and the observed ERP scalp distribution for the attend left minus attend right difference waveform (note that a lower value on the residual variance graph represents a better goodness of fit). Dipole models were constrained by the PET activations (left and right fusiform gyri, and left and right middle occipital gyri) elicited by the attend left versus attend right comparison. The fusiform gyrus model (indicated by the solid line in the graph) produced a better fit than the middle occipital model (1.2% versus 6.0%, respectively) in the latency range of 110–140 ms, corresponding to the P1 ERP attention effect. In contrast, at a latency range of 260–300 ms, the middle occipital gyrus model (indicated by the thick dashed line) produced a better fit than did the fusiform model (8.0% versus 12.3%). *(b–d)* Recorded topographic maps of attention effects *(b)* corresponding to the attend left minus attend right difference waveform, and model data topographic maps *(c, d)* for dipoles placed at the location of the PET defined fusiform gyrus attention effects *(c)* or the location of the PET defined middle occipital gyrus attention effects *(d)*. The maps are for the time period of the P1 component (110–140 ms) in the left column, and for a later sustained positivity (260–300 ms) in the right column. The difference between the recorded and model data, expressed as percent residual variance (RV), is shown below each model head. The view of the heads is from the rear (left on left). The locations of electrodes are indicated by gray disks. (Reprinted from Hopfinger et al., 2001, with permission from Elsevier Science.) See chapter 15.

7 Source Localization of ERP Generators

Scott D. Slotnick

Researchers use ERP source localization techniques to identify the loci of neural activity that give rise to a particular voltage distribution measured on the surface of the scalp. For example, when a small stimulus is presented in the upper right visual field (figure 7.1a), activity occurs in left occipital cortex (figure 7.1b), resulting in a measurable voltage response on the scalp (figure 7.1c) (see plate 3). One can use simple analysis of this voltage topography to make course statements about the location of the underlying cortical source—for example, the voltage maximum is over left occipital cortex. In contrast, however, one can use source localization techniques to identify the actual location of the voltage source in cortex—for example, left ventral primary visual cortex (V1).

Source localization is not a trivial undertaking. As Helmholz (1853) pointed out, a specific cortical source configuration produces a unique scalp voltage topography, but an infinite number of different cortical source configurations can produce the same given scalp voltage topography. This difficulty in determining source configuration from scalp topography—where a given scalp topography has an infinite number of source configurations—is formally known as the "inverse problem." Fortunately, however, there is also an "inverse solution" that one can use to localize cortical activity, and which is dependent upon the "forward solution."

The Forward Solution

The forward solution to source localization relies on modeling two key factors. First, given that a voltage measured at the surface of the scalp reflects a field potential that has traveled through a three-dimensional space (the head) that varies in its conductive properties (the brain, dura, skull, etc.), a model of the head is assumed that takes into account some or all of these factors. Second, because only certain anatomical configurations of neurons can lead to field potentials measurable at the surface of the scalp (known as far-field potentials), one must also assume a specific model of cortical source activity. The following section expands on both of these model assumptions.

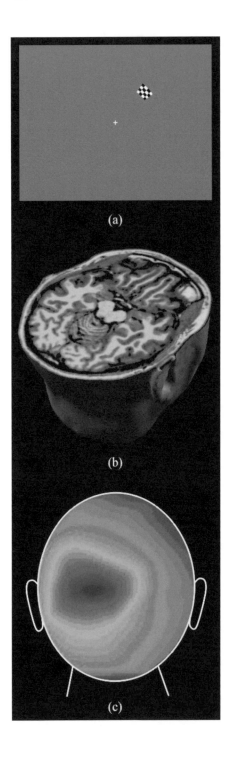

(a)

(b)

(c)

Modeling the Head as a Sphere

Although it is obvious that the human head is not shaped like a sphere (compare figure 7.1b to figure 7.2a), such a simplifying assumption is useful in deriving the mathematical expressions used for source localization. A spherical head model has homogeneous conductance and its surface represents the scalp.

A somewhat more realistic head model consists of three concentric spheres, or shells, where the regions corresponding to the brain, skull, and scalp each have a unique conductance. Given that a simple correction can convert solutions obtained using a homogeneous sphere to those obtained using a three-shell sphere (Ary, Klein, and Fender, 1981), only the former is considered in detail. We consider more realistic head models below.

Modeling Cortical Activity as a Dipole

An active patch of cortex can be modeled as a dipole current sheet, which consists of positive and negative layers of abutting charges (Nunez, 1981). This model can be reduced to an effective dipole point source (i.e., dipole source), as this term is dominant in the mathematical expansion of the dipole sheet. To test whether this model reduction was warranted, de Munck, van Dijk, and Spekreijse (1988) fit a dipole source to extended sources (e.g., a dipole disk) using a simulation, and found a dipole source was adequate. Thus, as long as the active patch of cortex is small enough that the dipole term is dominant, cortical activity appears to be well modeled by a dipole source.

A dipole current source can be described by its location, r, and moment, M (figure 7.2b). Dipole location is typically reported in reference to the center of the head model, whereas dipole moment uses dipole location as its origin. For convenience, dipole location is described in Cartesian coordinates and dipole moment is described in spherical coordinates; both coordinate systems are interchangeable.

Model-Generated Scalp Potentials

Wilson and Bayley (1950) were the first to formulate the electrical activity of a dipole within a homogeneous sphere, followed by Frank (1952), who restricted the solution

◄ **Figure 7.1**

(a) Stimulus display with fixation cross at center and checkerboard probe at 4° visual angle in the upper right visual field, measuring 1° along each edge. (b) High-resolution anatomic MRI, with reconstructed skin surface. Only elements below a selected axial slice are shown. The head volume is rotated clockwise and the view is from posterior and above. The cortical activity in left ventral visual area V1 elicited by the stimulus is shown in yellow with a red outline, as assessed using functional MRI (fMRI). (c) Posterior view of scalp voltage topography elicited 100 ms following probe onset. Red, yellow, cyan, and blue indicate progressively decreasing voltage amplitudes, respectively. The left posterior voltage maximum is due to the underlying left ventral V1 activity. (See plate 3 for color version.)

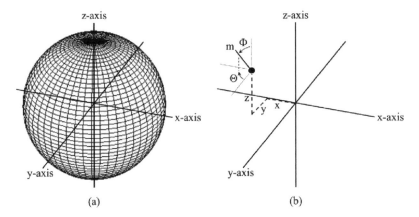

Figure 7.2
(*a*) Spherical head model with center at Cartesian coordinate $(0,0,0)$. (*b*) Dipole with Cartesian coordinate location parameters (x, y, z), r, and spherical coordinate moment parameters (m, Θ, Φ), M. Parameter m depicts dipole magnitude and parameters Θ and Φ describe dipole orientation.

to voltages generated on the surface of a sphere (i.e., the scalp). However, the latter equations were not determinate for all dipole and electrode locations, which were ultimately derived by Brody, Terry, and Ideker (1973). Their weighting matrix, W, is defined by

$$W(e,r) = \frac{e + \dfrac{2(e-r)}{d^2} + \dfrac{e(e \cdot r) - r}{d + 1 - e \cdot r}}{d} \quad \text{where } d = |r - e| \tag{7.1}$$

where e is a matrix containing electrode locations on the surface of the sphere, r represents dipole location, and d is the distance matrix between the dipole location and electrode locations. The voltage at each electrode is given by

$$V_{\text{model}}(e) = W(e,r) \cdot M \tag{7.2}$$

(Brody, Terry, & Ideker, 1973) where M represents dipole moment and $\cdot$ is the dot product operator. Because superposition of electric fields can be assumed, these equations also apply if multiple dipoles are simultaneously active.

Equation 7.2 can be modified to include changes in scalp potential over time

$$V_{\text{model}}(e,t) = W(e,r) \cdot M(t) \tag{7.3}$$

where t refers to time. In equation 7.3, dipole moment, M, which is defined by magnitude, m, and orientation parameters (Θ, Φ), can vary over time; however, it is reasonable to assume the cortical patch underlying a particular dipole is invariant in location and orientation (Scherg, 1990; implemented in the software package BESA). In this framework, one can imagine the dipole in figure 7.2b fixed in location and orientation with only magnitude, m, fluctuating over time.

It is also possible to define a new parameter T that describes temporal variation, while dipole location, orientation, and magnitude remain fixed

$$V_{\text{model}}(e, t) = W(e, r) \cdot MT(t) \tag{7.4}$$

(Slotnick et al., 1999). Parameter T is normalized to unity over time. By isolating a time-invariant estimate of dipole magnitude, useful magnitude comparisons can be made across experimental conditions (Slotnick et al., 2001; Slotnick et al., 2002).

The Inverse Solution

Solving the inverse problem via the forward solution can be reduced to model fitting. A nonlinear model-fitting algorithm iteratively modifies the input parameters in such a way as to minimize the sum-of-squares error (SSE) between the data and model (figure 7.3). Parameter fitting routines include the Levenberg-Marquardt method (Marquardt, 1963), the simplex method (Nelder & Mead, 1965), simulated annealing (Kirkpatrick, 1984; Khosla, Singh, & Don, 1997), and genetic algorithms (McNay et al., 1996). See Press et al. 1992 for a description of the first three techniques.

In dipole source localization, the to-be-fit data are the voltages measured with scalp electrodes, V_{data}, and the corresponding model voltages, V_{model}, are generated using the forward solution. Iteratively adjusted model parameters include dipole location, orientation, magnitude, and timecourse. Certain parameters, such as dipole timecourse, can be fit outside of the dipole fitting routine using linear regression.

Although there is a best solution in source localization in terms of SSE minimization, less optimal solutions are possible. Specifically, the fitting algorithm can settle on a set of parameters that minimizes SSE in the local sense, but not in the global sense (i.e., it gets caught in a local minimum). If different initial dipole parameters were set, the global minimum may have been found. Thus, initial conditions are an important factor when conducting dipole source localization. The following section considers factors essential for optimizing the obtained inverse solution.

Number of Recording Electrodes Because an increase in electrode number provides more information about the underlying neural source, it is not surprising that simulation results have shown an increase in electrode number is associated with an increase in localization accuracy (Laarne et al., 2000). Gevins (1990) has reported that the cortex-to-scalp point spread function is approximately 2.5 cm. Taking this value into account, approximately a hundred electrodes are required to adequately sample the voltage topography across the scalp. It would follow that the spatial resolution of

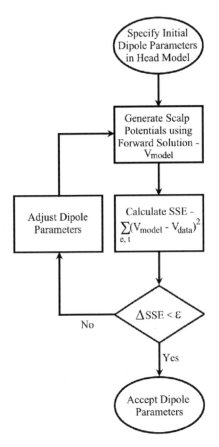

Figure 7.3
Flowchart of inverse solution. First, the initial parameters for the dipole(s) are specified. Then, a fitting procedure is used to minimize the change in sum-of-squares error (ΔSSE) between scalp voltages produced by the model (V_{model}) and those measured (V_{data}).

source localization may suffer if one uses fewer electrodes and may remain unchanged if one uses more electrodes.

Constraining the Solution   Researchers have used a number of constraints to increase the accuracy of source localization. One obvious constraint is to reject dipole solutions that are located outside of the head, a scenario that is physiologically impossible.

Perhaps the most important user defined constraint is the number of dipoles; which is matched to the expected number of neural sources. This knowledge can come from detailed analysis of ERP waveforms, mathematical methods such as principle component analysis or reduced chi-square analysis (Supek & Aine, 1993), results from the literature, or neuroimaging data.

To avoid local minima, one frequently used technique is to vary the initial dipole parameters randomly, within reasonable limits, and accept the most convergent results, which should represent the global minimum. Such a procedure can be automated to reduce user involvement (Huang et al., 1998). A priori knowledge extracted from the literature can also be used to specify initial conditions (Tarkka et al., 1995). The locus of neuroimaging activity, during the same task as for ERP recording, has also been used for initial locations in source localization (Heinze et al., 1994; Mangun, Hopfinger, & Heinze, 1998; Mangun et al., 2001; see also chapter 15 of this volume). In these visual attention studies, two dipoles were first fixed at the loci of activation in extrastriate cortex, fit using an inverse solution (equation 7.3 with fixed location and orientation), and then, using these parameters as starting points, the fixed location constraint was released and the fit was conducted again. In all cases, the dipoles moved only slightly during the second fit.

The time window relative to stimulus onset within which one conducts source localization can also be restricted. In a visual perception study, Clark, Fan, and Hillyard (1995) restricted their two dipole analysis to 50–80 ms following stimulus onset, arguing, based on the polarity of ERP waveforms, that the ERP C1 and P1 components within this temporal window could be attributed to striate and extrastriate cortical activity. Some have used a stepwise temporal constraint approach (Plendl et al., 1993; Gomez Gonzalez et al., 1994; Martinez et al., 2001; Di Russo et al., 2001). The Gomez Gonzalez et al. (1994) study on visual attention fit one V1 dipole and two lateral occipital dipoles within the 75- to 125-ms range, fit two inferotemporal dipoles separately within the 125- to 175-ms range, and then using these solutions as initial conditions, allowed all five dipoles to vary within the 75- to 175-ms range.

When a pair of dipoles is fit, one spatial constraint that has been implemented is to force the solutions to have hemispheric symmetry (Scherg & Berg, 1991). Although this constraint is common (Gomez Gonzalez et al., 1994; Martinez et al., 2001; Di Russo et al., 2001), its anatomic validity has not been tested.

Head Models The brain consists of white and gray matter, contains ventricals, and is surrounded by cerebrospinal fluid, the skull, and the scalp (figure 7.1b). The skull has varying thickness and openings (e.g., at the ears). Even within a given tissue type, there can be large differences in conductance (i.e., anisotropy); white matter conductance can vary by a factor of 15 (Geddes & Baker, 1967). All of these complexities make spherical models, including three- or four-shell renditions, a bit too simplistic. To improve on the homogeneity assumption of spherical models, de Munck (1988) formulated an anisotropic multilayered spherical model.

More realistic head modeling has also been implemented using the boundary element method (BEM; Menninghaus, Lütkenhöner, & Gonzalez, 1994; Fuchs, Wagner, & Kaster, 2001). The BEM approximates a realistic head shape (or brain, skull, and scalp shapes) using thousands of triangles. If modeling multiple compartments, the BEM method assumes they have homogeneous conductivity (a limitation that the related finite element method, FEM can address, in principle). The major drawback of the BEM, and even more so the FEM, is computation burden, which will become less of an issue as more efficient algorithms are produced (Yvert, Crouzeix-Cheylus, & Pernier, 2001) and computational speed increases.

A FEM simulation study claimed that an accurate head model, including the appropriate conductivities, is necessary in order to achieve a localization accuracy of within a few millimeters (Awada et al., 1998). However, head models created using the BEM or FEM methods are far from an accurate representation of a real head, and are perhaps closer to their spherical counterparts than their proponents would like to admit. In support of this latter position, a recent simulation showed that if one uses a sufficient number of recording electrodes and assumes correlated noise, the importance of real head modeling over spherical head modeling is limited (Vanrumste et al., 2002). Furthermore, in a recent empirical study, BEM results were similar to those obtained using a four-shell spherical model (Schaefer et al., 2002). These examples indicate that the best head models in use are still poor approximations of a real head, a problem known as model misspecification (i.e., when the head model is not accurate).

Model misspecification necessarily results in source localization errors; these effects are magnified when multiple dipoles are simultaneously active (Zhang & Jewett, 1993; Mosher et al., 1993; Zhang, Jewett, & Goodwill, 1994; Jewett & Zhang, 1995). Therefore, the effects of model misspecification can be minimized by assuming a single dipole source.

Source Localization Accuracy   Given the numerous assumptions involved in dipole source localization, it is crucial to quantify the accuracy of this technique. Cuffin et al. (1991) used electrodes implanted into the human brain to create artificial dipole sources by passing current between pairs of depth electrodes. Sixteen scalp electrodes were used for single dipole source localization, with a four-shell spherical head model. In three participants using 28 dipoles, the average dipole localization error was equal to 1.1 cm. This value replicated a previous localization error of 1 centimeter using similar techniques (Cohen, Cuffin, & Yunokuchi, 1990) and also provided empirical support for Cuffin (1990), who argued that a source localization error of less than 1 cm is achievable using a spherical head model. Also using depth electrodes and up to 41 scalp electrodes, Krings et al. (1999) localized artificial dipole sources and Merlet and Gotman (1999) localized epileptic spikes. Both used four-shell spherical head models, and reported average localization errors of 1.3 and 1.1 cm, respectively. The results of these studies show a surprising degree of convergence, suggesting that dipole source localization can be accurate to approximately 1 cm using a four-shell spherical head model. Employing additional scalp electrodes may further improve accuracy. Still, these results indicate that a spherical head model can be used to obtain source localization results that are reasonably accurate.

Empirical Examples

I present two examples from my own work, as they demonstrate the techniques described and also illustrate two different uses of source localization results: analysis of dipole locations and analysis of dipole magnitudes.

Estimating Cortical Magnification Factor

Cortical magnification refers to the relative increase in cortical area allocated to processing an object at fixation compared to when that same object is presented at an eccentric location. Numerous techniques have been used to estimate human cortical magnification, including psychophysics (Beard, Levi, & Klein, 1997), scaling monkey results from single-cell recording (Horton & Hoyt, 1991), direct cortical stimulation (Cowey & Rolls, 1974), and fMRI (Sereno et al., 1995; Engel, Glover, & Wandell, 1997). We recently estimated cortical magnification using dipole source localization (Slotnick et al., 2001).

In this study, the stimulus display consisted of 60 checkerboard probes (figure 7.4a). All probes were modulated with a binary *m*-sequence (Zierler, 1959; Golumb, 1982) at a frame rate of 75 Hz. A binary *m*-sequence is a pseudo-random series of zeros and ones that define the state of a given probe on each frame (e.g., 0 indicates a particular black/ white checkerboard configuration and 1 indicates the reverse white/black contrast). Because the *m*-sequence of each probe was orthogonal to the *m*-sequences of all other probes (i.e., the *m*-sequences were mathematically independent), all probes were modulated simultaneously. The flash response elicited by any given probe was calculated through cross-correlation of that probe's *m*-sequence with the response at any given electrode (see Sutter, 1992). This method of stimulation primarily activates visual area V1 such that a single dipole source was assumed generated by each stimulus probe (Slotnick et al., 1999).

The voltage response was recorded at 48 posterior scalp electrodes (43 for one participant) placed according to the standard 10–20 convention (Jasper, 1958) with additional electrodes placed at intermediate positions such that all electrodes were spaced approximately 2.5 cm apart (see electrode configuration in figure 7.5b and plate 4). For each probe, the voltage response across the electrode array for 333 ms following stimulus onset was subjected to dipole source localization. To conduct source localization, a single dipole current source, fixed in location, orientation, and magnitude, within a

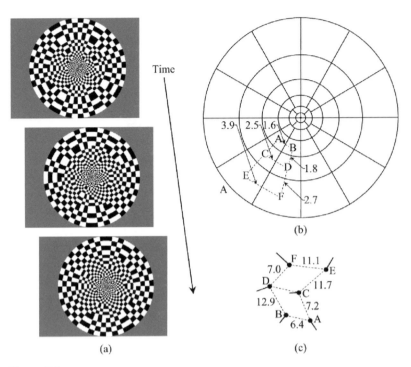

Figure 7.4

(*a*) Three frames of a stimulus display consisting of 60 checkerboard stimulus probes. Every 27 ms, on average, each probe reversed in contrast according to an independent *m*-sequence. The stimulus had an outer diameter of 18.2° visual angle. Participants maintained fixation at the center of the display. (*b*) Outline of each probe within the stimulus display. Six probes, labeled A through F, were selected to illustrate the procedure used to estimate cortical magnification. Distances between probes, indicated by dotted lines, were measured in degrees of visual angle. Probes A and B were located 2.6° visual angle from the center of the display. (*c*) Dipole sources in visual area V1, corresponding to the select probes, as if viewed from above (the anterior of the head is toward the top of the page). The distance between each pair of dipoles, indicated by dotted lines and reported in millimeters, represents cortical distance. Cortical magnification can be computed using the distances between probe pairs and the distances between corresponding dipole pairs at various eccentricities.

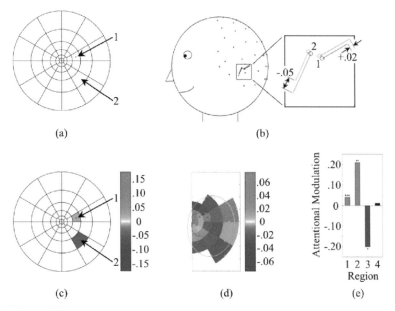

(a)   (b)

(c)   (d)   (e)

Figure 7.5
(*a*) Outline of checkerboard stimulus identical to that shown in figure 7.4a, except using an outer diameter of 15.6° visual angle. While maintaining central fixation, participants attended to a small color reversing circle, indicated by the black dot, located 2.6° in eccentricity. Probe 1, at the attended location, and probe 2 were selected to illustrate the procedure used to quantify attentional modulation. The response to these probes during attention to the left visual field served as baseline. (*b*) Left: profile of a head model with electrodes and best-fit dipoles corresponding to probe 1 and probe 2 in the attend right and attend left conditions, shown in red and black, respectively. Right: the dipole magnitude corresponding to probe 1 is larger in the attend right than the attend left condition; this difference of magnitude is a measure of attentional modulation. A positive difference of magnitude indicates attentional facilitation, whereas a negative difference of magnitude indicates attentional inhibition, as with probe 2. (*c*) The difference of dipole magnitude values corresponding to probe 1 and probe 2 were projected onto the stimulus display using the color bar. Red indicates attentional facilitation and blue attentional inhibition. (*d*) Mean difference of magnitude values across all participants. Magenta asterisks demarcate the outer boundary of the contiguous facilitatory region and cyan asterisks demarcate the outer boundary of the contiguous inhibitory region. These boundaries were fit with elliptical models that defined a facilitatory region and inhibitory region. (*e*) Statistical significance of attentional modulation within region 1, the attended probe; region 2, probes within the facilitatory region; region 3, probes within the inhibitory region (excluding probes from regions 1 and 2); and region 4, probes outside of the inhibitory region. ***$p < 0.001$, **$p < 0.01$, *$p < 0.05$. (See plate 4 for color version.)

homogeneous spherical head model were used in the forward solution (equation 7.4). A one-shell to three-shell correction was applied to the results (Ary, Klein, & Fender, 1981). The Levenberg-Marquardt algorithm was used for the inverse solution. Initial dipole locations were randomly selected from a 3×3 grid placed 30 percent in depth from the surface of the sphere and contralateral to the probe under analysis. Dipole orientation was initially set to be radial with a magnitude of 1, which were arbitrary settings, and the initial timecourse was obtained using linear regression. During the fitting procedure, both dipole magnitude and timecourse were computed using linear regression. All source localization was conducted using custom software written in MATLAB (The MathWorks, Inc., Natick, MA).

Dipole solutions were invariant to different initial dipole parameters, indicating that local minima were not a significant factor. Figure 7.4 shows a subset of stimulus probes and their corresponding dipole locations, orientations, and magnitudes. Cortical magnification is defined in terms of cortical distance (in millimeters) and visual field distance (in degrees of visual angle) at a given eccentricity. Thus, the distance between each pair of probes and the distance between the corresponding pair of dipoles was used to estimate human cortical magnification (Slotnick et al., 2001). The estimate was similar to previous estimates based upon psychophysics, cortical stimulation, and fMRI (Beard, Levi, & Klein, 1997; Cowey & Rolls, 1974; Sereno et al., 1995). The concordance of source localization results with fMRI, a technique known to have spatial resolution on the order of millimeters, suggests source localization can have excellent spatial resolution.

The Spatial Distribution of Visual Attention

Slotnick et al. (2002) used the same method of stimulation described in the previous example to study visual attention. While maintaining central fixation, participants attended to a $0.1°$ visual angle diameter circle that alternated in color between red and green at random time intervals ranging from 1 to 10 s. The attended circle was centered on a probe 2.6 degrees from fixation and adjacent to the horizontal meridian in the right visual field or on the analogous probe in the left visual field (figure 7.5a).

As before, a single dipole current source in a homogeneous sphere was used for the forward solution. The inverse solution was also the same, except dipoles for a given probe were constrained to have the same location and orientation in both attend-right and attend-left conditions. This constraint was imposed as a given probe was expected to activate the same patch of cortex but only change its magnitude of response with attention (Motter, 1993; Mangun & Hillyard, 1988; Heinze et al., 1994). The time window of analysis was also restricted to 50–110 ms following stimulus onset, which contained the dominant ERP response using this method of stimulation (Slotnick et al., 1999).

Figure 7.5a illustrates the stimulus display in the attend right condition. To quantify the effect of attention at a particular probe location, dipole magnitude with attention was compared to dipole magnitude without attention (figure 7.5b,c). Difference of magnitude values were projected within the outlines of the stimulus probes, such that the nature (i.e., facilitatory or inhibitory modulation) and spatial distribution of attention could be assessed. Figure 7.5d shows group results. The outer boundary of the contiguous facilitatory probes and the contiguous inhibitory probes were fit with an ellipse using a $(n + 1) - D$ fitting algorithm (Slotnick, 2003), as conventional fitting procedures could not provide a solution. Attentional facilitation occurred not only at the attended location, as expected, but also extended toward fixation. The facilitatory region was also surrounded by a region of attentional inhibition. This study provides unequivocal evidence that attention effects can be both facilitatory and inhibitory. The results also exemplify that dipole magnitude is a meaningful parameter that researchers can use to measure the magnitude of the cortical response.

Future Directions

One of the biggest weaknesses in dipole source localization relates to the forward problem—poor head models. Even the more realistic head models produced to date, using the BEM or FEM, do not fare much better than multilayer spherical head models. If one is to achieve localization accuracy on the order of millimeters, there must be better head models constructed. For this reason, realistic head modeling is an area of active investigation.

Another line of research is concerned with the inverse problem. Dale and Sereno (1993) describe a technique in which researchers place thousands of dipoles normal to an MRI surface, then obtain the strength of each dipole via linear error minimization. This method has the advantage that the user need not specify the number of dipoles in the solution, a concern of more conventional source localization procedures. Neural networks have also been proposed for use in source localization (Van Hoey et al., 2000). Other methods are also in use, and more will be developed.

Source localization has many complex aspects, including head modeling, iterative model fitting, and user specified constraints. For this reason, it is unlikely that there will ever be one correct method to conduct source localization. Rather, the field of source localization is expected to continue on its course of rapid evolution.

Acknowledgments

I am indebted to Stan Klein and Dr. Don Jewett for invaluable discussions concerning source localization. I also thank Lauren Moo for her adroit comments on this chapter.

References

Ary, J. P., Klein, S. A., & Fender, D. H. (1981). Location of sources of evoked scalp potentials: Corrections for skull and scalp thicknesses. *Biomedical Engineering, 28,* 447–452.

Awada, K. A., Jackson, D. R., Baumann, S. B., Williams, J. T., Wilton, D. R., Fink, P. W., & Prasky, B. R. (1998). Effect of conductivity uncertainties and modeling errors on EEG source localization using a 2-D model. *IEEE Transactions on Biomedical Engineering, 45,* 1135–1145.

Beard, B. L., Levi, D. M., & Klein, S. A. (1996). Vernier acuity with non-simultaneous targets: The cortical magnification factor estimated by psychophysics. *Vision Research, 37,* 325–346.

Brody, D. A., Terry, F. H., & Ideker, R. E. (1973). Eccentric dipole in a spherical medium: Generalized expression for surface potentials. *IEEE Transactions on Biomedical Engineering, 20,* 141–143.

Clark, V. P., Fan, S., & Hillyard, S. A. (1995). Identification of early visual evoked potential generators by retinotopic and topographic analyses. *Human Brain Mapping, 2,* 170–187.

Cohen, D., Cuffin, B. N., Yunokuchi, K., Maniewski, R., Purcell, C., Cosgrove, G. R., Ives, J., Kennedy, J. G., Schomer, D. L. (1990). MEG versus EEG localization test using implanted sources in the human brain. *Annals of Neurology, 28,* 811–817.

Cowey, A., & Rolls, E. T. (1974). Human cortical magnification factor and its relation to visual acuity. *Experimental Brain Research, 21,* 447–454.

Cuffin, B. N. (1990). Effects of head shape on EEGs and MEGs. *IEEE Transactions on Biomedical Engineering, 37,* 44–52.

Cuffin, B. N., Cohen, D., Yunokuchi, K., Maniewski, R., Purcell, C., Cosgrove, G. R., Ives, J., Kennedy, J., & Schomer, D. (1991). Tests of EEG localization accuracy using implanted sources in the human brain. *Annals of Neurology, 29,* 132–138.

Dale, A. M., & Sereno, M. I. (1993). Improved localization of cortical activity by combining EEG and MEG with MRI cortical surface reconstruction: A linear approach. *Journal of Cognitive Neuroscience, 5,* 162–176.

de Munck, J. C. (1988). The potential distribution in a layered anisotropic spheroidal volume conductor. *Journal of Applied Physics, 64,* 464–470.

de Munck, J. C., van Dijk, B. W., & Spekreijse, H. (1988). Mathematical dipoles are adequate to describe realistic generators of human brain activity. *IEEE Transactions on Biomedical Engineering, 35,* 960–966.

Di Russo, F., Martinez, A., Sereno, M. I., Pitzalis, S., & Hillyard, S. A. (2001). Cortical sources of the early components of the visual evoked potential. *Human Brain Mapping, 15,* 95–111.

Engel, S. A., Glover, G. H., & Wandell, B. A. (1997). Retinotopic organization in human visual cortex and the spatial precision of functional MRI. *Cerebral Cortex, 7,* 181–192.

Frank, E. (1952). Electric potential produced by two point current sources in a homogeneous conducting sphere. *Journal of Applied Physics, 23*, 1225–1228.

Fuchs, M., Wagner, M., & Kaster, J. (2001). Boundary element method volume conductor models for EEG source reconstruction. *Clinical Neurophysiology, 112*, 1400–1407.

Geddes, L. A., & Baker, L. E. (1967). The specific resistance of biological material: A compendium of data for the biomedical engineer and physiologist. *Medical & Biological Engineering, 5*, 271–293.

Gevins, A. S. (1990). Analysis of multiple lead data. In J. Rohrbaugh, R. Johnson, & R. Parasuraman (Eds.), *Event-Related Potentials of the Brain* (pp. 44–56). New York: Oxford University Press.

Golomb, S. W. (1982). *Shift register sequences.* Laguna Hills, CA: Aegean Park Press.

Gomez Gonzalez, C. M., Clark, V. P., Fan, S., Luck, S. J., Hillyard, S. A. (1994). Sources of attention-selective visual event-related potentials. *Brain Topography, 7*, 41–51.

Heinze, H. J., Mangun, G. R., Burchert, W., Hinrichs, H., Scholz, M., Münte, T. F., Gös, A., Scherg, M., Johannes, S., Hundeshagen, H., Gazzaniga, M. S., & Hillyard, S. A. (1994). Combined spatial and temporal imaging of brain activity during visual selective attention in humans. *Nature, 372*, 543–546.

Helmholz, H. (1853). Ueber Einiger Gezetze der Vertailung Elektrischer Strome in Korperlichen Leiter mit anwendung auf die Thierisch Elektrischeb Versuche. *Pogg. Ann. Physik. Chemie., 89*, 211–233.

Horton, J. C., & Hoyt, W. F. (1991). The representation of the visual field in human striate cortex: A revision of the classic Holmes map. *Archives of Ophthalmology, 109*, 816–824.

Huang, M., Aine, C. J., Supek, S., Best, E., Ranken, D., & Flynn, E. R. (1998). Multi-start downhill simplex method for spatio-temporal source localization in magnetoencephalography. *Electroencephalography and Clinical Neurophysiology, 108*, 32–44.

Jasper, H. H. (1958). Appendix to report to Committee on Clinical Examination in EEG: The ten-twenty electrode system of International Federation. *Electroencephalography and Clinical Neurophysiology, 10*, 371–375.

Jewett, D. L., & Zhang, Z. (1995). Multiple-generator errors are unavoidable under model misspecification. *Electroencephalography and Clinical Neurophysiology, 95*, 135–142.

Khosla, D., Singh, M., & Don, M. (1997). Spatio-temporal EEG source localization using simulated annealing. *IEEE Transactions on Biomedical Engineering, 44*, 1075–1091.

Kirkpatrick, S. (1984). Optimization by simulated annealing: Quantitative studies. *Journal of Statistical Physics, 34*, 975–986.

Krings, T., Chiappa, K. H., Cuffin, B. N., Cochius, J. I., Connolly, S., & Cosgrove, G. R. (1999). Accuracy of EEG dipole source localization using implanted sources in the human brain. *Clinical Neurophysiology, 110*, 106–114.

Laarne, P. H., Tenhunen-Eskelinen, M. L., Hyttinen, J. K., Eskola, H. J. (2000). Effect of EEG electrode density on dipole localization accuracy using two realistically shaped skull resistivity models. *Brain Topography, 12*, 249–254.

Mangun, G. R., & Hillyard, S. A. (1988). Spatial gradients of visual attention: Behavioral and electrophysiological evidence. *Electroencephalography and Clinical Neurophysiology, 70*, 417–428.

Mangun, G. R., Hinrichs, H., Scholz, M., Mueller-Gaertner, H. W., Herzog, H., Krause, B. J., Tellman, L., Kemna, L., & Heinze, H. J. (2001). Integrating electrophysiology and neuroimaging of spatial selective attention to simple isolated visual stimuli. *Vision Research, 41*, 1423–1435.

Mangun, G. R., Hopfinger, J. B., & Heinze, H. J. (1998). Integrating electrophysiological and neuroimaging in the study of human cognition. *Behavior Research Methods, Instruments, & Computers, 30*, 118–130.

Marquardt, D. W. (1963). An algorithm for least-squares estimation of non-linear parameters. *Journal of the Society for Industrial and Applied Mathematics, 11*, 431–441.

Martinez, A., DiRusso, F., Anllo-Vento, L., Sereno, M. I., Buxton, R. B., & Hillyard, S. A. (2001). Putting spatial attention on the map: Timing and localization of stimulus selection processes in striate and extrastriate visual areas. *Vision Research, 41*, 1437–1457.

McNay, D., Michielssen, E., Rogers, R. L., Taylor, S. A., Akhtari, M., & Sutherling, W. W. (1996). Multiple source localization using genetic algorithms. *Journal of Neuroscience Methods, 64*, 163–172.

Menninghaus, E., Lütkenhöner, B., & Gonzalez, S. L. (1994). Localization of a dipolar source in a skull phantom: Realistic versus spherical model. *IEEE Transactions on Biomedical Engineering, 41*, 986–989.

Merlet, I., & Gotman, J. (1999). Reliability of dipole models of epileptic spikes. *Clinical Neurophysiology, 110*, 1013–1028.

Mosher, J. C., Spencer, M. E., Leahy, R. M., & Lewis, P. S. (1993). Error bounds for EEG and MEG dipole source localization. *Electroencephalography and Clinical Neurophysiology, 86*, 303–321.

Motter, B. C. (1993). Focal attention produces spatially selective processing in visual cortical areas V1, V2, and V4 in the presence of competing stimuli. *Journal of Neurophysiology, 70*, 909–919.

Nelder, J., & Mead, R. (1965). A simplex method for function minimization. *Computer Journal, 4*, 308–313.

Nunez, P. L. (1981). *Electric fields of the brain: The neurophysics of EEG.* New York: Oxford University Press.

Plendl, H., Paulus, W., Bötzel, K., Towell, A., Pitman, J. R., Scherg, M., & Halliday, A. M. (1993). The time course and location of cerebral evoked activity associated with the processing of colour stimuli in man. *Neuroscience Letters, 150*, 9–12.

Press, W. H., Teukolsky, S. A., Vetterling, W. T., & Flannery, B. P. (1992). *Numerical recipes in C: The art of scientific computing*, 2d ed. Cambridge: Cambridge University Press.

Schaefer, M., Mühlnickel, W., Grüsser, S. M., & Flor, H. (2002). Reproducibility and stability of neuroelectric source imaging in primary somatosensory cortex. *Brain Topography, 14*, 179–189.

Scherg, M. (1990). Fundamentals of dipole source potential analysis. In F. Grandori, M. Hoke, G. L. Romani (Eds.), *Auditory evoked magnetic fields and electric potentials* (pp. 40–69). Basel: Karger.

Scherg, M., & Berg, P. (1991). Use of prior knowledge in brain electromagnetic source analysis. *Brain Topography, 4*, 143–150.

Sereno, M. I., Dale, A. M., Reppas, J. B., Kwong, K. K., Belliveau, J. W., Brady, T. J., Rosen, B. R., & Tootell, R. B. (1995). Borders of multiple visual areas in humans revealed by functional magnetic resonance imaging. *Science, 268*, 889–893.

Slotnick, S. D. (2003). Model fitting in $(n + 1)$ dimensions. *Behavior Research Methods, Instruments, & Computers, 35*, 322–324.

Slotnick, S. D., Hopfinger, J. B., Klein, S. A., & Sutter, E. E. (2002). Darkness beyond the light: Attentional inhibition surrounding the classic spotlight. *NeuroReport, 13*, 773–778.

Slotnick, S. D., Klein, S. A., Carney, T., Sutter, E., & Dastmalchi, S. (1999). Using multi-stimulus VEP source localization to obtain a retinotopic map of human primary visual cortex. *Clinical Neurophysiology, 110*, 1793–1800.

Slotnick, S. D., Klein, S. A., Carney, T., & Sutter, E. E. (2001). Electrophysiological estimate of human cortical magnification. *Clinical Neurophyisology, 112*, 1349–1356.

Supek, S., & Aine, C. J. (1993). Simulation studies of multiple dipole neuromagnetic source localization: Model order and limits of source resolution. *IEEE Transactions on Biomedical Engineering, 40*, 529–540.

Sutter, E. E. (1992). A deterministic approach to nonlinear systems analysis. In R. B. Pinter & B. Nabet (Eds.), *Nonlinear Vision: Determination of Neural Receptive Fields, Function, and Networks* (pp. 171–220). Boca Raton, FL: CRC Press.

Tarkka, I. M., Stokic, D. S., Basile, L. F. H., & Papanicolaou, A. C. (1995). Electric source localization of the auditory P300 agrees with magnetic source localization. *Electroencephalography and clinical Neurophysiology, 96*, 538–545.

Van Hoey, G., De Clercq, J., Vanrumste, B., Van de Walle, R., Lemahieu, I., D'Havé, M., & Boon, P. (2000). EEG dipole source localization using artificial neural networks. *Physics in Medicine and Biology, 45*, 997–1011.

Vanrumste, B., Van Hoey, G., Van de Walle, R., D'Have, M. R., Lemahieu, I. A., & Boon, P. A. (2002). Comparison of performance of spherical and realistic head models in dipole localization from noisy EEG. *Medical Engineering & Physics, 24*, 403–418.

Wilson, F. N., & Bayley, R. H. (1950). The electric field of an eccentric dipole in a homogeneous spherical conducting medium. *Circulation, 1*, 84–92.

Yvert, B., Crouzeix-Cheylus, A., & Pernier, J. (2001). Fast realistic modeling in bioelectromagnetism using lead-field interpolation. *Human Brain Mapping, 14*, 48–63.

Zhang, Z., & Jewett, D. L. (1993). Insidious errors in dipole localization parameters at a single time-point due to model misspecification of number of shells. *Electroencephalography and Clinical Neurophysiology, 88*, 1–11.

Zhang, Z., Jewett, D. L., & Goodwill, G. (1994). Insidious errors in dipole parameters due to shell model misspecification using multiple time-points. *Brain Topography, 6*, 283–298.

Zierler, N. (1959). Linear recurring sequences. *Journal of the Society for Industrial and Applied Mathematics, 7*, 31–49.

8 High-Resolution EEG: Theory and Practice

Ramesh Srinivasan

The primary motivation for using EEG to investigate brain function is the excellent (millisecond) temporal resolution. The event-related potential (ERP) paradigm, for example, provides a method for connecting the chronology of mental processes to the neural events following a sensory stimulus. Other paradigms emphasize using EEG to measure aspects of neural population dynamics; for instance, one can investigate functional integration or segregation between cortical areas during cognitive or perceptual processes by analyzing the correlation (or coherence) between EEG electrodes (Singer, 1999; Srinivasan et al., 1999; Sarnthein et al., 1998; von Stein and Sarnthein, 2000; Mima et al., 2001). Here I use the term EEG to encompass all phenomenon recorded with scalp electrodes, including spontaneous EEG, ERP, or evoked potentials (EP), with the chapter focusing on the spatial information inherent in EEG measures.

Importantly, the spatial information available in EEG is limited. EEG electrodes are separated from current sources in the brain by the tissues of the head: cerebrospinal fluid (CSF), skull, and scalp. As a consequence, EEG has poor spatial resolution. Toward addressing this limitation, one approach has been to model the location of dipole current sources (see chapter 7 of this volume). In practice, many spatial patterns of EEG can be reasonably fit (in a least squares sense) by a few equivalent dipoles. However, these dipoles may only reflect "centers" of a complex pattern of activity distributed throughout many regions of the brain. The limited evidence available from intracranial recordings in humans does not support the contention that only a few sites in the brain are active in generating EEG signals (Aoki et al., 2001; Towle et al., 1998; Menon et al., 1996; Ragavachari et al., 2001). Nevertheless, converging evidence from other methods, such as fMRI or PET, is often provided as support for inverse solutions (Vittaco et al., 2002), or even used to seed inverse solutions (Ahlfors et al., 1999), even though there may be little theoretical basis to make such a connection (Nunez & Silberstein, 2000; Horwitz & Poeppel, 2002).

Given the potential limitations of traditional dipole modeling, an alternative approach for locating the generators of EEG is to improve the spatial resolution of the

EEG rather than making assumptions about the nature or number of sources. Such *high-resolution EEG* methods have been developed to estimate the dura surface (inner skull surface) potential from scalp potentials. Unlike the inverse problem, which has an infinite number of potential solutions, *the scalp potential is uniquely related to the dura surface potential*, assuming (reasonably) that there are no sources between the dura and the scalp.

Two entirely distinct high-resolution EEG methods have been developed independently: (1) skull current density estimates by means of a surface Laplacian algorithm (Babiloni et al., 1996; Nunez 1988, 1989, 1990, 1995; Nunez et al., 1991, 1994; Law et al., 1993; Perrin, Bertrand, & Echalier, 1989; Perrin et al., 1987; Srinivasan, 1999; Srinivasan et al., 1996, 1998). (2) Estimates of dura surface potential by a spatial deconvolution algorithm (Silberstein & Cadusch, 1992; Edlinger, Wach, & Pfurtscheller, 1998; Gevins et al., 1991, 1994; Sidman, 1991). Dura surface potential estimates obtained by spatial deconvolution (also known as deblurring, cortical imaging, or dura imaging) do not require assumptions about the sources of the EEG, but do require the specification of an electrical model of the head. The surface Laplacian (or second spatial derivative) of the scalp potentials is an estimate of current density entering (or exiting) the scalp through the skull. The surface Laplacian method only requires a geometric model of the head. Despite the independent theoretical basis of the two methods, which are estimates of different physical quantities, both methods yield robust estimates of dura surface potential in simulation studies and consistent estimates in applications to EEG data (Nunez, 1990; Nunez et al., 1994). However, the surface Laplacian offers the advantage of requiring less information about volume conduction in the head and will be the emphasis of this chapter.

The theory and examples presented here will demonstrate that the surface Laplacian method isolates those aspects of the EEG attributable to sources that are spatially localized in superficial areas of the cortex. The remainder of the EEG is not as easily localized; it may be generated by coherent sources distributed over larger areas on the lobeal or even bigger scales. In this case, the question of source localization of EEG is somewhat meaningless, as the underlying phenomenon is not local, but instead regional or perhaps even global (Nunez, 2000).

This chapter begins by examining the nature of spatial information available in the EEG through simulations and analysis of EEG data and develops quantitative measures of the spatial resolution of EEG. We review the theoretical basis of the surface Laplacian estimate of skull current density, to establish the relationship between skull current density, dura surface potential, and the underlying source distribution. We also consider practical issues such as the required number of electrodes and the choice of surface Laplacian algorithm. Finally, we analyze some real EEG data.

Are EEG Phenomena Local?

The existence of localized generators is not a general property of EEG data. Some EEG signals may be generated by neurons in only one compact area of the brain. Other EEG signals may be generated regionally or even globally, involving neural populations acting in concert, distributed throughout the brain (Bressler et al., 1993; Bressler, 1995; Nunez, 1995, 2000). In general, the underlying generators of most EEG phenomena are not known, and large-scale theoretical models suggest that we should anticipate a mixture of local, regional, and global sources (Nunez, 1989, 1995, 2000). In limited cases, such as early sensory EPs, the assumption that a single focal region of the cortex is the generator may sometimes be justified in modeling the EEG with a dipole source. By contrast, in studies of EEG signals related to cognitive processes, we can expect that distributed areas of cortical tissue, perhaps in multiple brain regions, generate the measured potentials. In this case, the assumption of a small number of dipoles, although generating excellent fits to the data, is not as well justified.

The dipole approximation to cortical current sources is based on the idea that at a large distance, any complex current distribution in a region of the cortex can be approximated by a dipole. In this context, a large distance is at least three or four times the distance between the positive and negative poles of the dipole (Nunez, 1981). Superficial gyral surfaces are at a distance of roughly 1.5 cm from scalp electrodes. Thus, the dipole approximation appears to be valid only for superficial cortical tissue with a maximum extent in any dimension of 0.5 cm or less! If extended areas of the cortical surface are active, a dipole layer, oriented perpendicular to the cortical surface, is the appropriate model of the source distribution underlying the EEG (Nunez, 1981).

The use of dipoles that represent small regions of the cortex, such as macrocolumns, rather than fitting point dipoles (that can represent arbitrary volumes of tissue) allows for a quantitative approach to model the spatial resolution of EEG. The sources of the EEG are then several thousand dipoles, mainly oriented perpendicular to the cortical surface. In recordings within the brain, one can observe high correlation between neurons or neuronal populations extending over the cm scale (Ragavachari et al., 2001; Bressler et al., 1993; Bressler, 1995). Dipole layers of varying size, shape, and degree of correlation among its functional units are apparently possible in the cortex.

Within this framework, we can operationally define localization of the sources of the EEG. A localized EEG current source is a dipole layer of finite extent and *relatively segregated from the rest of the cortex.* In the context of any EEG time series, segregation not only refers to spatial separation, but also implies that the source activity is temporally uncorrelated from the surrounding cortex.

Volume conduction of currents through the tissues of the head—cerebrospinal fluid (CSF), skull, and scalp (Nunez, 1981)—critically influence the relative contribution of different cortical current sources to scalp EEG. Theoretical studies of the head transfer function, using multilayered spherical models of the head, suggest that the head acts as a low-pass spatial filter, reducing the EEG generated by small dipole layers in comparison to larger dipole layers (Srinivasan et al., 1996, 1998). Thus, large magnitude EEG signals, such as alpha oscillations, are likely to be generated by large dipole layers distributed over many cortical areas, whereas very small EEG signals, such as early sensory EPs, might be generated by a small dipole layer in the primary sensory cortex. In general, EEG signals will be generated by the mixture of contributions of dipole layers of different sizes, location, and orientation.

Spatial Resolution of EEG

Analyses of the spatial resolution of EEG (and comparisons to MEG) are often carried out in the context of the accuracy of localization of a single dipole source. For example, researchers have demonstrated in using implanted sources in epilepsy surgery patients that the dipole location can be fit with an accuracy of less than 1 cm (Cohen et al., 1990; Cuffin et al., 1991). Comparisons of scalp recordings to intracranial recordings in animal models suggest that localization accuracy will depend on the nature of the sources (Okada et al., 1999). In general, localization accuracy is not a useful measure of the spatial resolution of EEG because the results cannot be generalized to a wide variety of EEG signals.

One measure of the spatial resolution of EEG is the distance between two electrodes at which the signals are identical except for additive noise, such as electrode or amplifier noise. Figure 8.1 shows sample EEG and ERP recorded from a single subject to visual stimuli (see figure caption for details of the recording). The ERP data is average-referenced, an approach to the problem of the reference electrode that has some theoretical basis (Bertrand et al., 1986), and provides a reasonable estimate of reference-independent potentials in simulation studies (Srinivasan, Nunez, & Silberstein, 1998). The figure shows ERP data at 12 neighboring electrodes with average nearest-neighbor spacing of 2.7 cm, on the basis of a best-fit sphere to the electrode positions. It is immediately apparent that adjacent channels are more similar to each other than widely separated electrodes. The observation that closely spaced electrodes are very similar to each other is consistently observed in ERP recordings with dense arrays of electrodes (>64) and is equally evident in raw EEG traces. In simulation studies and analytic derivations with a multilayered spherical model of the head, artificial correlation between electrodes results from volume conduction even when the underlying sources in the brain are entirely uncorrelated, as with spatial white noise (Srinivasan, Nunez, & Silberstein, 1998). This correlation falls off with separation distance between electrodes, and in part accounts for the similarity of neighboring electrodes.

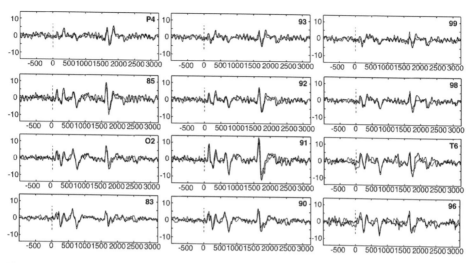

Figure 8.1

Event-related potentials recorded in a cued-spatial orienting paradigm. Event-related potentials were obtained at 128 electrodes by averaging time-locked to stimulus presentation. The stimuli consisted of a cueing arrow presented for 500 ms, followed by a target that was presented in either the left or right visual fields, at an interval of 200 or 1,000 ms after the cue offset. The data shown consists of only those trials where the cue was valid and the target arrived 1,000 ms after the cue offset in the left (thick lines) and right (thin lines) visual field. The EEG was recorded from a 10-year-old boy, and 48 trials were averaged in each condition. ERP waveforms were transformed to an average reference. The 12 figures correspond to 12 neighboring electrodes over the right posterior hemisphere, including the 10/20 electrodes O2, P4, and T6, and electrodes that are adjacent or intermediate to these electrodes. The average electrode spacing is 2.7 cm on the scalp.

Approximating the continuous potential distribution on the scalp with discrete samples—the electrodes—is subject to a Nyquist criterion, analogous to time domain sampling (Srinivasan et al., 1999). In analog to digital conversion, the Nyquist criterion, $f_{dig} > 2 * f_{max}$, indicates that the digitization of the time series must be done at a rate f_{dig} at least twice the highest frequency f_{max} present in the signal. In practice, the EEG signal is low-pass filtered prior to analog-to-digital conversion (by hardware as an analog signal) at the appropriate frequency to avoid aliasing at the sampling frequency selected by the experimenter. The Nyquist criterion applies to any discrete representation of a continuous signal, including the spatial distribution of EEG. Unlike temporal sampling, spatial sampling in EEG is inherently digitized by the placement of the electrodes. As a consequence, any aliasing on the account of undersampling cannot be undone, and it is critical that an adequate sampling of the potential be accomplished at the outset. Fortuitously, the skull acts as an analog low-pass spatial filter, which limits the spatial resolution of EEG, but makes the discrete spatial sampling problem manageable. Theoretical (Srinivasan et al., 1996, 1999) and experimental studies (Srinivasan et al., 1999; Spitzer et al., 1989) by different groups using different types of EEG signals suggest that an electrode separation of 2–3 cm is required to meet the Nyquist requirement for spatial sampling.[1] Note that sampling with a widely spaced electrodes does not "alias" the EEG time series: it simply means that in this case, the EEG record cannot be considered an accurate discrete representation of a continuous spatial signal and hence is not a candidate for high-resolution EEG analysis (or, for that matter, source localization). The EEG record obtained at each channel remains an accurate representation of the potential difference between that electrode position and the reference electrode position.

A clear physical interpretation of these results can be obtained using the framework of half-sensitivity volumes (Malmivuo & Plonsey, 1995). The signal recorded at each electrode is a spatial average of active current sources distributed over a volume of space. The size and shape of this volume depend on a number of factors, including the volume conduction properties of the head and choice of reference electrode. The contribution of each source to the average depends on the distance between source and electrode, source orientation, and source strength. When two electrodes are very closely spaced, they record the same signal, because they are recording the average activity in almost identical volumes of tissue. The goal of high-resolution EEG methods is to reduce the volume of tissue that each electrode averages, thereby improving the spatial resolution of EEG. Clearly, simply increasing the number of electrodes will not improve the spatial resolution of EEG.

Physical Basis of Surface Laplacian Estimates

The critical feature of volume conduction in real heads is the poorly conductive skull layer between highly conductive brain (and CSF) and scalp (Nunez, 1981). Concentric spheres models of the head can incorporate this feature and be used to compute potential anywhere in the volume and develop our intuition about the path of current flow in the head. Figure 8.2A shows potential as a function of radial position above a radial dipole source in a homogeneous sphere, three spheres (brain, skull, and scalp), and four spheres (brain, CSF, skull, and scalp). In the one-sphere model, the potential gradually falls off toward the boundary of the outer sphere ($r = 9.2$ cm). Within the thickness of the skull the potentials fall off by two orders of magnitude in both the three and four concentric spheres model because of the poor conductivity of the skull. By comparison, the potential variation across the thickness of the scalp is negligible in both models. The addition of the CSF layer in the four-spheres model lowers the potential due to its higher conductivity than the brain.

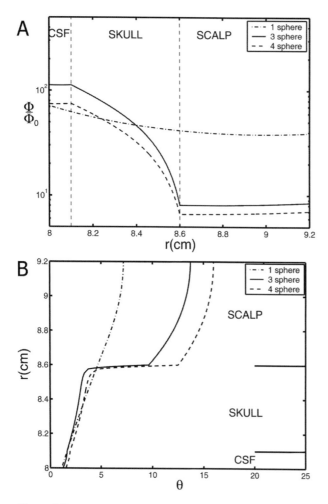

Figure 8.2

Variation of potential due to a single radial dipole source in a one-, three-, and four-concentric spheres model of the head. The four-concentric spheres model consists of brain, CSF, skull, and scalp spheres, with radii of 8, 8.1, 8.6, and 9.2 cm respectively. The three-spheres model excludes the CSF layer. In the one-sphere model, all the layers are assumed to be homogeneous. The sphere is surrounded by air with zero conductivity. The conductivities of the tissue compartments are expressed as ratios. Brain and scalp are assumed to have the same conductivity; CSF is five times as conductive as brain, and the skull is 80 times less conductive than the brain. (*A*) Variation of potential with radial position through the layers of model. (*B*) Fifty percent of peak of potential in each layer.

Figure 8.2B shows the dependence of the distribution of potentials with angular distance on radial position within the four concentric spheres model. At each radial position r, the potentials at each angular position were normalized with respect to the potential directly above the dipole, as given in figure 8.2A. The contour line shown corresponds to 50 percent of the peak potential. Within the thickness of the CSF and skull the potentials are only slightly smeared as radial position increases. The main spreading of potentials occurs at the skull/scalp boundary. A similar but smaller effect occurs in the four concentric spheres model at the brain/CSF boundary, and accounts for the greater angular spread of the potentials in the four-sphere model in comparison to the three-sphere model. In both cases, the main factor that determines the spatial smearing of scalp potentials is the poor conductivity of the skull in comparison to the scalp.

From these simulations we can develop an intuitive picture of current flow in the scalp due to dipole sources in the brain. In regions of the head with high source activity, current flows mainly in the radial direction through the skull into the scalp and spreads outward, whereas in other regions, for instance an area with less source activity, current converges and flows through the skull into the brain. There can also be regions that neither inject nor accept scalp current. Thus, different regions of the skull are "sources," "sinks," or "quiet" with respect to the scalp, as a consequence of source activity in the brain. Of course, in real heads the picture is more complicated as the conductivity and thickness of the skull and scalp are not uniform, but the general principle is valid.

In order to determine whether a given point serves as a source or a sink for scalp currents, one must evaluate the change in current density along the two-dimensional scalp surface. The only reason that scalp currents can change as they pass over a point on the scalp is the presence of a source or sink of scalp current in the skull directly below the scalp. The divergence along the scalp of current density at a point is proportional to radial current density into or out of the skull (Katznelson, 1981). Current density in the scalp is proportional to the spatial gradient of the potential (Ohm's Law). Thus, the radial current density in the skull is proportional to the second spatial derivative of scalp potentials along the scalp, that is, the surface Laplacian of the potential along the scalp. *The surface Laplacian can be used to detect sources of sinks of current flow into the scalp from the skull.*

The physical basis for relating the surface Laplacian of the scalp potential to the dura surface potential is based on Ohm's Law and the assumption that most current flows only in the radial direction through the skull into the scalp. Simulations with a spherical model with a poorly conducting skull layer as figure 8.2 shows suggest that this assumption is reasonable. Very little smearing of the potential distribution takes place within the skull, indicating that little tangential current flow takes place there. In this case, following Ohm's law, the potential difference between the inner and outer surfaces of the skull is proportional to the radial current flow through the skull, which in turn is proportional the surface Laplacian of the scalp potential. Figure 8.2 indicates the potential on the inner surface of the skull is two or three orders of magnitude larger than the potential on the outer surface of the skull (or scalp). Thus, in the case of a single dipole, the magnitude of the scalp potential is negligible in comparison to the inner skull surface potential, and the surface Laplacian is roughly proportional to the potential on the inner surface of the skull (or equivalently, the outer surface of the dura matter). In the case of broadly distributed sources, the ratio of cortical to scalp potential is typically 2:4, and increases as the source becomes smaller in extent (Nunez, 1981). Thus, the surface Laplacian provides a good estimate of dura surface potential, if the underlying sources are localized.

To test the validity of this approximation, we can examine the scalp potential (Φ_S), scalp surface Laplacian (L_S), radial skull current density (J_K), and dura (inner skull) surface potential (Φ_c) due to a dipole source in a four-concentric spheres model of the head (Srinivasan et al., 1996). Figure 8.3 (upper) demonstrates the fall off of these quantities with distance for a radial (A) and tangential (B) dipole source demonstrating the close relationship among the scalp surface Laplacian, dura surface potential, and radial skull current density. The approximation improves if the quantities are averaged over regions of finite size to account for the finite size of the electrode (Srinivasan et al., 1996), thereby satisfying the large-scale approximation inherent in assuming purely radial current flow in the skull (Katznelson, 1981). As dipoles go deeper this approximation also improves, but the magnitude of the surface Laplacian is dramatically reduced in comparison to the potential as the middle row of figure 8.3 (C and D) shows. Figure 8.3C and D also show that the magnitudes of the potential and Laplacian due to radial dipoles is much larger than that due to tangential dipoles located at the same radial position. At the macrocolumn scale dipoles in the cortex are generally oriented perpendicular to the cortical surface, implying that tangential dipoles are located mainly on the sulcal surfaces and thus further from the EEG electrodes than radial dipoles on the gyral surfaces. The sum of these effects indicates that surface Laplacian is dominated by cortical sources oriented in the radial direction with respect to the scalp surface and principally on the superficial gyral surfaces of the cortex.

The spatial resolution of the surface Laplacian can also be characterized as a bandpass spatial filter (Srinivasan et al., 1996; Srinivasan, Nunez, & Silberstein, 1998). The effect of volume conduction by the head is a low-pass spatial filtering of the underlying source distribution, biasing the EEG signal in favor of broad dipole layers. The surface Laplacian operator is a high-pass spatial filter; when combined with the low-pass spatial filtering by the head, the net effect is a bandpass spatial filtering characteristic. Thus, applying the surface Laplacian to scalp EEG has the effect of reducing the contribution of very broad dipole layers in favor of smaller dipole layers. Figure 8.4 (upper) shows the potential ratio between scalp and cortex as a function of dipole layer size. In

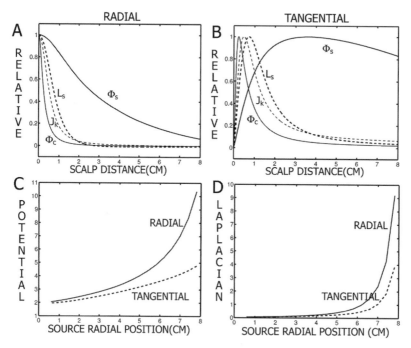

Figure 8.3
Simulations of scalp potential and Laplacian to verify theoretical basis of the surface Laplacian method. (*A*) Scalp potential (Φ_s), scalp Laplacian (L_s), radial skull current density (J_k), and cortical surface potential (Φ_c) due to a radial dipole source in the four concentric spheres model. Each quantity is normalized with respect to the peak value. (*B*) Same as (*A*) for a tangential dipole. (*C*) Maximum potential generated by a radial and tangential dipole source as a function of source position. (*D*) Same as (*C*) for Laplacian.

these simulations, radial dipole layers forming a spherical cap of uniform transcortical potential V_0 are the source distributions. The potential ratio between scalp potential and transcortical potential is maximum for a dipole layer of angular extent of approximately 60 degrees. By contrast, the ratio between surface Laplacian and transcortical potential is maximum for a spherical cap of angular extent of 20 degrees. Thus, the surface Laplacian is sensitive to source activity at a spatial scale that is different from the sensitivities of scalp potentials, and primarily reflects activity within a short distance (2–3 cm) of the electrode.

Algorithms for Surface Laplacian Estimates

Methods to estimate the surface Laplacian have evolved considerably since the simple nearest-neighbor Laplacian (Hjorth, 1975; Nunez, 1981; Gevins et al., 1983; Gevins &

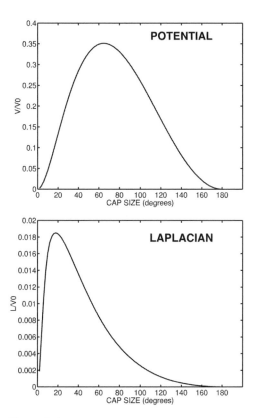

Figure 8.4
Potential and Laplacian due to dipole layer of varying angular extent forming a superficial spherical cap in a four concentric spheres model of the head. Each plot shows the ratio between the
scalp potential and the surface Laplacian with respect to transcortical potential (V0) as a function
of cap size. Note that potentials are primarily sensitive to broad dipole layers, whereas Laplacians
are sensitive to smaller dipole layers.

Cutillo, 1986). Although we now consider these simple local Laplacian methods crude,
they were very useful at the time and often provided a more accurate picture of cortical
source distributions than conventional EEG by eliminating volume conducted signals
from distant regions of the head and removing reference electrode effects (Nunez and
Pilgreen, 1991). They remain the most practical way to improve the spatial resolution
of EEG in circumstances where a limited number of electrodes are available.

    Surface Laplacian algorithms in common use today are based on fitting the scalp
potentials to a spline function, and then evaluating the surface Laplacian of the fitted
function. There are various forms of the spline function; the most commonly used
are spherical spline functions that can be readily used to obtain the surface Laplacian

along the best-fit sphere to the scalp surface (Perrin et al., 1989). The spherical spline functions employ a regularization parameter to smooth the data prior to the surface Laplacian calculation. The value of the regularization parameter is somewhat arbitrary in this algorithm. In practice, one of the main factors that determine the choice of smoothing is the electrode separation, which determines the upper limit for spatial information available in the EEG record (Srinivasan et al., 1999).

There is a three-dimensional spline function for EEG interpolation and surface Laplacian estimates that offers several advantages over the spherical spline method (Perrin, Bertrand, & Pernier, 1987; Law, Nunez, & Wijesinghe, 1993; Srinivasan et al., 1996; Srinivasan, 1999). One can use the three-dimensional spline function to fit the scalp potential on any surface that passes through the electrodes. Futhermore, the regularization parameter in this spline function is fixed by the effective electrode diameter, including gel or saline interface with the scalp (Srinivasan et al., 1996), reflecting the fact that the potential is measured over an area of this size rather than at a point.

To contrast the three-dimensional spline to spherical splines (Perrin et al., 1989), the three-dimensional spline has been rewritten as a spherical harmonic expansion for the case of electrodes on a best-fit spherical surface (Srinivasan et al., 1996). The three-dimensional spline intrinsically smoothes the data at high spatial frequencies above the Nyquist limit implied by the electrode spacing (Srinivasan et al., 1996). Thus, both electrode size and electrode spacing determine the amount of smoothing applied.

The three-dimensional spline function has been used to calculate the surface Laplacian along best-fit spherical and ellipsoidal surfaces, showing very similar results (Law, Nunez, & Wijesinghe, 1993). In principle, the three-dimensional spline can be used to interpolate the potential along a realistic scalp surface, if both electrode positions and scalp surface position are accurately known. There can be improvements in the accuracy of Laplacian estimates by extracting the scalp surface from an MRI to use for constraining the spatial derivative estimates (Babiloni et al., 1996). However, as comparisons of spherical and ellipsoidal surface Laplacians show (Law, Nunez, & Wijesinghe, 1993), the surface Laplacian is a robust estimate of dura surface potentials, and is relatively insensitive to errors in specifying the geometry of the scalp.

Simulation Studies

We present here a simple example simulation of the performance of the surface-Laplacian estimate. We have carried out hundreds of simulations to test the algorithm (Law, Nunez, & Wijesinghe, 1993; Nunez et al., 1991, 1994; Srinivasan et al., 1996, 1998; Srinivasan, 1994d, 1999). In addition, some have made contrasts between the surface Laplacian and high-resolution EEG estimates based on spatial deconvolution (Nunez et al., 1994), yielding consistent estimates of dura surface potential in simulations and experimental studies.

Figure 8.5 shows a simple example of three superficial dipole sources, as indicated on the source map. Two radial dipoles are superficial at a depth of 1.4 cm below the scalp, corresponding to a gyral surface, one oriented with the positive pole up (filled circle) and one oriented with the negative pole up (open circle). The other dipole is tangential, as indicated by the positive (+) and negative (−) poles, and located at a depth of 2.2 cm below the scalp, corresponding to a sulcal wall. The scalp potential, surface Laplacian, and dura surface potential were calculated using a four concentric spheres model (see figure caption for details). The scalp potential is strongly influenced by the positive pole of the tangential dipole and the negative dipole source. The fields generated by the negative pole of the tangential dipole and the positive source in part cancel. The net effect is an apparent reversal of the field over the lower right portion of the sphere, which is not an area that contains a source. The surface Laplacian of this potential distribution clearly identifies the two radial sources. The surface Laplacian also detects a much smaller field that appears to have the structure of a tangential dipole, with sharp inversion of the sign of the field. However, this field is much smaller than the Laplacian field generated by the more superficial radial dipoles, in spite of the dipole having twice as large moment. The Laplacian map is also consistent with the dura surface potential map. Interestingly, a direct measurement of the dura surface potential, as in EcoG, would be even less sensitive to the deeper, stronger tangential source than the surface Laplacians.

In summary, both dura potential and the surface Laplacian give accurate representation of the superficial radial sources, and are relatively insensitive to the deeper, stronger tangential source. By contrast, the scalp potential is strongly influenced by the tangential source. This has several important implications in interpreting the surface Laplacian transformed data. Because each of these three sources is likely to have a distinct time series, we anticipate that Laplacian data can have distinct time series information in comparison to potential data. Furthermore, the Laplacian may remove the contribution of those sources that are of interest to the cognitive experiment. In this case, Laplacian data may show no difference between experimental conditions, whereas the potential data shows strong differences. Here, we can interpret the combined analysis of potential and Laplacian data as indicating that the generator of the signal of interest is either deep or broadly distributed, and hence contributes minimal signal to the Laplacian data.

High-Resolution ERP

In applications to EEG data the resolution the surface Laplacian method achieves depends mainly on electrode density and signal-to-noise ratio. Theoretical simulations suggest that an electrode spacing of about 2 cm is ideal, reaching the Nyquist limit of scalp recordings (Srinivasan et al., 1999). However, the actual limit has not been mea-

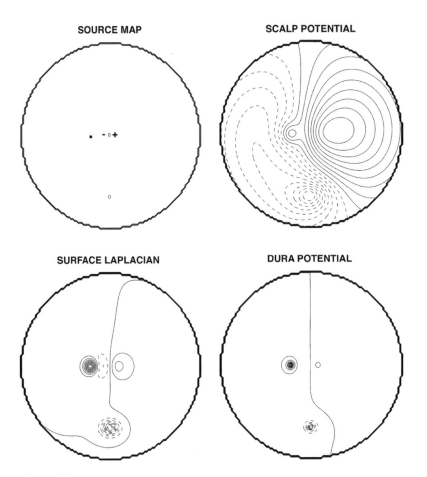

Figure 8.5
Simulation of scalp potentials and surface Laplacians due to dipole sources in a four concentric spheres model of the head. Two radial dipole sources—one positive (filled circle) and one negative (open circle)—are located at spherical coordinate positions (r, θ, ϕ): $(7.8, 20, 180)$ and $(7.8, 45, 270)$. The tangential dipole is oriented along the x axis ($\phi = 0$), as indicated by the positive $(+)$ and negative $(-)$ poles, and has twice the magnitude of the radial dipoles. The maps shown for scalp potential, surface Laplacian, and dura potential are calculated by placing the dipoles in a four-concentric-spheres model of the head. The model consists of four spherical layers: brian ($r = 8$), CSF ($r = 8.1$), skull ($r = 8.6$), and scalp ($r = 9.2$). Brain and scalp are assumed to have the same conductivity, CSF is five times as conductive as brain, and the skull is 80 times less conductive than the brain. The maps have been normalized to the maximum of each variable, in order to display relative values.

sured in real heads, and would in any case need to be measured in a variety of different EEG signals across different heads to be a comprehensive result. It is important to emphasize that without the use of a high-resolution EEG algorithm the information gained from additional electrodes is limited.

The effectiveness of the surface Laplacian as a tool to identify sources of EEG signals will depend strongly on the spatial structure of the signal. The surface Laplacian is a filter that will emphasize those aspects of the EEG signal that are generated by superficial sources that occupy a relatively small area of superficial cortical tissue, a source that is well localized. The EEG signal will also contain some activity generated by deep sources or by broad dipole layers. As figure 8.3C and D suggest, superficial sources will produce Laplacian magnitudes that are much larger than sources even 1 or 2 cm deeper. Given that the tangential dipoles produce smaller signals, the surface Laplacian detects primarily radial sources in the superficial gyral surfaces of the cortex. *If such sources are not present in the EEG signal, the surface Laplacian will simply filter out the entire record!* Furthermore, if sources at different depths or different spatial extent each have distinct time series, the surface Laplacian will also selectively filter aspects of the EEG time series.

To examine these issues, we applied the three-dimensional spline-generated surface Laplacian algorithm to the example EEG and ERP data shown in figure 8.1, assuming a best-fit sphere to the electrode positions. The surface Laplacian was evaluated along this best fit sphere at each time point and at each of the electrode position. Figure 8.6 shows the waveforms obtained using the surface Laplacian at the same 12 electrodes as figure 8.1. A dramatic difference is apparent in the waveforms. At many of the channels the ERP waveform is no longer visible. Because the waveforms were present in the potential data but are absent in the Laplacian, we can only conclude that no *localized* generator of the ERP waveform is present in the superficial tissue directly beneath the electrode. This does not establish that there are no sources there. If ERP sources were distributed uniformly throughout this region, we would anticipate recording minimal signal in the Laplacian data as well.

The ERP waveform in the Laplacian transformed data is now largely found at electrodes 91 and T6. Both the early positive potentials after cue ($\sim$130 ms) and after target ($\sim$1650 ms) are found at electrode 91. This provides strong evidence that the generator of this potential lies directly beneath this electrode. Electrode T6 exhibits two distinct potentials only for the targets on the left visual field, approximately 1200 ms after the cue and 300 ms after the target. These two electrodes account for the majority of the components of the ERP waveform over this region of the head.

ERP waveforms are usually characterized in terms of components such as the P1, N1, P2, and so on. Comparing the ERP waveform for the potential and Laplacian data (figure 8.1 versus figure 8.5) at channels reveals some selective filtering of ERP components

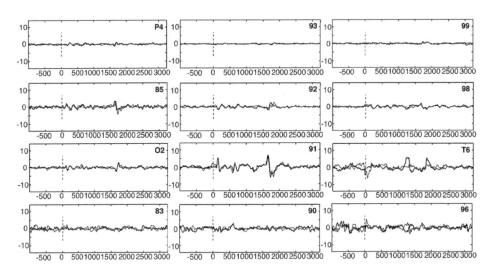

Figure 8.6
Laplacian ERP waveforms. See figure 8.1 for details on the ERP. The ERP at 128 channels was passed through a three-dimensional spline Laplacian algorithm. The potentials are in units of microvolts. Laplacians are in units of microvolts per squared centimeter.

by the Laplacian operator. For instance, in the potential data, the positive potential approximately 130 ms after the first stimulus (the cue) is comparable in magnitude to the second positive approximately 300 ms poststimulus. In the Laplacian data the later positive ERP component is reduced in comparison to the earlier ERP component. This implies that localized source activity under these electrodes makes a larger contribution to the earlier ERP potential than the later ERP potential. Finally, the ERP after the second stimulus (the target) differentiates between left (thick solid) and right (thin solid) visual field presentation. This difference is widespread in the potential data and is associated with at least one local source located under electrode 91. However, this effect is small, suggesting that the difference is not well localized in EEG recordings. By comparison, the late positive difference, localized to electrode T6, is a strong effect in both potential and Laplacian data, suggesting a localized generator directly beneath these electrodes. The interesting aspect of this difference is that it occurs both before and after the target.

Figure 8.7 (see plate 5) shows topographic maps of the potential and Laplacian data at selected time points following the presentation of the second stimulus (the target). These timepoints were selected based upon the maxima and minima of the potential ERP following the presentation of the target. Trials corresponding to left visual field targets are on the left, and right visual field targets are on the right. At the first time

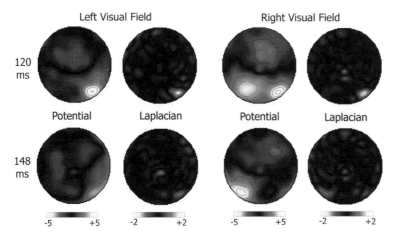

Figure 8.7
Topographic maps of potential and Laplacian of the ERP at two time points following the presentation of the target stimulus, 1000 ms after the offset of the cueing stimulus. Times shown on the figure are after the target stimulus arrives. Potentials are in units of microvolts. Laplacians are in units of microvolts per squared centimeter. (See plate 5 for color version.)

point, 120 ms poststimulus, the left side targets evoke a right posterior peak in the potential data. This peak is localized, as evidenced by the Laplacian map. At the same time point, right visual field targets elicit a more bilateral response, with positive peaks over both left and right posterior areas, although still larger over the right. The Laplacian map in this case is almost identical to the left visual field targets. Thus we must conclude that the left posterior potential generated by the right visual field target at this time point is not generated by a source localized to a region of the left posterior cortex. At the second time point shown, the left visual field target induces a potential that is peaked over the right posterior cortex and the right visual field target induces a potential over the left posterior cortex. At this time point, the Laplacian demonstrates a consistent lateralization, and indicates focal sources are present in the corresponding hemisphere.

This example also serves to highlight a crucial point in making effective use of Laplacian data to understand the generators of the EEG. When viewed in isolation, the Laplacian data entirely misses the differences in the first time point, which are only captured by the potential data. This reflects the fact that the differences at the first time point are not the result of focal superficial generators. Thus, there must be broad and/or deep generators of the potential. In the second time point, the potential and Laplacian give a consistent picture. *Thus, contrasting the potential and Laplacian data can clarify the nature of the generator of the EEG.* In isolation, neither measure is as informative.

Conclusion

The ERP, like most EEG phenomena is generated by coherent neural sources organized at macroscopic (centimeter) scales in the neocortex (Nunez, 1995, 2000). The source distribution underlying any particular ERP component or waveform need not be generated by a single dipole source located in a restricted cortical area. Such a simple model can explain very few EEG potentials, and ignores the possibility of dynamic interactions between the densely interconnected cortex and thalamic input from the sensory stimulus. Such interactions take place at many spatial and temporal scales, including macroscopic scales observable with EEG. When the ERP paradigm is applied to study higher cognitive processes the notion of a single brain area generating the potentials (or for that matter the behavior) is apparently too simplistic a model to be of general utility. In this context, source localization by fitting dipoles becomes not only technically unfeasible but also physiologically unrealistic.

High-resolution EEG methods apply spatial filters to the data rather than fitting the data to a model. This offers a number of advantages for ERP analysis. The results of spatial filtering with a surface Laplacian can be evaluated objectively, because the operation is not attempting to account for all of the EEG data. Instead, the filter isolates those aspects of the EEG that can be unambiguously associated with superficial cortical tissue in the immediate neighborhood, that is, 2–3 cm, surrounding the electrode. Potentials removed by applying this spatial filter are certainly not generated by a local source beneath the electrode. Thus the effect of the surface Laplacian is to reduce the sensitivity of each electrode to only superficial cortical sources near the electrode. The resultant waveforms and topography have not been compromised by assumptions inherent in modeling the data by fitting equivalent dipoles and can still be subject to a rigorous statistical analysis of experimental differences.

In this chapter we have emphasized the surface Laplacian algorithm for high-resolution EEG estimates rather than spatial deconvolution (also known as cortical imaging). This reflects both theoretical and practical advantages of the surface Laplacian. Spatial deconvolution methods require the assumption of an electrical head model. Although MRI data can be used to construct an exact geometrical model of the head, such models are only approximate models of volume conduction in the head due to uncertainty in the conductivity of the tissues of the head (Srinivasan et al., 2002). Tissue boundaries can be estimated for individual subjects using MRI and used to construct a computer model that incorporates the geometry of the cortical surface, inner and outer skull surfaces, and the scalp surface. (Gevins et al., 1994). Implicit in any of these models is that the effective resistance of each compartment depends on both the resistivity of the tissue layer and its thickness; a region of thicker skull has higher resistance. However, the impedance of 1-cm diameter skull plugs (in vitro) is independent of their thickness (Law, 1993). If the in vitro experimental results apply to living skulls, using MRI to determine the thickness of tissue compartments could yield a head model that is actually less accurate than using uniform tissue layers. In the absence of better information about heads, the surface Laplacian appears to be a more robust approach to obtain high-resolution EEG estimates than spatial deconvolution methods. However, should detailed information about tissue conductivity become available, perhaps by impedance imaging techniques (Ferree, Eriksen, & Tucker, 1999) or from MRI data (Ueno & Iriguchi, 1998), spatial deconvolution methods offer the potential to incorporate geometric and electrical information to obtain highly accurate estimates of dura surface potential, thereby dramatically improving the spatial resolution of the EEG.

Acknowledgments

The author wishes to thank to Michael Murias and Dr. James M. Swanson for making available evoked potential data used in the examples here. The author also wishes to thank Prof. Paul L. Nunez of Tulane University for many useful comments.

Note

1. All the simulations and EEG data presented here are based on an average sampling density of 2.7 cm, estimated along a best-fit sphere to the electrode positions. At this spacing, nearest neighbor electrodes appear nearly identical, and have high correlation coefficients obtained in both ERP and EEG signals. Although we cannot know for sure that this spatial sampling is adequate for all EEG phenomena, it appears reasonable considering that adjacent electrodes are close to redundant, within the limitations of noise and a finite amount of data.

References

Ahlfors, S. P., Simpson, G. V., Belliveao, J. W., Liu, A. K., Korvenoja, A., Virtanen, J., Huotilainen, M., Tootell, R. B., Aronen, H. J., & Iimoniemi, R. J. (1999). Spatiotemporal activity of a cortical network for processing visual motion revealed by MEG and fMRI. *Journal of Neurophysiology, 82*, 2545–2555.

Aoki, F., Fetz, E. E., Shupe, L., Lettich, E., & Ojemann, G. A. (2001). Changes in power and coherence of brain activity in human sensorimotor cortex during performance of visuomotor tasks. *Biosystems, 63*, 89–99.

Babiloni, F., Babiloni, C., Carducci, F., Fattorini, L, Onaratti, P., & Urbano, A. (1996). Spline Laplacian estimate of EEG potentials over a realistic magnetic resonance-constructed scalp surface model. *Electroencephalography and Clinical Neurophysiology, 98*, 204–215.

Bressler, S. L., Coppola, R., & Nakamura, R. (1993). Episodic multiregional cortical coherence at multiple frequencies during visual task performance. *Nature, 366*, 153–156.

Bressler, S. L. (1995). Large-scale cortical networks and cognition. *Brain Research Reviews, 20,* 288–304.

Cohen, D., Cuffin, B. N., Yunokuchi, K., Maniewski, R., Purcell, C., Cosgrive, G. R., Ives, J., Kennedy, J. G., & Schomer, D. L. (1990). MEG versus EEG localization test using implanted sources in the human brain. *Annals of Neurology, 28,* 811–817.

Cuffin, B. N., Cohen, D., Yunokuchi, K., Maniewski, R., Purcell, C., Cosgrove, G. R., Ives, J., Kennedy, J. G., & Schomer, D. L. (1991). Tests of EEG localization accuracy using implanted sources in the human brain. *Annals of Neurology, 29,* 132–128.

Edlinger, G., Wach, P., & Pfurtscheller, G. (1998). On the realization of an analytic high-resolution EEG. *IEEE Transactions on Biomedical Engineering, 45,* 736–745.

Ferree, T., Eriksen, K., & Tucker, D. M. (2000). Regional head tissue conductivity estimation for improved EEG analysis. *IEEE Transactions on Biomedical Engineering, 47,* 1584–1592.

Gevins, A. S., & Illes, J. (1991). Neurocognitive networks of the human brain. *Annals of the New York Academy of Sciences, 620,* 22–44.

Gevins, A. S., Schaffer, R. E., Doyle, J. C., Cutillo, B. A., Tannehill, R. L., & Bressler, S. L. (1983). Shadows of thought: Rapidly changing asymmetric brain-potential patterns of a brief visuo-motor task. *Science, 220,* 97–99.

Gevins, A. S., & Cutillo, B. A. (1986). Signals of cognition. In *Handbook of electroencephalography and clinical neurophysiology*, vol. 2. F. H. Lopes da Silva et al. (Eds.). Amsterdam: Elsevier.

Gevins, A. S., Le, J., Martin, N., Brickett, P., Desmond, J., & Reutter, B. (1994). High-resolution EEG: 124 channel recording, spatial enhancement and MRI integration methods. *Electroencephalography and Clinical Neurophysiology, 90,* 337–358.

Hjorth, B. (1975). An on line transformation of EEG scalp potentials into orthogonal source derivations. *Electroencephalography and Clinical Neurophysiology, 39,* 526–530.

Horwitz, B., & Poeppel, D. (2002). How can EEG/MEG and fMRI/PET data be combined? *Human Brain Mapping, 17,* 1–3.

Law, S. K. (1993). Thickness and resistivity variations over the upper surface of human head. *Brain Topography, 6,* 11–15.

Law, S. K., Nunez, P. L., & Wijesinghe, R. S. (1993). High-resolution EEG using spline-generated surface Laplacians on spherical and ellipsoidal surfaces. *IEEE Transactions on Biomedical Engineering, 40,* 145–152.

Malmivuo, J., & Plonsey, R. (1995). *Bioelectromagnetism.* New York: Oxford University Press.

Menon, V., Freeman, W. J., Cutillo, B. A., Desmond, J. E., Ward, M. F., Bressler, S. L., Laxer, K. D., Barbaro, N., & Gevins, A. S. (1996). Spatio-temporal correlations in human gamma band electrocorticograms. *Electroencephalography and Clinical Neurophysiology, 98,* 89–102.

Mima, T., Oluwatimilehin, T., Hiraoka, T., & Hallett, M. (2001). Transient interhemispheric neuronal synchrony correlates with object recognition. *Journal of Neuroscience, 21*, 3942–3948.

Nunez, P. L. (1981). *Electric fields of the brain: The neurophysics of EEG.* New York: Oxford University Press.

Nunez, P. L. (1988). Spatial filtering and experimental strategies in EEG. In D. Samson-Dolfus (Ed.). *Statistics and topography in quantitative EEG.* Paris: Elsevier.

Nunez, P. L. (1989). Estimation of large scale neocortical source activity with EEG surface Laplacians. *Brain Topography, 2*, 141–154.

Nunez, P. L. (1990). Localization of brain activity with electroencephalography. *Advances in Neurology, 54*, 39–65.

Nunez, P. L. (1995). *Neocortical dynamics and human EEG rhythms.* New York: Oxford University Press.

Nunez, P. L. (2000). Toward a quantitative description of large-scale neocortical dynamic function and EEG. *Behavioral and Brain Sciences, 23*, 371–437.

Nunez, P. L., & Pilgreen, K. L. (1991). The Spline-Laplacian is clinical neurophysiology: A method to improve EEG spatial resolution. *Journal of Clinical Neurophysiology, 8*, 397–413.

Nunez, P. L., & Silberstein, R. B. (2000). On the relationship of synaptic activity to macroscopic measurements: Does co-registration of EEG with fMRI make sense? *Brain Topography, 13*, 79–96.

Nunez, P. L., Silberstein, R. B., Cadusch, P. J., Wijesinghe, R. S., Westdorp, A. F., & Srinivasan, R. (1994). A theoretical and experimental study of high resolution EEG based on surface Laplacians and cortical imaging. *Electroencephalography and Clinical Neurophysiology, 90*, 40–57.

Nunez, P. L., Pilgreen, K. L., Westdorp, A. F., Law, S. K., & Nelson, A. V. (1991). A visual study of surface potentials and Laplacians due to distributed neocortical sources: Computer simulations and evoked potentials. *Brain Topography, 2*, 151–168.

Nunez, P. L., Silberstein, R. B., Cadusch, P. J., Wijesinghe, R. S., Westdorp, A. F., & Srinivasan, R. (1994). A theoretical and experimental study of high resolution EEG based on surface Laplacians and cortical imaging. *Electroencephalography and Clinical Neurophysiology, 90*, 40–57.

Nunez, P. L., Srinivasan, R., Westdorp, A. F., Wijesinghe, R. S., Tucker, D. M., Silberstein, R. B., & Cadusch, P. J. (1997). EEG coherency I: Statistics, reference electrode, volume conduction, Laplacians, cortical imaging, and interpretation at multiple scales. *Electroencephalography and Clinical Neurophysiology, 103*, 499–515.

Perrin, F., Bertrand, O., Pernier, J. (1987). Scalp current density mapping: Value and estimation from potential data. *IEEE Transactions on Biomedical Engineering, 34*, 283–289.

Perrin, F., Pernier, J., Bertrand, O., & Echalier, J. F. (1989). Spherical splines for scalp potential and current density mapping. *Electroencephalography and Clinical Neurophysiology, 72*, 184–187.

Raghavachari, S., Kahana, M. J., Rizzuto, D. S., Caplan, J. B., Kirschen, M. P., Bourgeois, B., Madsen, J. R., & Lisman, J. E. (2001). Gating of human theta oscillations by a working memory task. *Journal of Neuroscience, 21,* 3175–3183.

Sarnthein, J., Petsche, H., Rappelsberger, P., Shaw, G. L., & von Stein, A. (1998). Synchronization between prefrontal and posterior association cortex during human working memory. *Proceedings of the National Academy of Science USA, 95,* 7092–7096.

Sidman, R. D. (1991). A method for simulating intracerebral fields: The cortical imaging method. *Journal of Clinical Neurophysiology, 8,* 432–441.

Silberstein, R. B., & Cadusch, P. J. (1992). Measurement processes and spatial principal components analysis. *Brain Topography, 4,* 267–276.

Singer, W. (1999). Striving for coherence. *Nature, 397,* 391–393.

Spitzer, A. R., Cohen, L. G., Fabrikant, J., & Hallett, M. (1989). A method for determining optimal interelectrode spacing for cerebral topographic mapping. *Electroencephalography and Clinical Neurophysiology, 72,* 355–361.

Srinivasan, R. (1999a). Methods to improve the spatial resolution of EEG. *International Journal of Bioelectromagnetism, 1,* 102–111.

Srinivasan, R. (1999b). Spatial structure of the human alpha rhythm: Global correlation in adults and local correlation in children. *Clinical Neurophysiology, 110,* 1351–1362.

Srinivasan, R., Nunez, P. L., & Silberstein, R. B. (1998). Spatial filtering and neocortical dynamics: Estimates of EEG coherence. *IEEE Transactions on Biomedical Engineering, 45,* 814–826.

Srinivasan, R., Russell, D. P., Edelman, G. M., & Tononi, G. (1999). Increased synchronization of neuromagnetic responses during conscious perception. *Journal of Neuroscience, 19,* 5345–5348.

Srinivasan, R., Nunez, P. L., Tucker, D. M., Silberstein, R. B., & Cadusch, P. J. (1996). Spatial sampling and filtering of EEG with spline Laplacians to estimate cortical potentials. *Brain Topography, 8,* 355–366.

Towle, V. L., Syed, I., Grzeszczuk, R., Milton, J., Erickson, R. K., Cogen, P., Berkson, E., & Spire, J. P. (1998). Identification of sensory/motor and pathological areas using EcoG coherence. *Electroencephalography and Clinical Neurophysiology, 106,* 30–39.

Ueno, S., & Iriguchi, N. (1998). Impedance magnetic resonance imaging: A method for imaging impedance distributions based on magnetic resonance imaging. *Journal of Applied Physics, 83,* 6450–6452.

Vitacco, D., Brandeis, D., Pascual-Marqui, R., & Martin, E. (2002). Comparison of event-related potential tomography and functional magnetic resonance imaging during language processing. *Human Brain Mapping, 17,* 4–12.

von Stein, A., & Sarnthein, J. (2000). Different frequencies for different scales of cortical integration: From local gamma to long range alpha/theta synchronization. *International Journal of Psychophysiology, 38,* 301–313.

9 Principal Components Analysis of ERP Data

Joseph Dien and Gwen A. Frishkoff

Over the last several decades, researchers have developed a variety of methods for statistical decomposition of event-related potentials (ERPs). The simplest and most widely applied of these techniques is principal components analysis (PCA). It belongs to a class of factor-analytic procedures, which use eigenvalue decomposition to extract linear combinations of variables (*latent factors*) in such a way as to account for patterns of covariance in the data parsimoniously, that is, with the fewest factors.

In ERP data, the variables are the microvolt readings either at consecutive time points (*temporal PCA*) or at each electrode (*spatial PCA*). The major source of covariance is assumed to be the *ERP components*, characteristic features of the waveform that are spread across multiple time points and multiple electrodes (Donchin & Coles, 1991). Ideally, each latent factor corresponds to a separate ERP component, providing a statistical decomposition of the brain electrical patterns that are superposed in the scalp-recorded data.

PCA has a range of applications for ERP analysis. First, it can be used for *data reduction* and *cleaning or filtering*, prior to data analysis. By reducing hundreds of variables to a handful of latent factors, PCA can greatly simplify analysis and description of complex data. Moreover, the factors retained for further analysis are considered more likely to represent pure signal (i.e., brain activity), as opposed to noise (i.e., artifacts or background EEG).

Second, PCA can be used in *data exploration* as a way to detect and summarize features that might otherwise escape visual inspection. This is particularly useful when measuring ERPs over many tens or hundreds of recording sites; spatial patterns can then be used to constrain the decomposition into latent temporal patterns, as described below.

The use of such high-density ERPs (recordings at 50 or more electrodes) has become increasingly popular in the last several years. A striking feature of high-density ERPs is that the complexity of the data seems to grow exponentially as the number of recording sites is doubled or tripled. Thus, although increases in spatial resolution can lead to important new discoveries, subtle patterns are likely to be missed, as higher spatial sampling reveals more and more complex patterns, overlapping in both time and space. A rational approach to data decomposition can improve the chances of detecting these subtler effects.

Third, PCA can serve as an effective means of *data description*. In principle, PCA can describe features of the dataset more objectively and more precisely than is possible with the unaided eye. Such increased precision could be especially helpful when using PCA as a preprocessing step for ERP source localization (Dien, 1999; Dien et al., 1997, 2003; Dien, Spencer, & Donchin, 2003).

Despite the many useful functions of PCA, this method has had a somewhat checkered history in ERP research, beginning in the 1960s (Donchin, 1966; Ruchkin, Villegas, & John, 1964). An influential review paper by Donchin and Heffley (1979) promoted the use of PCA for ERP component analysis. A few years later, however, PCA entered something of a dark age in the ERP field with the publication of a methodological critique (Wood & McCarthy, 1984), which demonstrated that PCA solutions may be subject to *misallocation of variance* across the latent factors. Wood and McCarthy noted that the same problems arise in the use of other techniques, such as reaction time and peak amplitude measures. The difference is that PCA makes misallocation more explicit, which they argued should be regarded as an advantage. Yet this last point was often overlooked, and this seminal paper has, ironically, been cited as an argument against the use of PCA. Perhaps as a consequence, many researchers continued to rely on conventional ERP analysis techniques.

More recently, the emergence of high-density ERPs has revived the interest in PCA as a method of data reduction. Moreover, some recent studies have shown that statistical decomposition can lead to novel insights into well-known ERP effects, providing evidence to help separate ERP components associated with different perceptual and cognitive operations (Dien et al., 1997, 2003; Dien, Frishkoff, & Tucker, 2000; Spencer, Dien, & Donchin, 2001).

The present review presents a systematic outline of the steps in temporal PCA, and the issues that arise at each step in implementation. We discuss some problems and limitations of temporal PCA, including rotational indeterminacy, problems of misallocation, and latency jitter. We then compare some recent alternatives to temporal PCA, namely, spatial PCA (Dien, 1998a), sequential (spatiotemporal or temporospatial) PCA (Spencer, Dien, & Donchin, 2001), parametric PCA (Dien et al., 2003), multimode PCA (Möcks, 1988), and partial least squares (PLS) (Lobaugh, West, & McIntosh, 2001). Each technique has evolved to address certain weaknesses with the traditional PCA method. We conclude with questions for further research, and advocate a research program for systematic comparison of the strengths and limitations of different multivariate techniques in ERP research.

Steps in Temporal PCA

The two most common types of factor analysis are principal axis factors and principal components analysis. These methods are equivalent for all practical purposes when there are many variables and when the variables are highly correlated (Gorsuch, 1983), as in most ERP datasets. In the ERP literature, PCA is the more common method. Normally, one and the same term, "component," has been used for both PCA linear combinations and for characteristic spatial and temporal features of the ERP. To avoid confusion, we will use the term *factor* (or latent factor) to refer to PCA (latent) components, and the term *component* for spatiotemporal features of the ERP waveform.

The PCA process consists of three main steps: computation of the relationship matrix, extraction and retention of the factors, and rotation to simple structure. In the following sections, we perform PCA simulation to illustrate each step, using the PCA Toolkit (version 1.06), a set of Matlab functions for performing PCA on ERP data. This toolkit was written by the first author and is freely available upon request.

The Data Matrix

A key to understanding PCA procedures as applied to ERPs is to be clear about how multiple sources of variance contribute to the data decomposition. In temporal PCA, the dataset is organized with the variables corresponding to time points, and observations corresponding to the different waveforms in the dataset, as figure 9.1 shows.

The waveforms vary across subjects, electrodes, and experimental conditions. Thus, subject, spatial, and task variance are collectively responsible for covariance among the temporal variables. Although it may seem odd to commingle these three sources of variance, they provide equally valid bases for distinguishing an ERP component; in this respect, it is reasonable to treat them collectively. For example, the voltage readings tend to rise and fall together between 250 and 350 ms in a simple oddball experiment, because they are mutually influenced by the P300 that occurs during this period. Because individual differences, scalp location, and experimental task may all affect the recorded P300 amplitude, the amplitudes of these time points will likewise covary as a function of these three sources of variance. Figure 9.2 shows the grand-averaged waveforms (for $n = 10$ subjects) corresponding to the simulated data in figure 9.1. For simplicity, this example involves only one electrode site, ten subjects, and two experimental conditions. In subsequent sections, we will use these simulated data to help illustrate the steps in implementation of PCA for ERP analysis.

The Relationship Matrix

The first step in applying PCA is to generate a relationship (or association) matrix, which captures the interrelationships between temporal variables. The simplest such

		t1	t2	t3	t4	t5	t6
S01	A	0.077	0.136	0.075	0.095	0.188	0.097
S02	A	0.891	1.780	0.895	0.805	1.612	0.813
S03	A	0.014	0.018	0.013	0.040	0.066	0.035
S04	A	0.657	1.309	0.657	0.789	1.571	0.785
S05	A	0.437	0.864	0.432	1.007	2.002	1.003
S06	A	0.303	0.603	0.303	0.128	0.250	0.123
S07	A	0.477	0.951	0.483	0.418	0.841	0.418
S08	A	0.042	0.073	0.038	0.029	0.043	0.022
S09	A	0.538	1.061	0.533	0.628	1.254	0.626
S10	A	0.509	1.024	0.510	0.218	0.434	0.219
S01	B	1.497	2.987	1.500	0.384	0.769	0.386
S02	B	1.275	2.555	1.281	0.326	0.648	0.329
S03	B	0.666	1.321	0.666	1.026	2.051	1.029
S04	B	0.673	1.341	0.678	1.966	3.914	1.966
S05	B	0.284	0.564	0.292	0.511	1.012	0.507
S06	B	0.980	1.960	0.978	1.741	3.486	1.739
S07	B	0.367	0.721	0.365	1.470	2.934	1.472
S08	B	0.864	1.729	0.866	1.342	2.680	1.337
S09	B	0.568	1.134	0.575	0.210	0.423	0.215
S10	B	0.149	0.287	0.151	0.433	0.860	0.433

Figure 9.1
Data matrix, with dimensions 20 × 6. Variables are time points, measured in two conditions for 10 subjects.

matrix is the sum-of-squares cross-products (SSCP) matrix. For each pair of variables, the two values for each observation are multiplied and then added together. Thus, variables that tend to rise and fall together will produce the highest values in the matrix. The diagonal of the matrix (the relationship of each variable to itself) is the sum of the squared values of each variable. For an example of the effect of using the SSCP matrix, see Curry et al., 1983. SSCP treats mean differences in the same fashion as differences in variance, which has odd effects on the PCA computations. In general, we do not recommend using the SSCP matrix in ERP analyses.

An alternative to the SSCP matrix is the covariance matrix. This matrix is computed in the same fashion as the SSCP matrix, except that the mean of each variable is subtracted out before generating the relationship matrix. Mean correction ensures that variables with high mean values do not have a disproportionate effect on the factor solution. The effect of mean correction on the solution depends on the EEG reference site, a topic that is beyond the scope of this review (cf. Dien, 1998a).

A third alternative is to use the correlation matrix as the relationship matrix. The correlation matrix is computed in the same fashion as the covariance matrix, except

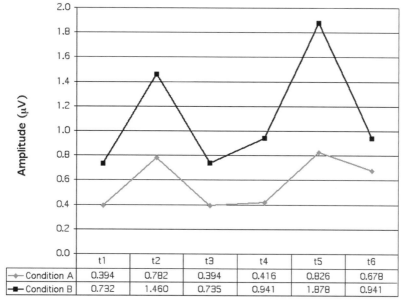

	t1	t2	t3	t4	t5	t6
Condition A	0.394	0.782	0.394	0.416	0.826	0.678
Condition B	0.732	1.460	0.735	0.941	1.878	0.941

Samples (timepoints)

Figure 9.2
Waveforms for grand-averaged data ($n = 10$), corresponding to data in figure 9.1. Graph displays two non-overlapping correlated components, plotted for two hypothetical conditions (A and B).

that the variable variances are standardized. This is accomplished by first mean correcting each variable, and then dividing each variable by its standard deviation, which ensures that the variables contribute equally to the factor solution. Because time points that do not contain ERP components have smaller variances, this procedure may exacerbate the influence of background noise. Simulation studies indicate that covariance matrices can yield more accurate results (Dien, Beal, & Berg, submitted). We therefore recommend using covariance matrices.

In figure 9.3a, the simulated data are converted into a covariance matrix. Observe how the time points containing the two components (t2 and t5) result in larger entries than those without. The entries with the largest numbers will have the most influence on the next step in the PCA procedure: factor extraction.

Factor Extraction
In the extraction stage, a process called eigenvalue decomposition is performed, which progressively removes linear combinations of variables that account for the greatest variance at each step. Each linear combination constitutes a latent factor. In figure 9.3,

	t1	t2	t3	t4	t5	t6
t1	0.157	0.314	0.157	0.077	0.155	0.077
t2	0.314	0.632	0.315	0.154	0.310	0.155
t3	0.157	0.315	0.158	0.077	0.155	0.077
t4	0.077	0.154	0.077	0.336	0.672	0.336
t5	0.155	0.310	0.155	0.672	1.343	0.672
t6	0.077	0.155	0.077	0.336	0.672	0.336

(a) Original covariance matrix.

	t1	t2	t3	t4	t5	t6
t1	0.152	0.305	0.152	0.038	0.077	0.039
t2	0.305	0.613	0.306	0.076	0.156	0.078
t3	0.152	0.306	0.153	0.308	0.078	0.039
t4	0.038	0.076	0.038	0.010	0.019	0.010
t5	0.077	0.156	0.078	0.019	0.039	0.020
t6	0.039	0.078	0.039	0.010	0.020	0.010

(b) Covariance matrix after subtraction of Factor 1
(see text for details).

	t1	t2	t3	t4	t5	t6
t1	0.000	0.000	0.000	0.000	0.000	0.000
t2	0.000	0.000	0.000	0.000	0.000	0.000
t3	0.000	0.000	0.000	0.000	0.000	0.000
t4	0.000	0.000	0.000	0.000	0.000	0.000
t5	0.000	0.000	0.000	0.000	0.000	0.000
t6	0.000	0.000	0.000	0.000	0.000	0.0006

(c) Covariance matrix after subtraction of both
Factor 1 and Factor 2.

Figure 9.3
(*a*) Original covariance matrix. (*b*) Covariance matrix after subtraction of factor 1 (Varimax-rotated; see next section). (*c*) Covariance matrix after subtraction of factors 1 and 2. Because factors 1 and 2 together account for nearly all of the variance, the result is the null matrix.

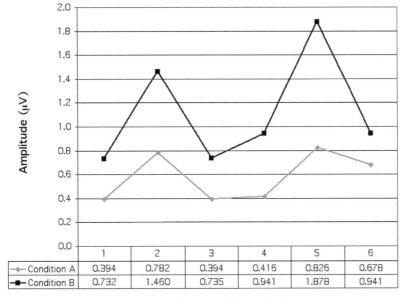

	1	2	3	4	5	6
—◆— Condition A	0.394	0.782	0.394	0.416	0.826	0.678
—■— Condition B	0.732	1.460	0.735	0.941	1.878	0.941

Samples (timepoints)

Figure 9.4
Reconstructed waveforms, calculated by multiplying the factor loadings by the factor scores, scaled to microvolts (i.e., multiplied by the matrix of standard deviations for the original data). Data reconstructed using Varimax-rotated factors for this example.

we demonstrate how this process iteratively reduces the remaining values in the relationship matrix to zero.

In general, PCA should extract as many factors as there are variables, as long as the number of observations is equal to or greater than the number of variables (i.e., as long as the data matrix is of full rank).

The initial extraction yields an unrotated solution, consisting of a *factor loading matrix* and a *factor score matrix*. The factor loading matrix represents correlations between the variables and the factor scores. The factor score matrix indexes the magnitude of the factors for each of the observations and thus represents the relationship between the factors and the observations. If the two matrices are multiplied together, they will reproduce the data matrix. By convention, the reproduced data matrix will be in standardized form, regardless of the type of relationship matrix that was entered into the PCA. To recreate the original data matrix, the variables of this standardized matrix are multiplied by the original standard deviations, and the original variable means are restored (figure 9.4).

For a temporal PCA, the loadings describe the time course of each of the factors. To accurately represent the time course of the factors, it is necessary to first multiply them by the variable standard deviations, which rescales them to microvolts (see proof in Dien, 1998a). Further, it is important to note that the sign of a given factor loading is arbitrary. This is necessarily the case, as a given peak in the factor time course will be positive on one side of the head, and negative on the other side, due to the dipolar nature of electrical fields (Nunez, 1981). Note further, that the dipolar distributions can be distorted or obscured by referencing biases in the data (Dien, 1998b). Only the product of the factor loading and the factor score corresponds to the original data in an unequivocal way. Thus, if the factor loading is positive at the peak, then the factor scores from one side of the head will be positive and the other side will be negative, corresponding to the dipolar field.

The factor scores, on the other hand, provide information about the other sources of variance (i.e., subject, task, and spatial variance). For example, to compute the amplitude of a factor at a specific electrode site for a given task condition, one simply takes the factor scores corresponding to the observations for that task at the electrode of interest and computes their mean (across subjects). If this mean value is computed for each electrode, the resulting values can be used to plot the scalp topography for that factor. If a specific time point is chosen, it is possible reconstruct the scalp topography with the proper microvolt scaling by multiplying the mean scores by the factor loading and the standard deviation for the time point of interest (see proof in Dien, 1998a).

Unlike the PCA algorithm in most statistics packages, the PCA Toolkit does not mean correct the factor scores. This maintains an interpretable relationship between the factor scores and the original data. If factor scores are mean corrected as part of the standardization, the mean task scores will be centered around zero, which can make factor interpretation more difficult. In an oddball experiment, for example, the P300 factor scores should be large for the target condition and small for the standard condition. However, if the factor scores are mean corrected, then the mean task scores for the two conditions will be of equal amplitude and opposite signs (because mean correction splits the difference).

Factor Retention

Most of the PCA factors that are extracted account for small proportions of variance, which may be attributed to background noise, or minor departures from group trends. In the interest of parsimony, only the larger factors are typically retained, because they are considered most likely to contain interpretable signal. A common criterion for determining how many factors to retain is the scree test (Cattell, 1966; Cattell & Jaspers, 1967), is based on the principle that the PCA of a random set of data will produce a set of randomly sized factors. Because factors are extracted in order of descending size, when graphed, they will form a steady downward slope. A dataset containing sig-

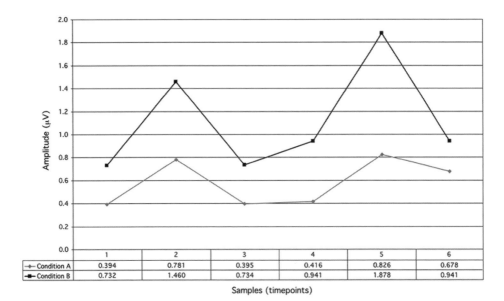

	1	2	3	4	5	6
Condition A	0.394	0.781	0.395	0.416	0.826	0.678
Condition B	0.732	1.460	0.734	0.941	1.878	0.941

Samples (timepoints)

Figure 9.5
Reconstructed waveforms, computed as in figure 9.4, using only factors 1 and 2. Because the first two factors account for nearly all of the variance, the reconstruction is nearly as good as the original data (cf. figure 9.2).

nal, in addition to the noise, should have initial factors that are larger than would be expected from random data alone. The point of departure from the slope (the elbow) indicates the number of factors to retain. Factors beyond this point are likely to contain noise and are best dropped. Figure 9.5 plots the reconstructed grand-averaged data, using the retained factors in order to verify that meaningful factors have not been excluded.

In practice, the scree plot for ERP datasets often contains multiple elbows, which can make it difficult to determine the proper number of factors to retain. Part of the problem is that the noise contains some unwanted signal (remnants of the background EEG). One can use a modified version of the parallel test to address this issue (Dien, 1998a). The parallel test determines how many factors represent signal by comparing the scree produced by the full dataset to that produced when only the noise is present. The noise level is estimated by generating an ERP average with every other trial inverted, which has the effect of canceling out the signal while leaving the noise level unchanged. The results of the parallel test should be considered a lower bound because retaining additional factors to account for major noise features can actually improve the analysis (for an example, see Dien, 1998a), although in principle if too many additional factors are retained it can result in unwanted distinctions being made (such as

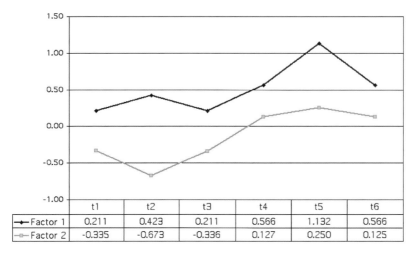

	t1	t2	t3	t4	t5	t6
—●—Factor 1	0.211	0.423	0.211	0.566	1.132	0.566
—□—Factor 2	-0.335	-0.673	-0.336	0.127	0.250	0.125

Figure 9.6
Graph of unrotated factors. Only factors 1 and 2 are graphed, because factors 3–6 are close to 0.

between subject-specific variations of the component). In general, the experience of the first author is that between eight and sixteen factors is often appropriate, although this may depend, among other things, on the number of recording sites.

Factor Rotation
A critical step, after deciding how many factors to retain, is to determine the best way of allocating variance across the remaining factors. Unfortunately, there is no transparent relationship between the PCA factors and the latent variables of interest (i.e., ERP components). Eigenvalue decomposition blindly generates factors that account for maximum variance, which may be influenced by more than one latent variable; however, the goal is to have each factor represent a single ERP component.

As figure 9.6 shows, there is not a one-to-one mapping of factors to variables after the initial factor extraction. Rather, the initial extraction has maximized the variance of the first factor by including variance from as many variables as possible. In doing so, it has generated a factor that is a hybrid of two ERP components, the linear sum of roughly 10 percent of the P1 and 90 percent of the P3. The second factor contains the leftover variance of both components. This example demonstrates the danger of interpreting the initial unrotated factors directly, as some advocate (e.g., Rösler & Manzey, 1981).

Factor rotation restructures the allocation of variables to factors to maximize the chance that each factor reflects a single latent variable. The most common rotation is Varimax (Kaiser, 1958). In Varimax, each of the retained factors is iteratively rotated pairwise with each of the other factors in turn, until changes in the solution become

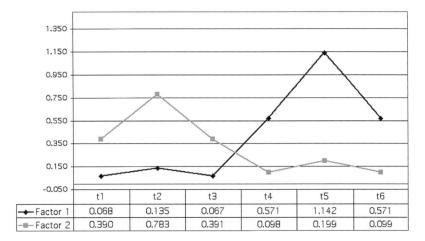

	t1	t2	t3	t4	t5	t6
◆ Factor 1	0.068	0.135	0.067	0.571	1.142	0.571
■ Factor 2	0.390	0.783	0.391	0.098	0.199	0.099

Figure 9.7
Graph of Varimax-rotated factor loadings. Only factors 1 and 2 are graphed, because factors 3–6 are close to 0.

negligible. More specifically, the Varimax procedure rotates the two factors such that the sum of the factor loadings (raised to the fourth power) is maximized. This has the effect of favoring solutions in which factor loadings are as extreme as possible with a combination of near-zero loadings and large peak values. Because ERP components (other than DC potentials) tend to have zero activity for most of the epoch with a single major peak or dip, Varimax should yield a reasonable approximation to the underlying ERP components (figure 9.7). Temporal overlap of ERP components raises additional issues, which we address in the following section.

Simulation studies demonstrate that several situations influence the accuracy of a rotation, including component overlap and component correlation (Dien, 1998a). Component overlap is a problem, because the more similar two ERP components are, the more difficult it is to distinguish them (Möcks & Verleger, 1991). Further, correlations between components may lead to violations of statistical assumptions. The initial extraction and the subsequent Varimax rotation maintain strict orthogonality between the factors (so the factors are uncorrelated). To the extent that the components are in fact correlated, the model solution will be inaccurate, producing misallocation of variance across the factors. Component correlation can arise when two components respond to the same task variables (an example is the P300 and slow wave components, which often co-occur), or when both components respond to the same subject parameters (e.g., age, sex, or personality traits), or share a common spatial distribution. Further, these two components can be measured at some of the same electrodes due to their similar scalp topographies.

One can effectively address component correlation by using an oblique rotation, such as Promax (Hendrickson & White, 1964), allowing for correlated factors (Dien, 1998a). In Promax, the initial Varimax rotation is succeeded by a "relaxation" step, in which each individual factor is further rotated to maximize the number of variables with minimal loadings. A factor is adjusted in this fashion without regard to the other factors, allowing factors to become correlated, and thus relaxing the orthogonality constraint in the Varimax solution. The Promax rotation typically leads to solutions that more accurately capture the large features of the Varimax factors while minimizing the smaller features. As a result, Promax solutions tend to account for slightly less variance than the original Varimax solutions, but may also give more accurate results (Dien, 1998a). Figure 9.8 shows a typical result.

Spatial versus Temporal PCA

A limitation of temporal PCA is that factors are defined solely as a function of component time course, as instantiated by the factor loadings. This means that ERP components that are topographically distinct, but have a similar time course, will be modeled by a single factor. A sign that this has occurred is when temporal PCA yields condition effects characterized by a scalp topography that differs from the overall factor topography.

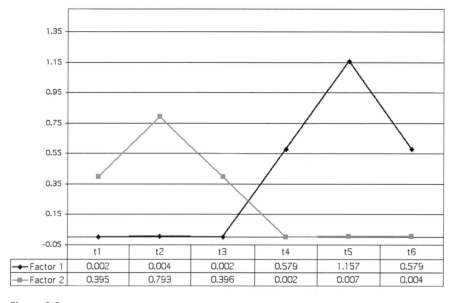

	t1	t2	t3	t4	t5	t6
—♦—Factor 1	0.002	0.004	0.002	0.579	1.157	0.579
—■—Factor 2	0.395	0.793	0.396	0.002	0.007	0.004

Figure 9.8
Graph of Promax-rotated factor loadings. Only factors 1 and 2 are graphed, because factors 3–6 are close to 0.

To address this problem, one may use spatial PCA as an alternative to temporal PCA (Dien, 1998a). In a spatial PCA, the data are arranged such that the variables are electrode locations, and observations are experimental conditions, subjects, and time points. The factor loadings therefore describe scalp topographies, instead of temporal patterns. This approach is less likely to confound ERP components with the same time course, as long as they are differentiated by the task or subject variance. On the other hand, it will be subject to the converse problem, confusing components with similar scalp topographies, even when they have clearly separate time dynamics.

The choice between spatial versus temporal PCA should depend on specific analysis goals. A rule of thumb is that if time course is the focus of an analysis, then one should use spatial PCA, and vice versa. The reason is that the factor loadings are constrained to be the same across the entire dataset (i.e., the same time course for temporal PCA, and the same scalp topography for spatial PCA). The factor scores, on the other hand, are free to vary between conditions and subjects. Thus, one can examine latency changes with spatial, but not temporal, PCA, and vice versa. In particular, this implies that temporal, rather than spatial, PCA should be more effective as a preprocessing step in source localization, because these modeling procedures rely on the scalp topography to infer the number and configuration of sources.

All other things being equal, temporal PCA is in principle more accurate than spatial PCA, because component overlap reduces PCA accuracy and volume conduction ensures that all ERP components will overlap in a spatial PCA. Furthermore, the effect of the Varimax and Promax rotations is to minimize factor overlap, which is a more appropriate goal for temporal than for spatial PCA. A caveat in either case is that ERP component separation can be achieved only if subject or task variance (or both) can effectively distinguish the components. In other words, the three sources of variance associated with each observation must collectively be able to distinguish the ERP components, regardless of whether the components differ along the variable dimension (time for temporal PCA, or space for spatial PCA).

Recent Alternatives to PCA

In recent years, researchers have developed a variety of multivariate statistical techniques that are increasingly making their way into the ERP literature. One such method, independent components analysis (Makeig et al., 1996), is discussed elsewhere in this volume.

In this section, we present four multivariate techniques in ERP analysis, which share a common basis in their use of eigenvalue decomposition. Each technique has been claimed to address one or more problems with conventional PCA. The application these techniques in ERP research is very recent, and more work is needed to characterize their respective strengths and limitations for various ERP applications. Future developments of these techniques may lead to a powerful suite of tools that can address a range of problems in ERP analysis.

Sequential Spatiotemporal (or Temporospatial) PCA

A recent procedure for improved separation of ERP components is spatiotemporal (or temporospatial) PCA (Spencer, Dien, & Donchin, 1999, 2001). This procedure separates ERP components that were confounded in the initial PCA by applying a second PCA, which separates variance along the other dimension. For a temporospatial PCA this is accomplished by rearranging the factor scores resulting from the temporal PCA so that each column contains the factor scores from a different electrode. A spatial PCA can then be conducted using these factor scores as the new variables. Although the initial PCA has collapsed the temporal variance, the observations still express subject and task variance, and can thus be used to separate ERP components that were confounded in the initial PCA.

Spencer, Dien, and Donchin (1999, 2001) followed the initial spatial PCA with a temporal PCA, with the factor scores from all the factors combined within the same analysis (number of observations equal to number of subjects x number of tasks x number of spatial factors). This procedure led to a clear separation of the P300 from the Novelty P3. However, it also had an important drawback: the application of a single temporal PCA to all the spatial factors could result in loss of some of the finer distinctions in time course between different spatial factors. This analytic strategy was necessary because the generalized inverse function, used by SAS to generate the factor scores, requires that there be more observations than variables.

The PCA Toolkit has bypassed this requirement by directly rotating the factor scores (Möcks & Verleger, 1991), allowing each initial factor to be subjected to a separate PCA (following the example of Scott Makeig's ICA toolbox and an independent suggestion by Bill Dunlap). In a more recent study (Dien et al., 2003), an initial spatial PCA yielded 12 factors; each spatial factor was then subjected to a separate temporal PCA (each retaining four factors for simplicity's sake). For analyses using this newer approach (it makes little difference for the original approach), temporospatial PCA is recommended over spatiotemporal PCA, because temporal PCA may lead to better initial separation of ERP components. Subsequent application of a spatial PCA can then help separate components that were confounded in the temporal PCA. On the other hand, if latency analysis is a goal of the PCA, then one should do spatial PCA first (because latency analysis cannot be done on the results of a temporal PCA), with the succeeding temporal PCA step used to verify whether multiple components are present in the factor of interest, as another recent study demonstrated (Dien, Spencer, & Donchin, in press).

The full equation to generate the microvolt value for a specific time point t and channel c for a spatiotemporal PCA is $L1 * V1 * L2 * S2 * V2$ (where $L1$ is the spatial

Principal Components Analysis of ERP Data

Please return this book to:
DEB JENSEN
deb.jensen04@post.harvard.edu

203

PCA factor loading for c, $V1$ is the standard deviation of c, $L2$ is the temporal PCA factor loading for t, $S2$ is the mean factor scores for the temporal factor, and $V2$ is the standard deviation of the spatial factor scores at t. The temporal and spatial terms are reversed for temporospatial PCA.

Parametric PCA

Another recent method involves the use of parametric measures to improve PCA separation of latent factors, which differ along one or more stimulus dimension (Dien et al., 2003). This more specialized procedure can only be conducted on datasets containing observations with a continuous range of values. Dien et al. (2003) averaged ERP responses to sentence endings for each stimulus item (collapsing over subjects) rather than averaging over subjects (collapsing over items in each experimental condition). This item-averaging approach resulted in 120 sentence averages, which were rated on a number of linguistic parameters, such as meaningfulness and word frequency. After an initial temporal PCA, it was then possible to correlate the parameter of interest with the mean factor score at each channel, to determine the influence of the stimulus parameter on a given ERP component, such as the N400. This had the effect of highlighting the relationship between ERP components and stimulus parameters, while factoring out the effects of ERP components unrelated to the parameters of interest. In this fashion, parametric PCA can lead to scalp topographies that reflect only the parameters of interest, providing a new approach to functional separation of ERP components. This approach thus provides an alternative method to sequential PCA for deconfounding components. These components can be then be subjected to further analyses, such as dipole and linear inverse modeling.

Partial Least Squares

Partial least squares (PLS), like PCA, is a multivariate technique based on eigenvalue decomposition. Unlike PCA, PLS operates on the covariance between the data matrix and a matrix of contrasts that represents features of the experimental design (McIntosh et al., 1996). Similar to parametric PCA procedures, the decomposition is focused on variance due to the experimental manipulations (condition differences). A recent paper (Lobaugh, West, & McIntosh, 2001) applied PLS to ERP data for the first time. Simulations showed that the PLS analysis led to accurate modeling of the spatial and temporal effects that were associated with condition differences in the ERP waveforms. Lobaugh, West, and McIntosh also suggest that PLS may be an effective preprocessing method, identifying time points and electrodes that are sensitive to condition differences and can therefore be targeted for further analyses.

One cautionary note concerning PLS arises from the use of difference waves, which are created by subtracting the ERP waveform in one experimental condition from the response in a different condition, in order to isolate experimental effects prior to factor extraction. This approach, based on the *logic of subtraction*, can lead to incorrect conclusions when the assumption of pure insertion is violated, that is, when two conditions are different in kind rather than in degree. It can also produce misleading results when a change in latency appears to be an amplitude effect or when multiple effects appear to be a single effect.

Neuroimaging measures, such as ERP and fMRI, may be particularly subject to such misinterpretations, because both spatial (anatomical) and temporal, variance can lead to condition differences. If these multiple sources of variance are not adequately separated, a temporal difference between conditions may be erroneously ascribed to a single anatomical region or ERP component (e.g., Zarahn, Aguirre, & D'Esposito, 1999). Spencer, Abad, and Donchin (2000) used PCA to examine the claim that recollection (as compared with familiarity) is associated with a unique electrophysiological component. They concluded that the effect was more accurately ascribed to differences in latency jitter, or trial-to-trial variance in peak latency of the P300 across the two conditions.

For this reason, condition differences, although useful, should only be interpreted in respect to the overall patterns in the original data. Further, one should fully analyze both spatial and temporal variance between conditions to rule out differences in latency jitter or other electrophysiological effects that may be hidden or confounded through cognitive subtraction. This recommendation also applies to the interpretation of results from the use of partial variance techniques, such as PLS.

Multimode Factor Analysis

The techniques discussed in previous sections were all based on two-mode (defined as a dimension of variance) analysis of ERP data. In temporal PCA, for instance, time points represent one dimension (variables axis), and the other dimension combines the remaining sources of variance—that is, subjects, electrodes, and experimental conditions (observations axis). By contrast, multimode procedures analyze the data across three or more dimensions simultaneously. For example, in trilinear decomposition (TLD), the subject data matrix X_i is expressed as the cross-product of three factors, as equation 9.1 shows:

$$X_i = B * A_i * C \tag{9.1}$$

where B is a set of spatial components and C is a set of temporal components. A_i represents the subject loadings on B and C. B and C are calculated in separate, spatial and temporal, singular value decompositions of the data and are then combined to yield a new decomposition of the data, for any fixed dimensionality (Wang, Begleiter, & Porjesz, 2000). Because tri-mode PCA is susceptible to the same rotational indeterminacies as regular PCA, rotational procedures will need to be developed and evaluated.

It has been claimed that tri-mode PCA can effectively remove "nuisance" sources of variance, as described by Möcks (1985), providing greater sensitivity as compared with conventional, two-dimensional PCA. Further, Achim has described the use of multi-modal procedures to help address misallocation of variance (Achim & Bouchard, 1997). These reports point to the need for thorough and systematic comparison of multimode methods such as TLD with other methods, such as parametric PCA and PLS. This can only be done for algorithms that are made available to the rest of the research community, either through open source or through commercial software packages.

Conclusion

PCA and related procedures can provide an effective way to preprocess high-density ERP datasets, and to help separate components that differ in their sensitivity to spatial, temporal, or functional parameters. This brief review has attempted to characterize the current state of the art in PCA of ERPs. Ongoing research will continue to refine and optimize statistical procedures and will aim to determine the optimal procedures for statistical decompositions of ERP data. Ultimately, it is likely that we will require a range of statistical tools, each best suited to different applications in ERP analysis.

References

Achim, A., & Bouchard, S. (1997). Toward a dynamic topographic components model. *Electroencephalography and Clinical Neurophysiology, 103*, 381–385.

Cattell, R. B. (1966). The scree test for the number of factors. *Multivariate Behavioral Research, 1*, 245–276.

Cattell, R. B., & Jaspers, J. (1967). A general plasmode (No. 3010-5-2) for factor analytic exercises and research. *Multivariate Behavioral Research Monographs, 67–3*, 1–212.

Curry, S. H., Cooper, R., McCallum, W. C., Pocock, P. V., Papakostopoulos, D., Skidmore, S., & Newton, P. (1983). The principal components of auditory target detection. In A. W. K. Gaillard & W. Ritter (Eds.), *Tutorials in ERP research: Endogenous components* (pp. 79–117). Amsterdam: North-Holland Publishing Company.

Dien, J. (1998a). Addressing misallocation of variance in principal components analysis of event-related potentials. *Brain Topography, 11*(1), 43–55.

Dien, J. (1998b). Issues in the application of the average reference: Review, critiques, and recommendations. *Behavioral Research Methods, Instruments, and Computers, 30*(1), 34–43.

Dien, J. (1999). Differential lateralization of trait anxiety and trait fearfulness: Evoked potential correlates. *Personality and Individual Differences, 26*(1), 333–356.

Dien, J., Beal, D., & Berg, P. (submitted). Optimizing principal components analysis for event-related potential analysis.

Dien, J., Frishkoff, G. A., Cerbonne, A., & Tucker, D. M. (2003). Parametric analysis of event-related potentials in semantic comprehension: Evidence for parallel brain mechanisms. *Cognitive Brain Research, 15*, 137–153.

Dien, J., Frishkoff, G. A., & Tucker, D. M. (2000). Differentiating the N3 and N4 electrophysiological semantic incongruity effects. *Brain & Cognition, 43*, 148–152.

Dien, J., Spencer, K. M., & Donchin, E. (2003). Localization of the event-related potential novelty response as defined by principal components analysis. *Cognitive Brain Research, 17*, 637–650.

Dien, J., Spencer, K. M., & Donchin, E. (in press). Parsing the "Late Positive Complex": Mental chronometry and the ERP components that inhabit the neighborhood of the P300. *Psychophysiology*.

Dien, J., Tucker, D. M., Potts, G., & Hartry, A. (1997). Localization of auditory evoked potentials related to selective intermodal attention. *Journal of Cognitive Neuroscience, 9*(6), 799–823.

Donchin, E. (1966). A multivariate approach to the analysis of average evoked potentials. *IEEE Transactions on Bio-Medical Engineering, BME-13*, 131–139.

Donchin, E., & Coles, M. G. H. (1991). While an undergraduate waits. *Neuropsychologia, 29*, 557–569.

Donchin, E., & Heffley, E. (1979). Multivariate analysis of event-related potential data: A tutorial review. In D. Otto (Ed.), *Multidisciplinary perspectives in event-related potential research (EPA 600/9-77-043)* (pp. 555–572). Washington, DC: U.S. Government Printing Office.

Gorsuch, R. L. (1983). *Factor analysis* (2nd ed.). Hillsdale, NJ: Lawrence Erlbaum Associates.

Hendrickson, A. E., & White, P. O. (1964). Promax: A quick method for rotation to oblique simple structure. *The British Journal of Statistical Psychology, 17*, 65–70.

Kaiser, H. F. (1958). The varimax criterion for analytic rotation in factor analysis. *Psychometrika, 23*, 187–200.

Lobaugh, N. J., West, R., & McIntosh, A. R. (2001). Spatiotemporal analysis of experimental differences in event-related potential data with partial least squares. *Psychophysiology, 38*, 517–530.

Makeig, S., Bell, A. J., Jung, T., & Sejnowski, T. J. (1996). Independent component analysis of electroencephalographic data. *Advances in Neural Information Processing Systems, 8*, 145–151.

McIntosh, A. R., Bookstein, F. L., Haxby, J. V., & Grady, C. L. (1996). Spatial pattern analysis of functional brain images using Partial Least Squares. *Neuroimage, 3*, 143–157.

Möcks, J. (1988). Topographic components model for event-related potentials and some biophysical considerations. *IEEE Transactions on Biomedical Engineering, 35*, 482–484.

Möcks, J., & Verleger, R. (1991). Multivariate methods in biosignal analysis: Application of principal component analysis to event-related potentials. In R. Weitkunat (Ed.), *Digital Biosignal Processing* (pp. 399–458). Amsterdam: Elsevier.

Nunez, P. L. (1981). *Electric fields of the brain: The neurophysics of EEG*. New York: Oxford University Press.

Rösler, F., & Manzey, D. (1981). Principal components and varimax-rotated components in event-related potential research: Some remarks on their interpretation. *Biological Psychology, 13*, 3–26.

Ruchkin, D. S., Villegas, J., & John, E. R. (1964). An analysis of average evoked potentials making use of least mean square techniques. *Annals of the New York Academy of Sciences, 115*, 799–826.

Spencer, K. M., Abad, E. V., & Donchin, E. (2000). On the search for the neurophysiological manifestation of recollective experience. *Psychophysiology, 37*, 494–506.

Spencer, K. M., Dien, J., & Donchin, E. (1999). A componential analysis of the ERP elicited by novel events using a dense electrode array. *Psychophysiology, 36*, 409–414.

Spencer, K. M., Dien, J., & Donchin, E. (2001). Spatiotemporal analysis of the late ERP responses to deviant stimuli. *Psychophysiology, 38*, 343–358.

Wang, K., Begleiter, H., & Porjesz, B. (2000). Trilinear modeling of event-related potentials. *Brain Topography, 12*, 263–271.

Wood, C. C., & McCarthy, G. (1984). Principal component analysis of event-related potentials: Simulation studies demonstrate misallocation of variance across components. *Electroencephalography and Clinical Neurophysiology, 59*, 249–260.

Zarahn, E., Aguirre, G. K., & D'Esposito, M. (1999). Temporal isolation of the neural correlates of spatial mnemonic processing with fMRI. *Cognitive Brain Research, 7*, 255–268.

10 Averaging, Detection, and Classification of Single-Trial ERPs

Kevin M. Spencer

ERP Averaging

Variability of the ERP Signal

The first main assumption of signal averaging is that the detected signal in each single trial has stable characteristics, such as constant waveform morphology, amplitude, and latency across all single trials. The problem is that the ERP does not constitute a unitary signal. Instead, it consists of multiple components whose amplitude and latency can vary independently as a result of many factors. If the entire ERP waveform had a constant morphology and only varied in its amplitude, the average ERP would at least present an unbiased estimate of the mean of the distribution of single-trial ERPs, but this is not the case. The average ERP may present only a gross picture of the neural processes elicited by the event of interest. Lumping together single trials in the average obscures the intertrial variability of ERP components and their inter-relationships.

A common example of the confounding effect of intertrial variability on ERP estimation is latency jitter (cf. Brazier, 1964). If the latency of an ERP component varies from trial to trial, the amplitude of the component in the average will be reduced and its shape distorted. Then the average ERP will not be a valid estimate of the component's amplitude and morphology. Figure 10.1 presents an example of a component that varies in amplitude but not latency. Here, the peak (0.902) and average (0.0901) amplitudes of the simulated component in the average ERP are identical to the mean peak and average amplitude computed from the single-trial distributions (30 trials). However, when single-trial latency is varied, the average ERP becomes less valid. Figure 10.2 presents two examples. The top left plot shows the average that results when the latency of the simulated ERP component is jittered with random values drawn from a Gaussian distribution having a standard deviation of ± 10 time points. The bottom left plot shows the effect of latency jitter on the average with a latency jitter of ± 20 time points. The top and bottom plots on the right show the respective single-trial distributions (data sets consisted of 30 trials each). From these examples it is clear that as

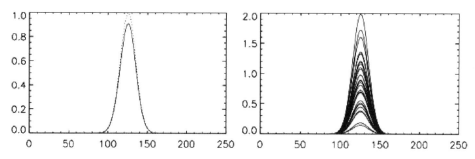

Figure 10.1
Effect of amplitude variability. (*Left*) The simulated ERP component is drawn with a dotted line and the average with a solid line. (*Right*) Simulated component on each single trial (the *y*-axis differs from the left plot). The single-trial amplitudes were drawn from a Gaussian distribution with a mean of 1.0 and a standard deviation of 1.0.

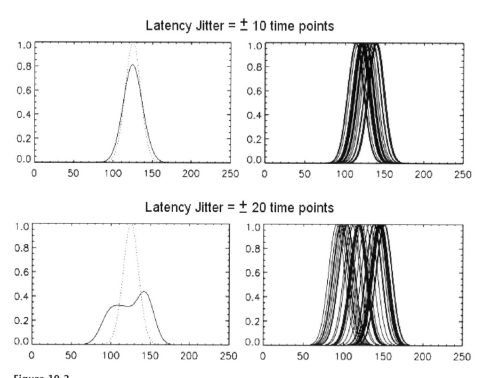

Figure 10.2
Effects of latency variability. (*Left*) The simulated ERP component is drawn with a dotted line and the average with a solid line. (*Right*) Simulated component on each single trial.

latency jitter across single trials increases, the degree of distortion of the component in the average ERP increases, and the peak amplitude of the component decreases.

An important implication of latency jitter is that a difference in the amplitude of an ERP component between experimental conditions or subject groups could result not from a real difference in component amplitude, but from a difference in the amount of latency jitter. Note that latency jitter is likely to affect endogenous ERP components more than exogenous ones, because the latencies of endogenous components will vary as a result of cognitive processes (e.g., stimulus evaluation in the case of the P300; Kutas, McCarthy, & Donchin, 1977) that are less time-locked to the event onset and are more dependent on the demands of the task. For example, Spencer, Vila Abad, and Donchin (2000) examined the contribution of latency jitter to the late ERP components elicited by "remembered" and "known" words in a recognition memory task. They found that the difference in the amplitude of the ERPs elicited by remembered and known items could be accounted for by differences in the amount of latency jitter between conditions. Thus, it can be problematic to compare the amplitudes of ERPs computed over trials with varying degrees of latency jitter. Below I will present methods for estimating and correcting for latency jitter.

In comparing the distributions of single-trial peak latencies and the corresponding average ERPs in figure 10.2, one can see that the morphology of the average ERP is determined by the latency distribution of single-trial waveforms. One question is the degree to which the peak latency of the average waveform, which is commonly used as a measure of the latency of an ERP component across single trials, corresponds to measures of the central tendency of the distribution of single-trial peak latencies. To explore this question, we conducted a simulation experiment that computed correlations between peak latency in the average ERP and the mean and median of single-trial latencies. One thousand data sets of 30 trials each were constructed for latency jitter standard deviations of ±5–45 time points (Gaussian distribution). Figure 10.3 presents the results of this experiment.

At a latency jitter of five time points, there is a high correspondence ($r = \sim0.92$) between the peak latency in the average ERP and the mean of the single-trial latency distributions, whereas the median has a lower correlation (~0.75) than the mean. But as the degree of latency jitter increases, the correlation with peak latency in the average ERP decreases sharply for the mean single-trial latency and much less so for the median. At the asymptotic values, the median and mean correlations are approximately 0.65 and 0.40, respectively. When amplitude variability is added to make the simulation more realistic (figure 10.4), the asymptotic values of the correlations decrease to ~0.55 for the median and ~0.33 for the mean. Hence, one can conclude that the latency of a component's peak in the average ERP is more closely related to the median of single-trial peak latencies, not the mean. This result implies that if one were to make

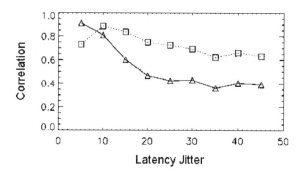

Figure 10.3
Correlations between the peak latency of a simulated component in the average ERP and the mean (triangles) and median (squares) of single-trial latencies when amplitudes are held constant and single-trial latency varies.

a comparison between the peak latency of a component in the average ERP and a re-action time measure, the median reaction time would be the most appropriate.

So far we have been considering the hypothetical case of the ERP consisting of a single component that is present on every trial. Of course, the ERP actually consists of a multitude of components, which can be influenced by very different factors. When experimental hypotheses consider effects on more than one ERP component, and measurements are based on the average ERP, there is an implicit assumption that the average ERP captures the relationship between the two components. For instance, average ERPs in an oddball task will show that the N2 and P300 components are both elicited by rare stimuli. What the average ERPs will not show, however, is the extent to which the amplitude and latency of these components covary across single trials. Do rare stimuli elicit the N2 and P300 together on every trial? Do rare items that elicit large N2s also elicit large P300s, or is there no relationship between the two compo-nents? Such information would be valuable if one is to understand the sequence in which areas of the brain process rare events.

Few studies have addressed the issue of ERP component interrelationships across single trials. One example is the examination of the latency variability of the N1, P2, N2, and P300 components in an auditory oddball task by Michalewski, Prasher, and Starr (1986). They used a single-trial detection technique to estimate the latency of each component on every trial, and found that the latencies of the N1 and P2 compo-nents were correlated, as were the latencies of the N2 and P300. This approach is nec-essary if one wishes to take full advantage of the temporal information available in the ERP to construct models of information processing in the brain.

One way to enhance the information derived from average ERPs is to selectively average trials based on overt performance measures, such as reaction time (RT) or ac-

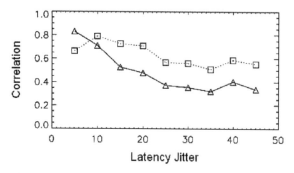

Figure 10.4
Same as in figure 10.3, but with both single-trial amplitude and latency variability. Single-trial amplitudes are drawn from a Gaussian distribution with a mean of 1.0 and a standard deviation of 0.5.

curacy. An early demonstration of this "outcome-related averaging" approach was by Donchin and Lindsley (1966), who reported that the amplitude of the "vertex potential" was larger on trials with short, compared to long, RTs. Outcome-related averaging has subsequently become a standard tool in ERP research. Some examples of its use are in averaging trials according to: recognition judgment (Sanquist et al., 1980) or subsequent recall (Karis, Fabiani, & Donchin, 1984) in memory paradigms; subthreshold motor response activation (Coles et al., 1985); correct or incorrect response (Gehring et al., 1993); and subjective confidence ratings of performance (Scheffers & Coles, 2000). When the dimension of a measure is continuous, such as RT, the trials can be ordered according to this measure and running averages constructed to illustrate trial-to-trial variability (e.g., Jung et al., 2001). Similarly, trials can be selectively averaged according to other EEG (e.g., Jasiukaitis & Hakerem, 1988) or physiological responses (e.g., Marinkovic, Halgren, & Maltzman, 2001).

Variability of the Background EEG
The second main assumption of signal averaging is that background EEG activity is random and uncorrelated with the ERP signal. Signal averaging will reduce the amplitude of background activity or noise[1] if it has a symmetric amplitude distribution that is stable across time, so that the mean across trials is the best estimate of the central tendency of the distribution.[2] But nearly a century of research has shown that the EEG is not entirely uncorrelated with event-related activity. First, the spectral content of the EEG varies widely depending on the individual's state of consciousness, from low-frequency delta activity during deep sleep, to alpha-range activity during a resting state, to high-frequency beta activity during alertness. Second, the early sensory components may reflect to some extent the reorganization of the phase of ongoing

rhythmic activity that is induced by the onset of a stimulus (e.g., Makeig et al., 2001). Third, a number of studies have provided evidence of non-stimulus-locked oscillations in the background EEG that relate to information processing (e.g., Spencer & Polich, 1999; Tallon-Baudry & Bertrand, 1999). For these reasons, it is inappropriate to assume that background EEG activity is uncorrelated with the ERP signal. These factors are also problematic for estimating the spectral properties of the EEG, from a theoretical perspective, because they mean that EEG signal is not stationary (i.e., its properties change over time).

We have discussed problems with using the average ERP as an estimate of event-related EEG activity. Variability in the ERP signal presents problems for using the average ERP to represent the distribution of single-trial ERPs, and the background EEG cannot be assumed to be uncorrelated with the ERP. Nevertheless, thousands of studies over decades of research have proven the average ERP to be a valuable tool for studying brain function. At the least, it is important for the ERP researcher to understand the limitations of the averaging method, and to be aware of other possible methods for extracting information from single-trial ERPs. Next we will discuss single-trial detection and classification techniques, which promise to unlock the wealth of information contained in single-trial ERPs.

Measurement of Single-Trial ERPs

Given the problems inherent in averaging, it would be ideal to be able to measure ERP components in single-trial epochs. Furthermore, being able to measure ERP components in single trials would maximize the amount of information that can be obtained from the ERP, as it would enable researchers to study the trial-by-trial variability among individual ERP components and between ERP components and overt performance measures. The low signal-to-noise ratio (SNR) of ERPs in relation to the ongoing EEG and artifacts (line noise, muscle and ocular artifacts) makes this a difficult problem, but there has been a great deal of research done in this area, and effective methods for single-trial analysis have been developed. The ERP component most often studied with single-trial methods is the P300 (cf. Donchin & Coles, 1988), for two main reasons. First, understanding the relationships between P300 latency and reaction time has been of theoretical importance; second, the relatively high amplitude and long latency of the P300 make it easier to distinguish from the background EEG than other components. Because most of the single-trial analysis literature concerns the P300, the examples we present here will focus on the problems associated with measuring this component.

This part of the chapter contains sections concerning preprocessing, detection, and classification methods. These distinctions are somewhat artificial, because there is considerable overlap and circularity among the methods. For instance, accurate detection and classification require filtering, but devising an optimal filter requires knowledge of the single-trial ERP distribution.

Preprocessing

The goal of preprocessing methods is to isolate the ERP component of interest from noise sources (background EEG and artifacts), thus improving the SNR. These methods fall into two domains, frequency and spatial. Frequency domain methods include various types of digital filters, which separate the component of interest from other signals by parsing the frequency spectrum. In an analogous manner, spatial domain methods attempt to separate signal from noise on the basis of scalp topography.

Frequency Domain Filters   The simplest method to improve SNR is to apply a low-pass digital filter to the single-trial epochs (e.g., Ruchkin & Glaser, 1978). The P300 is particularly amenable to low-pass filtering, because its long time course (~ 300 ms) means that the spectral power of the component is concentrated in low-frequency bands, below alpha waves (~ 8–13 Hz) and higher frequency noise. Given that the P300 typically has a large amplitude, a low-pass filter of 0–6 Hz will remove much of the background activity in a single trial without seriously attenuating or distorting the component. However, smaller ERP components with shorter durations (such as sensory evoked potentials) tend to overlap with the alpha band, making it much more difficult to improve the SNR with such a simple filtering scheme. Edgar, Stewart, and Miller discuss the issue of digital filters in depth in chapter 5 of this volume.

Although a low-pass filter with a passband determined a priori (as above) may improve SNR, it may not necessarily provide an optimal separation of signal from noise. Variations in EEG power spectra between individuals or experimental conditions make it unlikely that the same filter will work well under all conditions. One solution is to use an a posteriori (or Wiener) filter, which estimates the spectra of the signal and noise from existing data, and finds filter weights that provide optimal separation between signal and noise according to some criterion (usually minimizing mean-squared error). Researchers have proposed a number of methods of this type (e.g., de Weerd, 1981; Doyle, 1975; Walter, 1969; see also Cerutti et al., 1988). Generally they rely upon the average ERP as an estimate of the signal, and use the difference between this waveform and each single trial to obtain an estimate of the noise. This approach was originally devised for uncorrelated, stationary signals, whose power spectra can be determined exactly. Because these requirements are not met in ERP analysis, the optimality of a posteriori methods is questionable. For single-trial analysis, it is especially problematic to use the average ERP as an estimate of the signal, for reasons detailed above. However, a posteriori methods provide a more rigorous approach to filtering than simple low- or bandpass filters, especially because they are adaptable to different subjects and conditions.

Another problem with the basic a posteriori filter is that if the entire ERP epoch is used, the procedure for estimating filter weights will have to strike a balance between small, short-duration latency components (sensory evoked potentials) and large, long-duration components (P300 or CNV). The resulting filter will not be as optimal as possible for either type of component, due to their differing power spectra. Also, the spectrum of the background EEG can vary during the epoch. For these reasons, it would be better to determine filter weights for particular components and portions of the epoch. Time-adaptive a posteriori filters provide a solution to this problem (de Weerd, 1981), finding different weights for different portions of the epoch. Wavelet transforms (see chapter 11 of this volume) are especially well suited for this kind of filtering, because they are by nature time adaptive, and do not assume stationarity of signals. Orthogonal wavelet transforms represent a signal as a set of time-frequency components, each component represented by a coefficient indicating its amplitude. Several researchers have demonstrated promising results using wavelet transforms for a posteriori single-trial filtering, noise reduction, and artifact reduction (Bartnik, Blinowska, & Durka, 1992; Browne & Cutmore, 2002; Effern et al., 2000a, 2000b; Quian Quiroga & Garcia, 2003).

Spatial Domain Filters Compared to frequency methods for single-trial preprocessing, spatial methods are relatively unexplored. The simplest method is to use the electrode site or sites at which the ERP component of interest has the highest amplitude, such as Pz for the P300. However, one can obtain a much better isolation of the component by incorporating information from multiple sites into a weighted combination, which is used as a spatial filter. For example, because alpha waves mainly have an occipital scalp topography, a spatial filter for the P300 might have relatively larger weights at Fz and Cz, and a lower weight at Oz.

Three main methods have been proposed to find weights for spatial filtering. Gratton, Coles, and Donchin (1989a) proposed the "vector filter," which estimates weights using multiple regression. Gratton, Kramer, Coles, and Donchin (1989) demonstrated that with the appropriate set of weights, the vector filter could improve single-trial detection of the P300. Principal components analysis (see chapter 9 of this volume) and independent component analysis (Stone, 2002) decompose EEG data sets into representative spatial patterns based on variance patterns in the data. These spatial patterns typically represent one or a small number of ERP components, and make natural spatial filters for single-trial analysis (Jung et al., 2001; Kobayashi & Kuriki, 1999; Tang et al., 2002; Vigário et al., 2000). A comparison of the relative merits of these methods for single-trial filtering has yet to be reported.

Detection of Single-Trial ERPs

The most commonly used method for detecting ERP components in single trials and correcting for latency jitter between trials is template matching. Woody (1967) proposed this method for detecting epileptic spikes; Kutas, McCarthy, and Donchin (1977) first applied it to the detection of single-trial ERP components. Woody's method is as follows:

1. Take the initial template of the target component from the average ERP (e.g., the P300 waveform in the average), or use a simulated component (e.g., half-sine wave).
2. Compute the cross-correlation function between the template and each single-trial epoch. This involves computing the correlation between the template and a window of the same length, and moving this window across the epoch. Take the time point at which the cross-correlation is maximal as an estimate of the latency of the component.
3. Use the single-trial latency estimates to construct a new average ERP by shifting each epoch so that the estimated component latencies are aligned together, and then average the shifted single trials.
4. Repeat the cross-correlation step using a template from the new average until some criterion is reached.

In theory, this procedure will provide estimates of single-trial latency, as well as correcting for latency jitter. Woody's method has been extensively studied and compared with other methods, and several issues with template-matching methods have been identified.

Template Shape   The average ERP does not make a good template if there is much latency jitter, which results in a distorted waveform (see the previous discussion). Instead, investigators have used a half-sine wave to approximate the shape of an ERP component (e.g., Pfefferbaum & Ford, 1988; Smulders, Kenemans, & Kok, 1994). Note that if the shape of an ERP component were to vary from trial to trial (e.g., component width, rising and falling slopes could vary), it would compromise the performance of template-matching methods (also see below).

Number of Iterations   Although the iterative aspect of Woody's method is appealing, multiple iterations may degrade performance. Wastell (1977) reported that more than one iteration does not improve detection of the target component. This may occur because as the width of the template becomes narrower through successive iterations, the template becomes narrower than the target component (Gratton et al., 1989b), and spurious noise waveforms are detected instead (Pfefferbaum & Ford, 1988). However, a template that is too wide may also degrade detection (Gratton et al., 1989b; Smulders et al., 1994), so a moderate overestimation of component width may yield the best performance.

Comparison of Correlation, Covariance, and Peak-Picking   In computing the correlation between a template and a window of a single trial, amplitude information is lost, and only the shapes of the signals are compared. In the case of the P300, which has a relatively large amplitude, retaining amplitude information and combining it with shape information could yield better single-trial detection. This can be achieved by computing the covariance instead of the correlation, which appears to produce better results (Pfefferbaum & Ford, 1988; Smulders et al., 1994; Spencer & Donchin, 1996).

Investigators have also compared simple peak-picking with template-matching methods. (In a sense, peak-picking can be considered as a template-matching procedure in which the template is a single time point.) Surprisingly, peak-picking can perform as well or better than cross-correlation and cross-covariance methods under some conditions, such as when the SNR is high, the low-pass cutoff frequency is low, and/or the width of the true component is relatively narrow (Gratton et al., 1989b; Jaskowski & Verleger, 2000; Smulders, Kenemans, & Kok, 1994). In these cases it appears that the shape information taken into account by cross-correlation and cross-covariance is a hindrance.

Selection Criteria   As discussed previously, one cannot assume that an ERP component is in fact present on every trial. In single-trial detection, it is critical to have some means for determining whether or not the target component is present. Otherwise, the detection method will introduce false components into the single-trial estimates. Pfefferbaum and Ford (1988) proposed a screening procedure for P300 detection in which the cross-correlation and cross-covariance were computed between the template and the data in a "signal window" in which they expected P300, and in a later "noise window" in which they expected no P300. If they found the highest covariance in the signal window, and the correlation at this latency was statistically significant, they considered they had found a P300. Spencer, Vila Abad, and Donchin (2000) used a similar procedure with peak-picking, determining signal and noise windows for each subject and experimental condition. Their signal window began at the latency of the N400 component (between the P2 and P300) and ended when the P300 returned to baseline, or else at the end of the epoch. They discarded trials on which the largest positive peak fell outside the signal window as not containing P300s.

Another kind of selection criterion is to examine the distributions of single-trial measurements to see whether the results could be due to chance. One can assume that if a detection method is generally successful for a particular set of trials, the distribution of single-trial latencies for the target component will differ in shape from a rectangular distribution, which would result from randomly distributed, false-alarm detections. The chi-squared goodness-of-fit test is one statistical test useful for this purpose (Spencer, Vila Abad, & Donchin, 2000).

Although single-trial selection criteria are necessary to avoid introducing erroneous component estimates, there is a danger of biasing the selected trials in some manner, such as toward trials on which the component amplitude is relatively high. For an examination of this issue, see Smulders, Kenemans, and Kok, 1994.

Preprocessing Frequency and spatial filtering can of course improve the accuracy of single-trial detection methods, as noted above. For the P300 component, a small passband is advantageous, especially when using peak-picking, (Gratton et al., 1989b; Smulders, Kenemans, & Kok, 1994; cf. Spencer, Vila Abad, & Donchin, 2000). In a simulation study, Spencer and Donchin (1996) examined the combination of the wavelet transform with template matching. They computed cross-correlation and cross-covariance between the template and single-trial epochs after applying the discrete wavelet transform to both. Spencer and Donchin found that this technique eliminated the need for low-pass filtering, presumably because the wavelet transform represented the template and simulated component in both the time and frequency domains. A more thorough test of this technique remains to be done.

Other Methods A variety of more elaborate methods have been proposed for single-trial detection, although few of these have received much testing. Of these, the maximum-likelihood method proposed by Pham, Möcks, Köhler, and Gasser (1987) has been examined the most. Studies with simulated and real data suggest that this method can perform as well or better than template matching and peak-picking (Jaskowski & Verleger, 1999, 2000; Möcks et al., 1988; Puce et al., 1994a). However, it is much more complex to implement than standard template-matching or peak-picking schemes.

Sensitivity to SNR In general, all the single-trial detection methods that have been tested are highly sensitive to SNR. Studies show that as SNR decreases, so does the detection performance of these methods, with all reaching about the same asymptotic value. Hence, it may not be worthwhile for an investigator to implement a more complicated method in favor of a simpler one if the SNR is very low, because all methods will give approximately the same results.

This leads to the issue of estimating the SNR of a data set. In simulated data sets it is of course very easy to estimate the SNR, because the experimenter determines the amplitude of the simulated component and noise. With real data, SNR estimation becomes much more complicated, because there are multiple components present, and the background EEG (as well as artifacts) varies within and between trials, electrode sites, experimental conditions, and subjects. One simple approach is to use the amplitude of the target component in the average ERP as an estimate of signal amplitude (a conservative choice, because latency jitter will reduce the amplitude of the component in the average), and to estimate the noise amplitude by calculating the standard deviation of amplitudes across time points and trials. There are other approaches to SNR estimation; see papers by Raz, Turetsky, and Fein (1988), and Turetsky, Raz, and Fein (1988, 1989) for a thorough treatment of the problem.

Classification of Single-Trial ERPs

Single-trial classification methods aim to categorize single trials according to some criteria. There are two general types of methods, supervised and unsupervised learning. In discriminant analysis (DA), a supervised learning method, trials are classified according to whether they more closely match one or another category determined a priori. Donchin (1966; see also 1969) first proposed the use of DA for single-trial ERP classification. In DA, researchers use sets of single trials (training sets) to construct the discriminant function; the categories are typically defined by experimental conditions. The discriminant function is a linear combination of variables (time points) that maximally separate the categories. In the stepwise variant of DA, an iterative process removes all but the most important variables. (Fewer than six variables are usually needed.) Once the discriminant function has been computed, it can also be used to classify single trials not part of the original training set (the test set). To measure the degree to which a trial matches the category in which it has been classified, a discriminant score can be computed by multiplying the ERP amplitude at the selected time points by the discriminant function coefficients. The discriminant score can thus provide trial-by-trial measures of the ERP components upon which the discriminant function is based (e.g., Gehring et al., 1993). For more details on DA and its applications, see papers by Donchin and Herning (1975), Horst and Donchin (1980), and Squires and Donchin (1976).

Findings by Squires and Donchin (1976) demonstrate the potential usefulness of DA for single-trial analysis. Not all rare events elicit the P300 component, and some frequent events do. In their DA of single-trial ERPs from an oddball task, Squires and Donchin observed that the discriminant function incorrectly classified a small number of rare trials as frequents and frequents as rares. Selective averaging of the correct and incorrect classifications revealed that the incorrectly classified rare trials did not have P300s, and the incorrectly classified frequent trials did. Thus, although the discriminant function may not have classified the trials correctly according to their a priori categorization, it did correctly detect the presence of the P300 component, upon which the discriminant function was based. This observation led to the discovery of the influence of local stimulus probability on P300 amplitude (Squires et al., 1976).

As with single-trial detection methods, the performance of DA decreases as SNR decreases, so frequency and spatial domain filtering should be advantageous. A simple way to incorporate topographic information is to use time points from multiple electrode sites (Squires & Donchin, 1976; Childers et al., 1986). Parra et al. (2002) proposed a form of DA in which the variables are sensors (electrodes or MEG sensors) rather than time points, and have achieved successful single-trial classification with this technique.

Unsupervised learning procedures are the second type of single-trial classification methods. In these methods, trials are grouped according to some measure of their similarity to each other, not to predetermined categories. Hence, unsupervised learning methods present the opportunity to discover patterns in the data set that would not be detectable with averaging, nor with procedures that make assumptions about the contents of the single trials. Haig, Gordon, Rogers, and Anderson (1995) used a version of cluster analysis to examine single trials from an oddball task, and found that only about 40% of the trials resembled the average ERP. Inspection of the single-trial clusters revealed a large degree of intertrial variability among the components. Others reporting examples of the application of cluster analysis methods to single-trial analysis include Jansen, Nyberg, and Zouridakis (1994), Lagopoulos et al. (1998), Laskaris, Fotopoulos, Papathanasopoulos, and Bezerianos (1997), and Zouridakis, Jansen, and Boutros (1997). Lange, Siegelmann, Pratt, and Inbar (2000) used another unsupervised-learning procedure, the competitive-learning neural network, to classify single trials from an oddball task. Their results were similar to those of Squires and Donchin (1976). Classification methods are relatively unused in single-trial analysis, especially unsupervised learning techniques; one hopes that more researchers will begin to apply these methods in their research.

As mentioned at the beginning of this part of the chapter, single-trial measurement has most often been applied to the P300 component. Two additional examples are of note. In a series of classic experiments, Donchin and colleagues used single-trial detection to examine the relationship between P300 latency and reaction time, finding that P300 latency reflects the duration of stimulus evaluation processes prior to response selection (Kutas, McCarthy, & Donchin, 1977; McCarthy & Donchin, 1981; Magliero et al., 1984). Another area in which P300 single-trial detection has been applied is in the study of clinical populations and aging (e.g., Ford et al., 1994; Pfefferbaum et al., 1984a,b; Puce et al., 1994b; Unsal & Segalowitz, 1995). For instance, Ford et al. (1994) used single-trial detection to investigate the reduction of P300 amplitude in schizophrenia. They found that schizophrenia patients had fewer trials with P300s, and on those trials, P300 amplitude was reduced compared to healthy individuals. In sum, single-trial measurement methods can provide a richer picture of neural activity than average ERPs, which obscure the intra- and intertrial variability among ERP components.

Conclusion

The application of signal averaging to electroencephalography gave birth to the field of ERP research (e.g., Brazier, 1961), which has produced a wealth of knowledge about the relationships between brain activity and the mind, despite the problems inherent in the technique. Single-trial analysis methods can overcome the limitations of the average ERP and reveal new insights into the neural dynamics associated with mental activity. Although the technical procedures may appear demanding, the benefits are substantial, and advances in computing power and programming languages (e.g., array-based languages such as MATLAB and IDL) make single-trial analysis easier to perform than ever. In the future, the accuracy of single-trial analysis methods may be enhanced both with better techniques and with the combination of existing ones. For example, researchers could use classification methods to identify groups of single trials with similar morphologies for further processing by detection methods.

Acknowledgments

The author gratefully acknowledges Emanuel Donchin for his helpful comments on an earlier version of this chapter. Thanks are due to Emanuel Donchin and to Michael Coles, Judy Ford, Clay Holroyd, Gregory Miller, Leun Otten, and Marten Scheffers for their valuable discussions of these topics over the years. The author is also grateful to John Polich for providing the impetus and support for his initial forays into single-trial ERP analysis.

Notes

1. Here we will use the terms "background EEG activity" and "noise" interchangeably. However, it is not our intent to equate non-event-related EEG activity with a true random noise process.

2. But if this amplitude distribution is skewed, averaging will not eliminate noise, but introduce bias. In this case a better estimate of the EEG would be the median. Although to our knowledge no one has directly investigated this issue, Yabe, Saito, and Fukushima (1993) have examined the use of the median to estimate the ERP instead of the average.

References

Bartnik, E. A., Blinowska, K. J., & Durka, P. J. (1992). Single evoked potential reconstruction by means of wavelet transform. *Biological Cybernetics, 67*, 175–181.

Brazier, M. A. B. (1961). Computer techniques in EEG analysis. *Electroencephalography and Clinical Neurophysiology, 20 (Suppl.).*

Brazier, M. A. B. (1964). Evoked responses recorded from the depth of the human brain. In R. Katzman (Ed.), *Sensory evoked responses in man, Annals of the New York Academy of Science, 112,* 33–59.

Browne, M., & Cutmore, T. R. H. (2002). Low-probability event-detection and separation via statistical wavelet thresholding: An application to psychophysiological denoising. *Clinical Neurophysiology, 113,* 1403–1411.

Cerutti, S., Chiarenza, G., Liberati, D., Mascellani, P., & Pavesi, G. (1988). A parametric method of identification of single-trial event-related potentials in the brain. *IEEE Transactions on Biomedical Engineering, 35,* 701–711.

Childers, D. G., Fischler, I. S., Boaz, T. L., Perry, N. W., & Arroyo, A. (1986). Multichannel, single trial event related potential classification. *IEEE Transactions on Biomedical Engineering, 33,* 1069–1075.

Coles, M. G. H., Gratton, G., Bashore, T. R., Eriksen, C. W., & Donchin, E. (1985). A psychophysiological investigation of the continuous flow model of human information processing. *Journal of Experimental Psychology: Human Perception and Performance, 11,* 529–553.

De Weerd, J. P. C. (1981). A posteriori time-varying filtering of averaged evoked potentials. I. Introduction and conceptual basis. *Biological Cybernetics, 41,* 211–222.

Donchin, E. (1966). A multivariate approach to the analysis of averaged evoked potentials. *IEEE Transactions on Biomedical Engineering, 13,* 131–139.

Donchin, E. (1969). Discriminant analysis in average evoked response studies: The study of single trial data. *Electroencephalography and Clinical Neurophysiology, 27,* 311–314.

Donchin, E., & Coles, M. G. H. (1988). Is the P300 component a manifestation of context updating? *Behavioral and Brain Sciences, 11,* 355–425.

Donchin, E., & Herning, R. I. (1975). A simulation study of the efficacy of stepwise discriminant analysis in the detection and comparison of event related potentials. *Electroencephalography and Clinical Neurophysiology, 38,* 51–68.

Donchin, E., & Lindsley, D. B. (1966). Average evoked potentials and reaction times to visual stimuli. *Electroencephalography and Clinical Neurophysiology, 20,* 217–223.

Doyle, D. J. (1975). Some comments on the use of Wiener filtering in the estimation of evoked potentials. *Electroencephalography and Clinical Neurophysiology, 38,* 533–534.

Effern, A., Lehnertz, K., Fernandez, G., Grunwald, T., David, P., & Elger, C. E. (2000a). Single trial analysis of event related potentials: Non-linear de-noising with wavelets. *Clinical Neurophysiology, 111,* 2255–2263.

Effern, A., Lehnertz, K., Grunwald, T., Fernandez, G., David, P., & Elger, C. (2000b). Time adaptive denoising of single trial event-related potentials in the wavelet domain. *Psychophysiology, 37,* 859–865.

Ford, J. M., White, P., Lim, K. O., & Pfefferbaum, A. (1994). Schizophrenics have fewer and smaller P300s: A single-trial analysis. *Biological Psychiatry, 35*, 96–103.

Gehring, W. J., Goss, B., Coles, M. G. H., Meyer, D. E., & Donchin, E. (1993). A neural system for error detection and compensation. *Psychological Science, 4*, 385–390.

Gratton, G., Coles, M. G. H., & Donchin, E. (1989a). A procedure for using multi-electrode information in the analysis of components of the event-related potential: Vector filter. *Psychophysiology, 26*, 222–232.

Gratton, G., Kramer, A. F., Coles, M. G. H., & Donchin, E. (1989b). Simulation studies of latency measures of components of the event-related brain potential. *Psychophysiology, 26*, 233–248.

Haig, A. R., Gordon, E., Rogers, G., & Anderson, J. (1995). Classification of single-trial ERP subtypes: Application of globally optimal vector quantization using simulated annealing. *Electroencephalography and Clinical Neurophysiology, 94*, 288–297.

Horst, R. L., & Donchin, E. (1980). Beyond averaging. II. Single-trial classification of exogenous event-related potentials using stepwise discriminant analysis. *Electroencephalography and Clinical Neurophysiology, 48*, 113–126.

Jansen, B. H., Nyberg, H. N., & Zouridakis, G. (1994). Selective averaging of evoked potentials using trajectory-based clustering. *Methods on Information in Medicine, 33*, 49–51.

Jasiukaitis, P., & Hakerem, G. (1988). The effect of prestimulus alpha activity on P300. *Psychophysiology, 25*, 157–165.

Jaskowski, P., & Verleger, R. (1999). Amplitudes and latencies of single-trial ERP's estimated by a maximum-likelihood method. *IEEE Transactions on Biomedical Engineering, 46*, 987–993.

Jaskowski, P., & Verleger, R. (2000). An evaluation of methods for single-trial estimation of P3 latency. *Psychophysiology, 37*, 153–162.

Jung, T.-P., Makeig, S., Westerfield, M., Townsend, J., Courchesne, E., & Sejnowski, T. J. (2001). Analysis and visualization of single-trial event-related potentials. *Human Brain Mapping, 14*, 166–185.

Karis, D., Fabiani, M., & Donchin, E. (1984). "P300" and memory: Individual differences in the Von Restorff effect. *Cognitive Psychology, 16*, 177–216.

Kobayashi, T., & Kuriki, S. (1999). Principal component elimination method for the improvement of S/N in evoked field measurements. *IEEE Transactions on Biomedical Engineering, 46*, 951–958.

Kutas, M., McCarthy, G., & Donchin, E. (1977). Augmenting mental chronometry: The P300 as a measure of stimulus evaluation time. *Science, 197*, 292–295.

Lagopoulos, J., Gordon, E., Barhamali, H., Lim, C. L., Li, W. M., Clouston, P., & Morris, J. G. (1998). Dysfunctions of automatic (P300a) and controlled (P300b) processing in Parkinson's disease. *Neurological Research, 20*, 5–10.

Lange, D. H., Siegelmann, H. T., Pratt, H., & Inbar, G. I. (2000). Overcoming selective ensemble averaging: Unsupervised identification of event-related brain potentials. *IEEE Transactions on Biomedical Engineering, 47*, 822–826.

Laskaris, N., Fotopoulos, S., Papathanasopoulos, P., & Bezerianos, A. (1997). Robust moving averages, with Hopfield neural network implementation, for monitoring evoked signals. *Electroencephalography and Clinical Neurophysiology, 104*, 151–156.

Magliero, A., Bashore, T. R., Coles, M. G. H., & Donchin, E. (1984). On the dependence of P300 latency on stimulus evaluation processes. *Psychophysiology, 21*, 171–186.

Makeig, S., Westerfield, M., Jung, T.-P., Enghoff, S., Townsend, J., Courchesne, E., & Sejnowski, T. J. (2001). Dynamic brain sources of visual evoked responses. *Science, 295*, 690–694.

Marinkovic, K., Halgren, E., & Maltzman, I. (2001). Arousal-related P3a to novel auditory stimuli is abolished by a moderately low alcohol dose. *Alcohol and Alcoholism, 36*, 529–539.

McCarthy, G., & Donchin, E. (1981). A metric for thought: A comparison of P300 latency and reaction time. *Science, 211*, 77–80.

Michalewski, H. J., Prasher, D. K., & Starr, A. (1986). Latency variability and temporal interrelationships of the auditory event-related potentials (N1, P2, N2, and P3) in normal subjects. *Electroencephalography and Clinical Neurophysiology, 65*, 59–71.

Möcks, J., Köhler, W., Gasser, T., & Pham, D. T. (1988). Novel approaches to the problem of latency jitter. *Psychophysiology, 25*, 217–226.

Parra, L., Alvino, C., Tang, A., Pearlmutter, B., Yeung, N., Osman, A., & Sajda, P. (2002). Linear spatial integration for single-trial detection in encephalography. *NeuroImage, 17*, 223–230.

Pfefferbaum, A., & Ford, J. M. (1988). ERPs to stimuli requiring response production and inhibition: Effects of age, probability and visual noise. *Electroencephalography and Clinical Neurophysiology, 71*, 55–63.

Pfefferbaum, A., Ford, J. M., Wenegrat, B. G., Roth, W. T., & Kopell, B. S. (1984a). Clinical application of the P3 component of event-related potentials. I. Normal aging. *Electroencephalography and Clinical Neurophysiology, 59*, 85–103.

Pfefferbaum, A., Wenegrat, B. G., Ford, J. M., Roth, W. T., & Kopell, B. S. (1984b). Clinical application of the P3 component of event-related potentials. II. Dementia, depression and schizophrenia. *Electroencephalography and Clinical Neurophysiology, 59*, 104–124.

Pham, D. T., Möcks, J., Köhler, W., & Gasser, T. (1987). Variable latencies of noisy signals: Estimation and testing in brain potential data. *Biometrika, 74*, 525–533.

Puce, A., Berkovic, S. F., Cadusch, P. J., & Bladin, P. F. (1994a). P3 latency jitter assessed using 2 techniques. I. Simulated data and surface recordings in normal subjects. *Electroencephalography and Clinical Neurophysiology, 92*, 352–364.

Puce, A., Berkovic, S. F., Cadusch, P. J., & Bladin, P. F. (1994b). II. Surface and sphenoidal recordings in subjects with focal epilepsy. *Electroencephalography and Clinical Neurophysiology, 92,* 555–567.

Quian Quiroga, R., & Garcia, H. (2003). Single-trial event-related potentials with wavelet denoising. *Clinical Neurophysiology, 114,* 376–390.

Raz, J., Turetsky, B., & Fein, G. (1988). Confidence intervals for the signal-to-noise ratio when a signal embedded in noise is observed over repeated trials. *IEEE Transactions on Biomedical Engineering, 35,* 646–649.

Ruchkin, D. S., & Glaser, E. M. (1978). Simple digital filters for examining CNV and P300 on a single-trial basis. In D. Otto (Ed.), *Multidisciplinary perspectives in event-related brain potential (ERP) research* (pp. 579–581). Washington, D.C.: U.S. Government Printing Office, EPA-600/9-77-043.

Sanquist, T. F., Rohrbaugh, J. W., Syndulko, K., & Lindsley, D. B. (1980). Electrocortical signs of levels of processing: Perceptual analysis and recognition memory. *Psychophysiology, 17,* 568–576.

Scheffers, M. K., & Coles, M. G. H. (2000). Performance monitoring in a confusing world: Error-related brain activity, judgments of response accuracy, and types of errors. *Journal of Experimental Psychology: Human Perception and Performance, 26,* 141–151.

Smulders, F. T. Y., Kenemans, J. L., & Kok, A. (1994). A comparison of different methods for estimating single-trial P300 latencies. *Electroencephalography and Clinical Neurophysiology, 92,* 107–114.

Spencer, K. M., & Donchin, E. (1996). A simulation study of single-trial ERP latency estimation methods. *Psychophysiology, 33,* S80.

Spencer, K. M., & Polich, J. (1999). Poststimulus EEG spectral analysis and P300: Attention, task, and probability. *Psychophysiology, 36,* 220–232.

Spencer, K. M., Vila Abad, E., & Donchin, E. (2000). On the search for the neurophysiological manifestation of recollective experience. *Psychophysiology, 37,* 494–506.

Squires, K. C., & Donchin, E. (1976). Beyond averaging: The use of discriminant functions to recognize event related potentials elicited by single auditory stimuli. *Electroencephalography and Clinical Neurophysiology, 41,* 449–459.

Squires, K. C., Wickens, C., Squires, N. K., & Donchin, E. (1976). The effect of stimulus sequence on the waveform of the cortical event-related potential. *Science, 193,* 1142–1146.

Stone, J. V. (2002). Independent component analysis: An introduction. *Trends in Cognitive Science, 6,* 59–64.

Tallon-Baudry, C., & Bertrand, O. (1999). Oscillatory gamma activity in humans and its role in object representation. *Trends in Cognitive Sciences, 3,* 151–162.

Tang, A. C., Pearlmutter, B. A., Malaszenko, N. A., & Phung, D. B. (2002). Independent components of magnetoencephalography: Single-trial response onset times. *NeuroImage, 17,* 1773–1789.

Turetsky, B. I., Raz, J., & Fein, G. (1988). Noise and signal power and their effects on evoked potential estimation. *Electroencephalography and Clinical Neurophysiology, 71*, 310–318.

Turetsky, B. I., Raz, J., & Fein, G. (1989). Estimation of trial-to-trial variation in evoked potential signals by smoothing across trials. *Psychophysiology, 26*, 700–712.

Vigário, R., Särelä, J., Jousmäki, V., Hämäläinen, M., & Oja, E. (2000). Independent component approach to the analysis of EEG and MEG recordings. *IEEE Transactions on Biomedical Engineering, 47*, 589–593.

Unsal, A., & Segalowitz, S. J. (1995). Sources of P300 attenuation after head injury: Single-trial amplitude, latency jitter, and EEG power. *Psychophysiology, 32*, 249–256.

Walter, D. O. (1969). A posteriori Wiener filtering of average evoked response. *Electroencephalography and Clinical Neurophysiology, 27 (Suppl.)*, 61–70.

Wastell, D. G. (1977). Statistical detection of individual evoked responses: An evaluation of Woody's adaptive filter. *Electroencephalography and Clinical Neurophysiology, 42*, 835–839.

Woody, C. D. (1967). Characterization of an adaptive filter for the analysis of variable latency neuroelectric signals. *Medical and Biological Engineering, 5*, 539–553.

Yabe, H., Saito, F., & Fukushima, Y. (1993). Median method for detecting endogenous event-related brain potentials. *Electroencephalography and Clinical Neurophysiology, 87*, 403–407.

Zouridakis, G., Jansen, B. H., & Boutros, N. N. (1997). A fuzzy clustering approach to EP estimation. *IEEE Transactions on Biomedical Engineering, 44*, 673–680.

11 EEG Oscillations and Wavelet Analysis

Christoph S. Herrmann, Maren Grigutsch, and Niko A. Busch

Oscillations in the EEG

Both EEG and ERP measures can be investigated in the frequency domain, and it has been convincingly demonstrated that assessing specific frequencies can often yield insights into the functional cognitive correlations of these signals (Başar et al., 1999).

Analysis of EEG oscillations traces back to the beginning of EEG-based research, when the German neurophysiologist Berger (1929) first observed the dominant oscillations of approximately 10 Hz recorded from the human scalp. Berger coined the term alpha frequency, using the first letter of the Greek alphabet for activity in this frequency range. He dubbed the second type of rhythmic activity that he found in the human EEG as beta, the frequency range of approximately 12–30 Hz. Following this consecutive ordering, Adrian (1942) referred to oscillations around 40 Hz (more general, 30–80 Hz) observed after odor stimulation in the hedgehog as gamma waves. The slow oscillations below 4 Hz, which were discovered next, were labeled delta waves. Finally, waves that cycle 4–8 times per second (4–8 Hz) were named theta oscillations after the first letter of their assumed region of origin, the thalamus (table 11.1).

Evoked versus Induced Oscillations

Oscillations are characterized by their amplitude and phase. The amplitude of an EEG oscillation is typically between 0 and 10 µV. The (cyclic) phase ranges between 0 and 2π. At every point in time one can determine the amplitude and phase of an oscillation. According to a classification of different types of oscillatory activity by Galambos (1992), there are spontaneous, induced, and evoked rhythms, all of which are differentiated by their degree of phase-locking to the stimulus (emitted rhythms in response to omitted stimuli also have been observed, but we will not consider these here). In this framework, spontaneous activity is completely uncorrelated with the occurrence of an experimental condition. Induced activity is correlated with experimental conditions but is not strictly phase-locked to its onset. Evoked activity is strictly phase-locked to

Table 11.1
A list of well-established frequency bands and their names

Frequency	Name
0–4 Hz	Delta
4–8 Hz	Theta
8–12 Hz	Alpha
12–30 Hz	Beta
30–80 Hz	Gamma

the onset of an experimental condition across trials, that is, it has the same phase in every stimulus repetition.

Figure 11.1 (left) illustrates such evoked oscillations, which start at the same time after stimulation in every trial and have identical phases. In this case, the activity is called evoked, it sums, and it is visible in the averaged ERP. However, evoked oscillations are only visible in the ERP to the naked eye if they are of sufficient amplitude. Because high-frequency oscillations usually have lower amplitude than low-frequency oscillations, they are often not visible. Evoked oscillations usually result from any kind of sensory events, such as auditory, visual, or somatosensory stimulation.

If oscillations occur after each stimulation but with varying onset times and/or phase jitter, they are considered as being induced by the stimulus rather than evoked, and are not visible in the averaged ERP. Figure 11.1 (right) illustrates this outcome. One must apply special methods to analyze this type of activity (see below).

Delta and Theta Oscillations

An ERP constitutes a mixture of multiple waves of various frequencies. However, digital filters can selectively show single frequencies while filtering all others out. For example, a bandpass filter lets only a limited range of frequencies pass (see chapter 5 of this volume). When only theta frequencies are admitted (4–8 Hz), for instance, only such slow oscillations will remain in the event-related signal (figure 11.2). Evoked delta and theta oscillations represent the slow potentials in ERPs, such as P300, N400, P600, and so on (Basar-Eroglu et al., 1992). Researchers have described functional correlates of event-related theta oscillations for working memory functions (Tesche & Karhu, 2000; Jensen & Tesche, 2002). Moreover, event-related theta oscillations relating to memory performance have also been shown to interact with faster oscillations in the gamma frequency range (Fell et al., 2003). Note that these event-related signals are not identical to those that one can see with the naked eye in raw EEG, and usually relate to deep sleep (Steriade, McCormick, & Sejnowski, 1993) or malfunctions (Gloor, Ball, & Schaul, 1977).

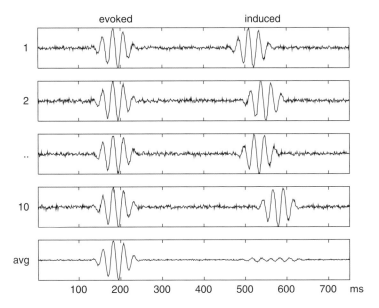

Figure 11.1
If oscillations occur at the same latency after stimulus onset and with the same phase relative to stimulus onset in multiple trials (rows 1–4), they are considered evoked by the stimulus (*left*). If latency or phase jitter relative to stimulus onset, the oscillations are considered to be induced by the stimulus (*right*). Evoked activity sums up in the average (bottom row), whereas induced activity is nearly cancelled out.

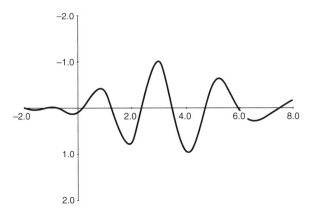

Figure 11.2
EROs in the theta band resulting from applying a 4–8-Hz bandpass filter to an ERP. An event-related theta oscillation emerges after stimulation that then decays over time.

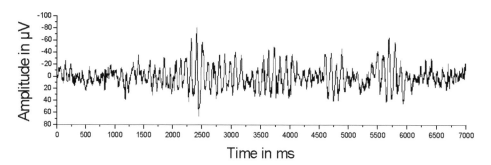

Figure 11.3

Ten seconds of unfiltered, spontaneous EEG showing alpha activity (8–12 Hz).

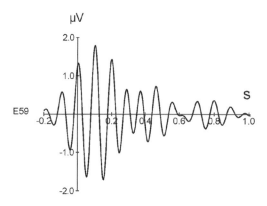

Figure 11.4

Short burst of 10-Hz oscillations evoked by visual stimulation.

Alpha Oscillations

The term alpha oscillation usually refers to the ongoing alpha rhythm. One can observe this rhythm, with approximately 10 Hz, in routine EEG recordings without averaging (cf. figure 11.3). Typically, the amplitude of the 10-Hz rhythm increases and decreases over time, which some have described as waxing and waning. Some authors have even hypothesized that there exist several independent rhythms in the alpha band with different functional properties (e.g., Niedermeyer, 1997). However, this is not the type of alpha activity we want to discuss here. We are interested in 10-Hz oscillations that occur in relation to an experimental condition—that is, evoked or induced 10-Hz oscillations.

Figure 11.4 shows a burst of 10-Hz oscillations after visual stimulation in an occipital electrode (Oz in the 10–20 system). In order to compute this evoked 10-Hz activity, an

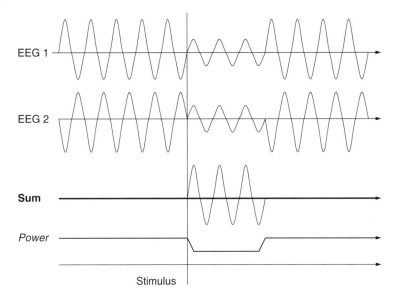

EEG 1

EEG 2

Sum

Power

Stimulus

Figure 11.5

A resetting of the phase of alpha oscillations at the time of stimulation leads to a short increase of evoked activity (sum) despite the fact that the amplitude (power) decreases.

ERP was first averaged and then bandpass-filtered in the alpha frequency range. Note that the burst of oscillatory activity seems to start before the onset of stimulation. This is an artifact of the filter algorithm. The filter uses time points of the past and future to compute each time point of the filtered signal. Therefore, the activity "leaks" into past and future events around its real peak (see chapter 5 of this volume).

Most any sensory stimulation—visual, auditory, and somatosensory—can evoke such bursts of alpha activity. The topography of this evoked alpha response is restricted to the primary sensory cortex that was stimulated. Interestingly, this burst of alpha activity is not due to an increase in amplitude. This becomes clear when one computes the total power of alpha activity following a visual stimulus. The total power contains both evoked and induced activity and typically decreases after visual stimulation. Thus, the amplitude of alpha oscillations is reduced after stimulation, whereas the evoked alpha activity is enhanced. Figure 11.5 schematically depicts this phenomenon, called the alpha paradox (Klimesch et al., 1998b). The first two traces show band-pass filtered alpha activity and its amplitude reduction after a visual stimulus. When these traces are simply added up as in the case of an average (third row), only those oscillations that are phase-locked (evoked) remain visible. Due to a so-called phase-resetting, the randomly distributed phase will be reset to start from the same value after stimulation for a short period of time (Brandt, 1997). This leads to the short burst of evoked alpha activity, because oscillations add up if they have identical phases across trials. However, the behavior of the amplitude is only reflected in the total power measure (bottom row), which is independent of the phase of the oscillations.

Alpha activity has been associated with a large number of cognitive processes. The most important of them are memory processes (Klimesch 1997; Klimesch, Schimke, & Pfurtscheller, 1993), attention (Klimesch et al., 1998a; Yordanova, Kolev, & Polich, 2001), and visual awareness (Sewards & Sewards, 1999; Strüber & Herrmann, 2002). For an overview, see Basar et al. 1997. Although researchers have assumed the generators of EEG alpha activity to reside in cortex, the generators are probably driven by thalamic cells (Steriade et al., 1990; Lopes Da Silva, 1991).

Beta Oscillations

The frequency range from 12 to 30 Hz constitutes the beta frequency band, which has been investigated in the context of motor actions. In particular, beta oscillations are suppressed during motor action but increase (a so-called rebound) approximately one second after movement, with a topography close to the primary sensorimotor regions representing the involved body part (Neuper & Pfurtscheller, 2001). They are also observed during imagined movements and can be elicited by median nerve stimulation (Salmelin & Hari, 1994). During somatosensory stimulation, beta activity is evoked together with gamma and alpha activity (Chen & Herrmann, 2001). Some have assumed that beta oscillations are induced by faster gamma oscillations (Haenschel et al., 2000) and perhaps they in turn induce slower alpha oscillations, a relationship that would explain the presence of all three frequencies in one experimental paradigm. In addition to motor and sensory processes, beta oscillations have also been associated with cognitive processes such as memory rehearsal (Tallon-Baudry, Bertrand, & Fischer, 2001).

Gamma Oscillations

In recent years technical improvements have revealed sensory-evoked oscillations of even higher frequencies. These have been reported up to about 600 Hz (Curio, 1999), the assumed theoretical limit of EEG activity due to the temporal width of single action potentials, which range between 1 and 2 ms. Among high-frequency oscillations, gamma waves (30–80 Hz, cf. figure 11.6) have received a considerable amount of attention because of their important correlates with higher brain functions (Engel, Fries, & Singer, 2001). Some have even assumed that they might be a neural correlate of consciousness (Llinás & Ribary, 1993).

The correlates of processes that are most frequently associated with gamma oscillations are binding phenomena (Müller et al., 1997; Tallon et al., 1995; Tallon-Baudry et al., 1996), perceiving meaningful objects (Keil et al., 1999; Tallon-Baudry et al.,

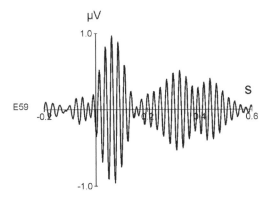

Figure 11.6
Evoked 40-Hz oscillations show a burst shortly after visual stimulation.

1997), and attention (Tiitinen et al., 1993; Müller, Teder-Sälejärvi, & Hillyard, 1998; Herrmann, Mecklinger, & Pfeiffer, 1999; Herrmann & Mecklinger, 2001; Debener et al., 2003).

Reviews related to the functional relevance of gamma oscillations include Başar-Eroglu et al. 1996b, Tallon-Baudry & Bertrand 1999, Müller et al. 2000, and Herrmann & Knight 2001.

Wavelet Analysis

Frequency Analysis Methods

In principle, every signal can be decomposed into sinusoidal oscillations of different frequencies. Such decomposition is usually computed using the Fourier transform to quantify the oscillations that constitute the signal (Dumermuth, 1977).

There are several methods to exclusively extract oscillations of a specific frequency from ERP data. Among the most popular are filtering, Fourier transformation, and wavelet analysis.

Figure 11.7 shows the results of these three methods to extract frequency information from an ERP. In the left panel, filtering two ERPs with a bandpass filter (35–45 Hz) shows a clear burst of 40-Hz activity around 100 milliseconds. This oscillatory activity is enhanced for the dotted as compared to the solid condition. The middle panel shows Fourier spectrum analyses of the two ERPs. An increase of activity for the dotted condition can be noticed around 40 Hz. However, it is unclear at what point this difference between conditions occurs. The right panel shows the absolute values of the wavelet coefficients of the ERP for a 40-Hz wavelet. The difference between conditions is very prominent and can be observed at every point in time due to the lack of oscillations in

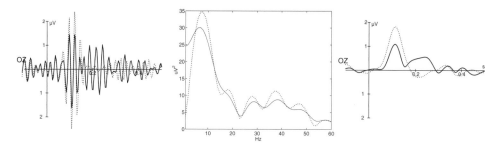

Figure 11.7

Three possibilities to extract frequency information from ERP data: two 35–45 Hz filtered ERPs (*left*), two FFT spectra of the ERPs (*middle*) and the wavelet transforms of the ERPs (*right*). Note that only the filtered signal and the wavelet transform still represent changes over time. The FFT spectra show the entire frequency range but no temporal information.

the signal. One can think of the wavelet transform as the envelope of the bandpass-filtered ERP. The wavelet transform is advantageous over the FFT, because the time course of frequency information can be observed. Although this is also true for the filtered signal, the wavelet transform directly yields the amplitude and the phase of the signal oscillations in the analyzed frequency band when one uses a complex wavelet function. The wavelet amplitude has only positive values and does not bear the problem that oscillations might cancel out when averaging across multiple subjects (negative values in figure 11.7 result from a baseline correction making the wavelet transform a relative measure with respect to the prestimulus interval). Samar et al. (1999) gives a review of using wavelets for EEG analysis.

The Wavelet Transform

To compute a wavelet transform, the original signal time series, $x(t)$, is convolved with a scaled and translated version of a mother wavelet function, $\psi(t)$. The convolution leads to a new signal of wavelet coefficients,

$$W_x^{\Psi}(b, a) = A_{\Psi} \cdot \int \Psi^* \left(\frac{t - b}{a} \right) \cdot x(t) \cdot dt$$

where Ψ^* denotes the complex conjugation of the wavelet function, b is the translation parameter, a is the wavelet's scaling parameter, and A_{Ψ} denotes a (wavelet-specific) normalization parameter. The wavelet coefficients quantify the similarity between the original signal and the wavelet function at a specific scale a and target latency b. Hence, the wavelet coefficients depend on the choice of the mother wavelet function.

The mother wavelet is constructed in such a way that it has zero mean and is localized in both time and frequency space. This is in contrast to the Fourier transform,

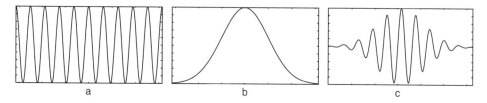

Figure 11.8

Multiplying a sinusoidal function (*a*) and an envelope function (*b*) results in a wavelet (*c*).

where the harmonic basis functions have a well-determined frequency but extend over the entire time axis. Due to its localization properties, the wavelet transform allows one to follow the time course of component structures in the signal. This feature is of crucial importance when analyzing nonstationary signals, but has to be paid for with a reduced frequency resolution.

Another important feature of the wavelet transform is its zooming property. Varying the scaling parameter, a, from high to low values, compresses the wavelet function, $\psi([t-b]/a)$. The corresponding wavelet transform zooms from coarser (i.e., low-frequency) to finer (i.e., high-frequency) signal structures.

In the case of Morlet's wavelets, also referred to as Gabor wavelets, the mother wavelet function is given by the formula

$$\Psi(t) = e^{j\omega_0 t} \cdot e^{-t^2/2}$$

where j denotes the imaginary unit, $(-1)^{1/2}$, and ω_0 is 2π times the frequency of the unshifted and uncompressed mother wavelet (if fewer than six cycles of a wavelet are used, a correction term $e^{-\omega_0/2}$ has to be subtracted from $e^{j\omega_0 t}$ to guarantee that the wavelet still has a mean value of zero). Morlet wavelets are complex functions. Both their real and imaginary parts consist of a harmonic oscillation windowed in time by a Gaussian envelope. Figure 11.8 illustrates this schematically.

Using sinusoidal wavelets such as the Morlet wavelet is ideally suited for detecting sinusoidal EEG activity, because the wavelet transform is similar to detecting whether the signal contains the used wavelet. Other wavelets that are more spiky can be used for detecting transient phenomena in EEG such as epileptic spikes (Schiff et al., 1994).

In the frequency domain, Morlet wavelets also have a Gaussian shape around their modulation frequency, that is, the wavelet scale can be directly interpreted in terms of a well-defined center frequency (we will use the terms scale and frequency synonymously here). Hence, we can write the scaled, unshifted wavelet as a function of frequency, f:

$$\Psi(t, f) = e^{j2\pi f t} \cdot e^{-t^2/2\sigma_t^2}$$

where the standard deviation σ_t of the Gaussian temporal envelope is reciprocally related to the frequency ($\sigma_t \sim 1/f$) in order to retain the wavelet's scaling properties. By this scaling one obtains the same number of significant wavelet cycles, $n_{co} = 6\sigma_t f$, at all frequencies. The standard deviation in the frequency domain is given by $\sigma_f = (2\pi\sigma_t)^{-1}$. It grows proportionally to the modulation frequency—that is, σ_f/f is constant. This implies that the Morlet wavelet transform has a different time and frequency resolution at each scale. If the number of significant cycles of the wavelet is kept constant, it varies in temporal width as a function of frequency, because the same number of cycles spread over a longer interval for lower frequencies. Therefore, at high frequencies the temporal resolution of a wavelet is better than at low frequencies. However, the inverse is true for the frequency resolution of the wavelet transform. At low frequencies the wide temporal extension of the wavelet results in a good frequency resolution, because the analysis considers many time points. At high frequencies, where the small width leaves fewer time points, the frequency resolution decreases. Figure 11.9 illustrates this.

In addition to this general trade-off between temporal and frequency resolution, wavelets also allow one to adjust their temporal and frequency width for any given center frequency. By using a wavelet with more cycles (i.e., larger n_{co}) the frequency resolution increases, because the frequency can be determined via more time points— but of course, the temporal resolution decreases at the same time. Using fewer cycles has the opposite effect.

Convolutions with Morlet wavelets can be computed for multiple frequencies in order to yield a time-frequency (TF, cf. figure 11.16) representation of the analyzed signal, $x(t)$. Because the Morlet wavelet function is complex, the wavelet transform, $W_x(t, f)$, is also a complex function that can be divided into its real part, $\Re\{W_x\}$, and its imaginary part, $\Im\{W_x\}$. Alternatively, using the polar notation, $W_x = |W_x| \exp\{j\theta_x\}$, the wavelet coefficients can be described by an amplitude, $|W_x| = [\Re\{W_x\}^2 + \Im\{W_x\}^2]^{1/2}$, and a phase angle, $\theta_x(t, f) = \tan^{-1}[\Im\{W_x\}/\Re\{W_x\}]$.

One can think of a wavelet function as a finite impulse response filter. In this context, the real part, $\Re\{W_x\}$, of the Morlet wavelet transform represents a bandpass-filtered signal, $x_f(t)$, whereas the imaginary part, $\Im\{W_x\}$, yields a 90-degree phase shifted signal (Hilbert transform). The amplitude, $|W_x(t, f)|$, corresponds to the envelope of the filtered signal, $x_f(t)$. It quantifies the instantaneous oscillatory strength of the signal with respect to the analyzed frequency band. Figure 11.10 shows a time-frequency representation of the signals depicted in figure 11.1. The TF representation has been obtained by gray-scale coding of the wavelet amplitudes. Positions on the horizontal axis correspond to different latencies, whereas different wavelet center frequencies have been mapped to the vertical axis.

In analogy to the Fourier power spectrum, the wavelet power spectrum is defined as $|W_x(t, f)|^2$. It is a measure for the signal energy (signal variance) contained in the time-

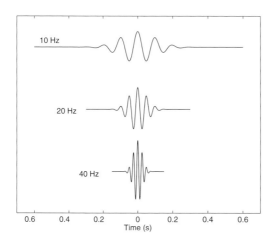

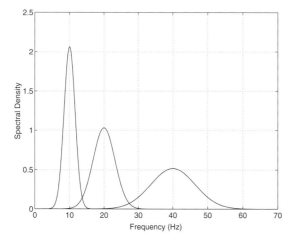

Figure 11.9

Three Morlet wavelets (*top*, only real part shown) with different central frequencies and the corresponding frequency spectra (*bottom*). A low-frequency wavelet of 10 Hz is very broad in the time domain but has a good frequency resolution, picking up only activity from adjacent frequencies in a wavelet analysis (left peak in frequency spectrum). A wavelet with a frequency of 40 Hz is more localized in time but has a lower frequency resolution, picking up frequencies from a wider range in a wavelet analysis (right peak in frequency spectrum).

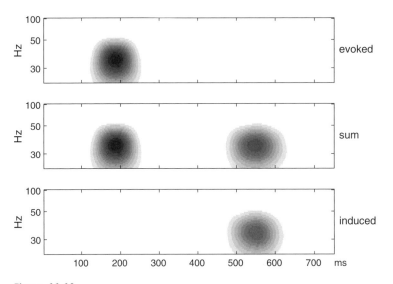

Figure 11.10

Multiple convolutions can be mapped in a time frequency representation. This is shown for the evoked gamma activity (*top*) of the example in figure 11.1, the sum of evoked and induced gamma activity (*middle*) and isolated induced gamma activity (*bottom*). The induced activity has been estimated by the difference of total and evoked activity.

frequency bin covered by the transform, centered around time point t and frequency f. The wavelet functions can be normalized prior to the convolution to have unit energy at all scales. In this case, the wavelet power spectra of an analyzed signal are then directly comparable to each other across all scales. For the Morlet wavelet transform this normalization is achieved with the factor $A_\psi = \sigma_t^{-1/2} \pi^{-1/4}$.

If, however, the wavelet transform should directly yield the amplitude of the analyzed signal, one needs to use a different normalization factor. The Morlet wavelet transform is very similar to the Gabor transform (windowed Fourier transform). The main difference is that in the wavelet method, the width of the data window is not fixed but adapted to the analyzed frequency. In analogy to the Gabor transform, the wavelet amplitude spectrum, $|W_x(t, f)|$, yields the instantaneous amplitude of an oscillation when using the Gabor normalization factor A_ψ:

$$A_\psi = \sigma_t^{-1}(2/\pi)^{1/2}$$

To represent phase-locked (evoked) activity in an ERP experiment, the wavelet transform is computed on the average over the single trials (i.e., on the ERP):

$$\text{Evoked} = \left| A_\Psi \int \Psi^* \left(\frac{t - b}{a} \right) \cdot \frac{1}{N} \sum_{i=1}^{N} eeg_i(t) \, dt \right|$$

Note that absolute value (or absolute power) is calculated. After calculating the evoked activity, the frequency-specific baseline activity can be subtracted to yield values that indicate oscillatory amplitude (or power) relative to baseline.

When wavelet transforms are computed, the convolution peaks at the same latency as the respective frequency component in the raw data, although the peak width will be smeared. Therefore, the baseline should be chosen to precede the stimulation by half the width of the wavelet (e.g., 75 ms for six 25-ms cycles of a 40-Hz wavelet) to avoid the temporal smearing of poststimulus activity into the baseline. To avoid distortions by the rectangular window function that can result from "cutting out" a single epoch from continuous raw data (edge effects), the convolution should start and end one-half of the wavelet length before the baseline and after the end of the assessed time interval, respectively.

The TF representation of the ERP contains only that part of the activity that is phase-locked to the stimulus onset. To compute the activity that is not phase-locked to stimulus onset (and is therefore cancelled out in the average), one can compute the total activity (sum of evoked and induced activity). To calculate the sum of all activity at one frequency, average the absolute values of the wavelet transforms of the single trials, which means that each single trial is at first transformed and the absolute values (or alternatively the power values) are averaged subsequently:

$$\text{Total} = \frac{1}{N} \sum_{i=1}^{N} \left| A_\Psi \int \Psi^* \left(\frac{t-b}{a} \right) \cdot eeg_i(t) \, dt \right|.$$

The corresponding TF representation (sum) contains all activity of one frequency that occurred after stimulus onset, no matter whether it was phase-locked to the stimulus or not (cf. figure 11.10). As above, the activity in a prestimulus interval can be subtracted to obtain a relative measure.

Necessary Conditions for Recording Oscillations

The analysis of EEG frequencies requires some precautions when data are recorded. We discuss these next.

Hardware Requirements

Two parameters of the recording equipment are critical for properly recording oscillatory activity. (1) The sampling rate has to be set to a value that is at least twice the highest frequency that should be analyzed (four times is better, and is required by some software). For example, to analyze gamma activity up to 80 Hz, one needs a minimum sampling rate of 160 Hz, and 320 is recommended. (2) The low-pass filter needs to be set to a value higher than the highest frequency that should be analyzed. The low-pass filter is usually integrated in the analog amplifier to prevent aliasing

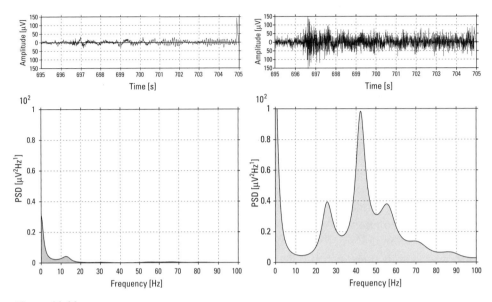

Figure 11.11
Clean EEG data and its frequency spectrum (*left*) and an epoch with EMG contamination leading to frequency peaks around 40 Hz.

errors when digitizing analog data. This step is sometimes overlooked when trying to record high-frequency oscillations for the first time.

Artifact Rejection

All artifacts that contaminate traditional ERP averages should be excluded from frequency analysis. In addition, there are several specific artifact conditions that are especially crucial when analyzing oscillatory activity.

When analyzing alpha activity, subjects should keep their eyes open even if they have no visual task to perform. When they close their eyes, strong alpha oscillations will appear in the EEG that show no correlation with the cognitive task and contaminate the analysis.

A potential confound of human gamma activity is electromyography (EMG). If subjects sit uncomfortably or chew during an EEG session and innervate their muscles, the EEG electrodes will record EMG activity. This high-frequency muscle-related activity (30–80 Hz) can be mistaken for gamma EEG activity. Therefore, all epochs that are subsequently averaged should be visually evaluated for the presence of such EMG artifacts, which should then be excluded from further analysis.

Figure 11.11 shows 10 s of clean EEG and the corresponding frequency spectrum with a 0-Hz and a 12-Hz alpha peak (left). EMG activity can easily be de-

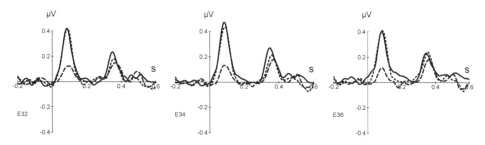

Figure 11.12
Evoked gamma responses in response to visual stimuli of different size. Large (solid) and medium (dotted) stimuli evoke strong gamma peaks, whereas small (dashed) stimuli evoke only weak responses.

tected in the time domain (right) but may be mistaken for gamma activity in the spectrum.

Stimulus Size

Exogenous parameters such as physical stimulus properties influence the amplitude of sensory evoked potentials. The same dependence upon exogenous parameters can be observed for oscillatory EEG activity. Especially for low-amplitude activity in the gamma range, it is crucial to present stimuli of sufficient size in order to evoke reliable responses. Cognitive differences between experimental conditions can only be observed when the amplitude is sufficiently high.

Figure 11.12 shows how the evoked gamma response depends upon stimulus size. Large (9° vis. angle) and medium (5° vis. angle) stimuli evoked gamma peaks of approx. 0.4 µV over occipital cortex that clearly differ from baseline activity. Small (1° vis. angle) stimuli, however, evoke only weak gamma responses that are only twice the amplitude of the baseline noise. The first peak of gamma activity is due to the onset of the visual stimuli and the second one due to their offset.

Stimulus Duration

Due to the fact that stimulus onsets as well as stimulus offsets evoke significant gamma bursts, the duration of a stimulus plays an important role in the observed pattern of oscillations.

When stimuli are sufficiently long in duration, their offset responses can clearly be differentiated from their onset peaks. Figure 11.13 illustrates this for stimuli of 250-ms duration (solid) and 150-ms duration (dotted). If, however, the duration is very short, onset peak and offset peak mix into each other and cannot be distinguished (50-ms duration, dashed). This is also true for ERP analysis, but is often disregarded. When analyzing late ERP components they should not be contaminated by offset responses.

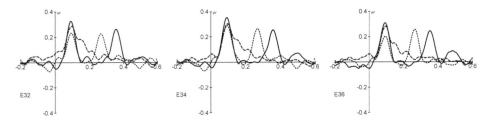

Figure 11.13
Stimuli of three different durations evoke approximately the same onset peak of gamma activity around 100 ms but different offset peaks. Stimulus durations: 250 ms (solid), 150 ms (dotted), and 50 ms (dashed).

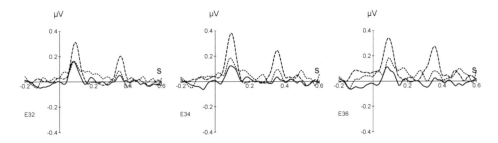

Figure 11.14
Influence of eccentricity on the evoked gamma response. Centrally presented stimuli (dashed) evoke much larger responses than stimuli of identical size and shape that are presented more eccentrically (dotted and solid).

Stimulus Eccentricity

Gamma oscillations are mainly generated over sensory cortices. In case of the visual cortex, the central visual field is represented by a greater number of neurons than the peripheral visual field. This leads to an influence of the eccentricity of visual stimuli on the evoked gamma response.

Figure 11.14 shows the responses to three identical stimuli at different eccentricity. A centrally presented stimulus (dashed) leads to the largest response. Already at 4 degrees eccentricity (dotted) the response is much lower. At an eccentricity of 8 degrees, it is even lower. Therefore, it is advantageous if one can apply central presentation.

Age of Subjects

Age influences the amplitude of ERPs (Polich, 1997). The same is true for evoked oscillations, especially in the gamma frequency range. Already at an age of around 45 years the amplitude of the response begins to decrease (Böttger, Herrmann, & von Cramon,

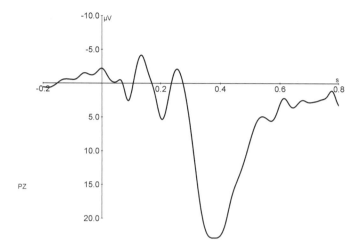

Figure 11.15
An ERP in response to a visual target stimulus exhibiting a series of components: P1, N1, P2, N2, and P3.

2002). Therefore, subjects must be chosen such that they represent a homogeneous age. Otherwise age might be a confound for cognitive parameters.

Analysis of an ERP

When all technical aspects have been taken care of, interesting new findings can be observed in the oscillatory EEG responses. As Makeig et al. (2002) nicely demonstrated, an ERP (figure 11.15) and the frequency representation of the ERP (figure 11.16) are two alternative ways of investigating the EEG in response to experimental stimulation.

Figure 11.16 shows the alternative representation of the ERP in figure 11.15 as a time-frequency plot. The early ERP components are visible as high-frequency blobs in the gamma and beta range, and the later components are visible as two overlapping big blobs in the theta and delta range. The earliest frequency component around 36 Hz has the shortest duration and terminates around 100 ms after stimulation. The subsequent oscillation around 18 Hz is already more widely spread across time and lasts approximately 150 ms after stimulation. The theta wave of about 7 Hz remains active until around 350 ms and a delta wave (approx. 3 Hz) can be observed up to 700 ms poststimulus. Such a shift from early high-frequency components to later low-frequency components is a typical finding (Chen & Herrmann, 2001; Haenschel et al., 2000). Sometimes they reveal a frequency relation of 4:2:1, suggesting underlying neural resonance circuits that trigger each other (Herrmann, 2001).

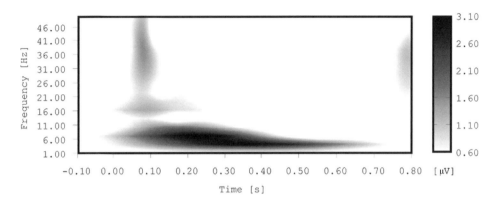

Figure 11.16
The time-frequency representation of the ERP in figure 11.15.

Wavelet-Based Dynamic Interdependence Measures

In the neuroscience community there has been growing interest not only in the modularization of brain functions (i.e., the functional specialization of local brain areas), but also in the cooperation between specialized and widely distributed areas that are a prerequisite of higher cognitive functions and large-scale integration. Such cooperation requires a certain degree of dynamic synchronization between the involved neuronal assemblies that in turn should be reflected in the EEG as a dynamic interrelation between the measured brain signals (von Stein et al., 1999; Schack et al., 1999).

Classical interrelation measures such as Fourier-based coherence and correlation depend on the stationarity of the measured signals, which is rarely fulfilled with concurrent brain signals. Recently, alternative tools based on wavelet analysis have been developed and successfully applied to EEG/MEG signals (e.g., Lachaux et al., 2002). They allow one to track the time course of coherence in nonstationary neuronal signals with good temporal and frequency resolution.

Wavelet Coherence

Analogous to classical coherence, wavelet coherence is defined as the cross-wavelet spectrum of two signals, x and y, normalized by their corresponding autospectra:

$$coh_w(t, f) = \frac{|W_{xy}(t, f)|}{\sqrt{W_{xx}(t, f) \cdot W_{yy}(t, f)}}$$

where $W_{xy}(t, f)$ is the cross-wavelet spectrum (see below) at latency t and frequency f, whereas W_{xx} and W_{yy} denote the auto-spectra of x and y, respectively. Wavelet coherence ranges between 0 and 1. It is a measure of the degree of linear relationship between x and y in a specific time-frequency bin. The instantaneous cross-wavelet spectrum can be estimated from the product of the corresponding univariate wavelet coefficients, $W_{xy}(t, f) = W_x(t, f) \cdot W_y^*(t, f)$. As is the case with Fourier cross-spectra, this estimate is inconsistent and has to be smoothed in an appropriate way in order to improve reliability.

In an event-related potential paradigm, the smoothing can be done across trials:

$$W_{xy}(t, f) = \frac{1}{N} \sum_{k=1}^{N} W_x^k(t, f) \cdot W_y^{k*}(t, f)$$

where N is the total number of trials and W^k means the wavelet coefficient calculated from a signal recorded during the kth trial. This method yields a coherence measure that is very similar to the event-related coherence introduced by Rappelsberger, Pfurtscheller, and Filz (1994). It does not require stationarity across time but is based on the (also questionable) assumption of stationarity across trials.

The wavelet coherence method introduced by Lachaux et al. (2002) estimates W_{xy} by averaging over a time period around the target latency,

$$W_{xy}(t, f) = \frac{1}{\delta} \int_{t-\delta/2}^{t+\delta/2} W_x(\tau, f) \cdot W_y^*(\tau, f) \, d\tau$$

Using Morlet wavelets, this approach corresponds to the WOSA (Welch overlapping segment averaging) estimate of the cross-spectrum (Welch, 1967), with the exception that, in the wavelet-based method, the length of the smoothing window can be varied in dependence upon the target frequency, f. The smoothing window can be chosen to contain the same fixed number of cycles, n_{cy}, at all frequencies, that is, $\delta = n_{cy}/f$. Due to the flexible integration window, the wavelet coherence measure yields a more consistent time-frequency resolution than the WOSA method. Moreover, the same statistical performance of the coherence estimator can be achieved at all frequencies. Bias and variance of the wavelet coherence estimator have been shown to depend only on the number of independent data epochs entering into the calculation of coherence (Lachaux et al., 2002). The ratio $n_{cy}:n_{co}$ gives the number of independent (non-overlapping) data segments, where n_{co} denotes the number of significant wavelet cycles. In order to gain statistical power, this ratio should be chosen as high as possible. However, a large n_{cy} (i.e., a large integration window) diminishes the temporal resolution for measuring coherence and decreases the probability of detecting short-lasting coherent epochs. Therefore, n_{cy} should be adapted to the length of the coherent epochs being searched for, using larger integration windows for longer epochs of coherency. By contrast, the parameter n_{co} has influence on the frequency resolution of the wavelet transform and thus, on the frequency selectivity of the coherence measure, which decreases for low values of n_{co}. Hence, n_{co} must be chosen in accordance to the frequency range of interest. Typical values Lachaux et al. (2002) proposed are $n_{co} \geq 3$ for wide frequency bands (more than 10 Hz) and values up to 8–10 for narrow bands.

Phase Synchronization

Coherence does not separate the effects of covariance of the amplitude waveforms and of the phases of two oscillatory signals. The recently developed concept of phase synchronization of chaotic (and/or noisy) systems (Rosenblum, Pikovsky, & Kurths, 1996) is more general. It implies the appearance of a certain relationship between the phases of oscillatory (sub)systems, but does not impose restrictions on their irregular amplitudes, which may remain noncorrelated. This concept is based on the well-known fact that weak coupling first affects the phases of oscillators, not their amplitudes. Hence, the detection of phase synchronization should be sufficient in order to reveal an interaction between two weakly coupled (sub)systems.

With respect to brain signals, phase synchronization in certain frequency bands is supposed to be a central mechanism in neuronal information processing (Varela et al., 2001). Based primarily on animal experiments, there is evidence that synchronization of neuronal activity within sensory cortex is involved in feature binding (Eckhorn et al., 1988; Gray et al., 1989). Transient synchronization between physically distant brain areas has also been reported (Roelfsema et al., 1997). This suggests a possible mechanism for large-scale integration, establishing a dynamic link between neural assemblies by temporarily adjusting their discharge frequencies. Recent experimental results from intracranial and scalp recordings support the assumption that magnitude and phase of brain signals might indeed be involved in a different manner during a cognitive process (Rodriguez et al., 1999; Bruns et al., 2000).

Instantaneous Phase Difference   The parameter for measuring phase synchronization is the relative phase angle between two oscillatory systems. Neuroelectrical recordings are broad-band signals and their phase cannot thoroughly be defined. Formally, one could apply the analytic signal approach (Gabor, 1946) and assign an instantaneous phase and an instantaneous amplitude via the Hilbert transform. However, the Hilbert phase and Hilbert amplitude have direct physical meaning only for band-limited signals.

As an alternative, the Morlet wavelet transform acts as a bandpass filter that, at the same time, yields separate values for the instantaneous amplitude $a(t, f)$ and the phase $\theta(t, f)$ of a time-series signal at a specific frequency f. Thus, the wavelet phases of two neuronal signals x and y can be utilized to determine their instantaneous phase difference in a given frequency band

$$\Delta\theta(t, f) = \theta_x(t, f) - \theta_y(t, f)$$

and to establish a synchronization measure that quantifies the coupling of phases independent from amplitude effects. (Note that according to the above equation, the phase difference has to be calculated from the unfolded univariate phase angles.)

Transient phase entrainment (phase locking) is observed if the phase difference remains approximately constant over some time period (typically hundreds of milliseconds in the context of neurocogniton). Due to the noisy and/or chaotic nature of neuronal signals, their relative phase is usually not bounded even when there exists some phase coupling between them. For weak noise, the phase difference fluctuates around some mean phase shift with occasional rapid phase jumps of $\pm 2\,\pi$. For strong and unbound noise (i.e., Gaussian noise), these phase slips occur irregularly. That means that phase locking can be detected in a statistical sense only (Tass et al., 1998; Rosenblum et al., 2001). One has to analyze the distribution of the relative phase angles on the unit circle (wrapped to the interval $[0, 2\pi]$). For independent signals, this distribution will be close to uniform, whereas synchrony shows up as the appearance of a dominating peak.

Figure 11.17 shows the phase difference between the 8-Hz oscillations recorded at electrodes O1 and F9 after visual stimulation. Although the phase difference varies over time before stimulation, it remains stable at a value of approx. $0.83\,\pi$ (2.6 rad) after stimulation for about 250 ms, as the plateau of the curves shows.

Phase-Locking Statistics   Researchers have proposed different synchronization measures based, for example, on the Shannon entropy, mutual information, a stroboscopic approach, or directional statistics (for reviews, see Tass et al., 1998; Rosenblum et al., 2001). According to directional statistics (Mardia & Jupp, 2000), the coherence of an angular distribution θ_i can be quantified by estimating the phase-locking index (PLI),

$$PLI = |\langle e^{j\theta} \rangle| = \sqrt{\langle \cos \theta \rangle^2 + \langle \sin \theta \rangle^2} = 1 - CV$$

where brackets denote the expectation operator and CV is the circular variance. It is easy to confirm that the PLI ranges between zero for uniformly scattered phases and one in the case of perfect phase locking.

In a repeated-stimulus design, one can estimate the PLI by averaging over trials (Lachaux et al., 1999):

$$PLI(t, f) = \frac{1}{N} \left| \sum_{k=1}^{N} \exp\{ j\Delta\theta^k(t, f) \} \right|$$

where N is the total number of trials and $\Delta\theta^k$ represents the instantaneous phase difference of the two brain signals recorded during the kth trial. The bivariate PLI measures the intertrial variability of the frequency-specific relative phase of two brain

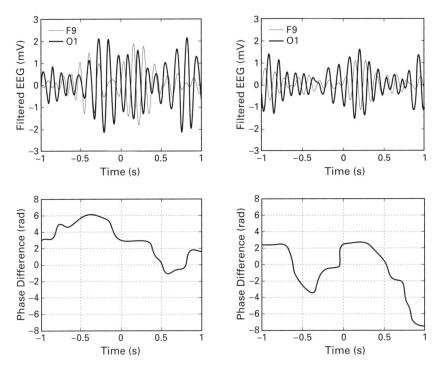

Figure 11.17
Two time courses of 8-Hz event-related oscillations after wavelet decomposition for two electrodes (*top*). The phase differences (*bottom*) reveal that after stimulation (at 0 ms) there is a stable phase relation between the two electrodes in both trials from 0 to approx. 250 ms.

signals at a given target latency—that is, it quantifies the stability of a linear phase relationship across trials.

Figure 11.18 shows the TF representation of the intertrial PLI for two EEG scalp recordings in a visual ERP experiment. A prominent epoch of transient phase coherence is detectable shortly after stimulus onset. The phase locking confines selectively to the alpha band.

Figure 11.19 shows how an experimental stimulus influences the phase of an oscillation. Before visual stimulation, the phase differences between the 8-Hz oscillations in electrodes O1 and F9 were almost randomly distributed (left panel). After a visual stimulus occurred, however, most phase differences showed a value of 150 degrees. This indicates that the stimulus affects the phase of the oscillations.

The PLI measure offers a good temporal resolution, limited only by the width of the wavelet function applied for the univariate phase estimation. Due to the trade-off be-

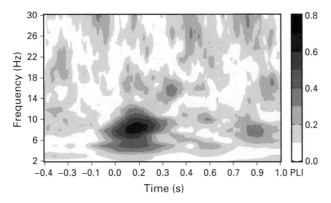

Figure 11.18

TF representation of the bivariate intertrial PLI estimated from two simultaneous EEG recordings (from an occipital [O1] and a frontal scalp electrode [F9]) during visual stimulation of a human subject (stimulus onset at time $t = 0$; $N = 59$ trials; $n_{co} = 6$ significant wavelet cycles). After stimulus onset, a transient period of phase coherence is selectively detected in the alpha band.

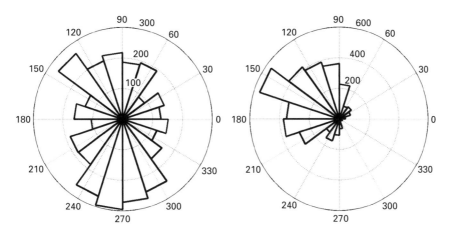

Figure 11.19

The phase distribution of the phase differences of the 8-Hz oscillations between electrodes O1 and F9. The numbers on the circle denote the phase difference in degrees and the extension of a wedge indicates how many single trials showed this phase difference. Before visual stimulation the phases were randomly distributed (*left*). In a time interval from 50 to 300 ms after stimulation the phases were clustered around a value of about 150 degrees (0.83π, *right*).

tween temporal and frequency resolution of the wavelet transform, it might be advantageous to prefilter the signals in a narrow frequency band around the target frequency prior to estimating their wavelet phases (Lachaux et al., 1999). This is recommended especially when dealing with high target frequencies in the gamma band, where the frequency resolution of the wavelet transform is rather poor.

When one estimates the PLI from a finite number of samples, as is always the case in real situations, a nonzero PLI value will be measured even if the samples are drawn from a uniform distribution. For N samples, the expected PLI value (i.e., the bias) is $N^{-1/2}$. One can apply the Rayleigh test (Mardia & Jupp, 2000) in order to assess significance of the detected phase locking against the null hypothesis of a uniform distribution.

Because the sampling distribution of the statistics is usually unknown for brain signals, Lachaux et al. (1999) have proposed a Monte Carlo approach based on the shuffling of trials. Surrogate values are computed from the same signals x and y used for original PLI estimation, except that the order of trials for y is permuted before calculating the relative phases. That means that the instantaneous phase difference is computed from signals that have been recorded during different trials and can thus be considered to be uncorrelated. For each permutation, the maximum PLI value is measured and compared against the original PLI value. The percentage of surrogate values that are greater than the original PLI at a given latency is called phase-locking statistics (PLS) (Lachaux et al., 1999). For PLS values that are smaller than a chosen significance level, the measured synchrony is considered significant. The number n of permutations needed for PLS calculation depends on the chosen significance level p; for a one-sided test it is given by $n = 1/p - 1$ (Theiler et al., 1992; Schreiber & Schmitz, 2000).

Although PLS is a powerful method, it has its caveats. Note that PLS fails to reject the null hypothesis in the important case when both univariate signals have constant phases across trials and thus, the bivariate phases are perfectly locked (Lachaux et al., 1999). PLS also cannot be applied to single trials (or averaged signals such as ERPs). Moreover, it fails to detect periods of synchrony that occur with varying phase delay across trials or at jittering latencies. As an alternative, Lachaux et al. (2000) proposed the single-trial phase-locking index

$$S - PLI(t, f) = \frac{1}{\delta} \left| \int_{t-\delta/2}^{t+\delta/2} \exp\{j\Delta\theta(\tau, f)\} \, d\tau \right|$$

also referred to as smoothed phase-locking index (S-PLI), where averaging of the phase vectors proceeds over adjacent time points. Time smoothing diminishes the temporal resolution of the S-PLI measure. As with wavelet coherence, the width of the smoothing window should be adapted to the target frequency, and to the expected length of the coherent epochs. Surrogate data for a statistical test can be obtained by data scrambling, that is, by the permutation of the temporal order of the samples in each of the two signals. For a review of surrogate data methods, see Paluš (1997) and Schreiber and Schmitz (2000).

Conclusion

We reviewed the nature of oscillations in human EEG and how to analyze them via wavelet analysis. We hope that we were able to convince the reader that oscillations are a valuable approach for looking at electrophysiological data that compliments the derivation of ERP signals. Our attempt to name a few of the many experiments investigating oscillations in the human EEG was by no means complete. However, the list gives a short overview of the different frequency bands and may give the interested reader a link to further articles. In addition to the frequency bands that we explicitly mentioned here, there are various others, ranging from oscillations close to 0 Hz up to 600 Hz (Curio, 1999).

We also hope that the reader has learned new ways to investigate oscillatory activity in EEG data. At the same time, we tried to show the limitations and caveats of the introduced methods. Wavelets are certainly not the only way to analyze oscillations, but they do have critical advantages over other methods. The possibility of investigating the time course of an oscillation and to compute time-frequency representations with variable resolutions are among the strengths of wavelet analysis, along with the analysis of phases and their temporal characteristics. However, one must take care with some of the analysis parameters, such as the number of cycles that determines the frequency resolution, as well as the temporal resolution of the analysis.

The interpretation of significant synchronies between brain signals that have been detected is not straightforward. Especially when dealing with EEG scalp recordings, spurious synchronies may arise from volume conduction and/or reference effects. Volume conduction leads to an artificially high synchrony, especially between adjacent electrodes because their recorded neuronal populations overlap in space (Srinivasan, Nunez, & Silberstein, 1998). The effect of the choice of a specific reference electrode can hardly be predicted without precise knowledge of the source locations and of the volume conductor (Nunez et al., 1997). It may lead to an increase as well as to a decrease of measured synchrony between EEG recordings due to adding or removing a common signal, respectively. To circumvent these problems, one can enhance the spatial resolution of EEG recordings by deblurring techniques (Le & Gevins, 1993), scalp current density (SCD) calculation (Pernier, Perrin, & Bertrand, 1988; Lagerlund et al., 1995), or cortical imaging (Nunez et al., 1994) prior to wavelet analysis. However, Biggins et al. (1991) argued that SCD estimation could also introduce spurious synchronies due to spatial interpolation inherent in the mathematical algorithm. A challenging approach could be to combine inverse methods and TF methods in order to reconstruct the sources of oscillatory neuroelectrical activity.

Of course, the approaches we focused on are not the only ones. There are a number of other fruitful applications of wavelets in neurophysiology, and some of them will probably gain more importance in the future.

One approach that is very promising is using a discrete wavelet analysis for denoising. An averaged ERP may be decomposed into wavelet coefficients by a discrete wavelet analysis. Then one can determine which coefficients yield significant activity at the corresponding frequency. In a second step only these significant coefficients are considered and others are set to zero. Now the ERP is reconstructed from the remaining wavelet coefficients. This procedure results in filtering out other frequencies that are considered noise for the cognitive task (e.g., Wang, Begleiter, & Pojesz, 1998; Quiroga & Garcia, 2003).

References

Adrian, E. (1942). Olfactory reactions in the brain of the hedgehog. *Journal of Physiology (London)*, *100*, 459–473.

Başar, E., Başar-Eroglu, C., Karakas, S., & Schürmann, M. (1999). Oscillatory brain theory: A new trend in neuroscience. *IEEE Engineering in Medicine and Biology*, *18*, 56–66.

Başar, E., Schürmann, M., Başar-Eroglu, C., & Karakas, S. (1997). Alpha oscillations in brain functioning: An integrative theory. *International Journal of Psychophysiology*, *26* (1–3), 5–29.

Başar-Eroglu, C., Strüber, D., Schürmann, M., Stadler, M., & Başar, E., (1996). Gamma-band responses in the brain: A short review of psychophysiological correlates and functional significance. *International Journal of Psychophysiology*, *24*, 101–112.

Başar-Eroglu, C., Başar, E., Demiralp, T., & Schürmann, M. (1992). P300-response: Possible psychophysiological correlates in delta and theta frequency channels. A review. *International Journal of Psychophysiology*, *13* (2), 161–179.

Biggins, C. A., Fein, G., Raz, J., & Amir, A. (1991). Artifactually high coherences result from using spherical spline computation of scalp current density. *Electroencephalography and Clinical Neurophysiology*, *79*, 413–419.

Böttger, D., Herrmann, C. S., & von Cramon, D. Y. (2002). Amplitude differences of evoked alpha and gamma oscillations in two different age groups. *International Journal of Psychophysiology*, *45* (3), 245–251.

Brandt, M. E. (1997). Visual and auditory evoked phase resetting of the alpha EEG. *International Journal of Psychophysiology*, *26* (1–3), 319–340.

Berger, H. (1929). Über das Elektrenkephalogramm des Menschen. *Archiv für Psychiatrie und Nervenkrankheiten*, *87*, 527–570.

Bruns, A., Eckhorn, R., Jokeit, H., & Ebner, A. (2000). Amplitude envelope correlation detects coupling among incoherent brain signals. *Cognitive Neuroscience, 11* (7), 1509–1514.

Chen, A. C. N., & Herrmann, C. S. (2001). Perception of pain coincides with the spatial expansion of human EEG dynamics. *Neuroscience Letters, 297* (3), 183–186.

Curio, G. (1999). High frequency (600 Hz) bursts of spike-like activities generated in the human cerebral somatosensory system. *Electroencephalography and Clinical Neurophysiology, 49*, 56–61.

Debener, S., Herrmann, C. S., Kranczioch, C., Gembris, D., & Engel, A. K. (2003). Top-down attentional processing enhances auditory evoked gamma band activity. *Neuroreport, 14* (5), 683–686.

Dumermuth, G. (1977). Fundamentals of spectral analysis in electroencephalography. In A. Remond (Ed.), *EEG informatics. A didactic review of methods and applications of EEG data processing* (pp. 83–105). Amsterdam: Elsevier.

Eckhorn, R., Bauer, R., Jordan, W., Brosch, M., Kruse, W., Munk, M., & Reitboeck, H. J. (1988). Coherent oscillations: A mechanisms of feature linking in the visual cortex? Multiple electrode and correlation analyses in the cat. *Biological Cybernetics, 60*, 121–130.

Engel, A. K., Fries, P., & Singer, W. (2001). Dynamic predictions: Oscillations and synchrony in top-down processing. *Nature Reviews Neuroscience, 2* (10), 704–716.

Fell, J., Klaver, P., Elfadil, H., Schaller, C., Elger, C. E., & Fernandez, G. (2003). *European Journal of Neuroscience, 17* (5), 1082–1088.

Fell, J., Klaver, P., Lehnertz, K., Grunwald, T., Schaller, C., Elger, C. E., & Fernandez, G. (2001). Human memory formation is accompanied by rhinal-hippocampak coupling and decoupling. *Nature Neuroscience, 4*, 1259–1264.

Gabor, D. (1946). Theory of communication. *Journal of IEE London, 93* (3), 429–457.

Galambos, R. (1992). A comparison of certain gamma band (40 Hz) brain rhythms in cat and man. In E. Başar & T. Bullock (Eds.), *Induced rhythms in the brain* (pp. 201–216). Boston: Birkhauser.

Gloor, P., Ball, G., & Schaul, N. (1977). Brain lesions that produce delta waves in the EEG. *Neurology, 27* (4), 326–333.

Gray, C. M., König, P., Engel, A. K., & Singer, W. (1989). Oscillatory responses in cat visual cortex exhibit intercolumnar synchronization which reflects global stimulus properties. *Nature, 338*, 334–337.

Haenschel, C., Baldeweg, T., Croft, R. J., Whittington, M., & Gruzelier, J. (2000). Gamma and beta frequency oscillations in response to novel auditory stimuli: A comparison of human electroencephalogram (EEG) data with in vitro models. *Proceedings of the National Academy of Sciences USA, 97* (13), 7645–7650.

Herrmann, C. S. (2001). Human EEG responses to 1–100 Hz flicker: Resonance phenomena in visual cortex and their potential correlation to cognitive phenomena. *Experimental Brain Research, 137*, 346–353.

Herrmann, C. S., & Knight, R. T. (2001). Mechanisms of human attention: Event-related potentials and oscillations. *Neuroscience and Biobehavioural Systems, 25* (6), 465–476.

Herrmann, C. S., & Mecklinger, A. (2001). Gamma activity in human EEG reflects attentional top-down processing. *Visual Cognition, 8,* 273–285.

Herrmann, C. S., Mecklinger, A., & Pfeiffer, E. (1999). Gamma responses and ERPs in a visual classification task. *Clinical Neurophysiology, 110,* 636–642.

Jensen, O., & Tesche, C. D. (2002). Frontal theta activity in humans increases with memory load in a working memory task. *European Journal of Neuroscience, 15* (8), 1395–1399.

Keil, A., Müller, M. M., Ray, W., Gruber, T., & Elbert, T. (1999). Human gamma band activity and perception of a gestalt. *The Journal of Neuroscience, 19,* 7152–7162.

Klimesch, W., Doppelmayr, M., Russegger, H., Pachinger, T., & Schwaiger, J. (1998a). Induced alpha band power changes in the human EEG and attention. *Neuroscience Letters, 13,* 73–76.

Klimesch, W., Doppelmayr, M., Rohm, D., Pollhuber, D., & Stadler, W. (1998b). Simultaneous desynchronization and synchronization of different alpha responses in the human electroencephalogram: A neglected paradox? *Neurocience Letters, 244,* 73–76.

Klimesch, W. (1997). EEG-alpha rhythms and memory processes. *International Journal of Psychophysiology, 26* (1–3), 319–340.

Klimesch, W., Schimke, H., & Pfurtscheller, G. (1993). Alpha frequency, cognitive load and memory performance. *Brain Topography, 5* (3), 241–251.

Lachaux, J.-P., Rodriguez, E., Martinerie, J., & Varela, F. J. (1999). Measuring phase synchrony in brain signals. *Human Brain Mapping, 8,* 194–208.

Lachaux, J.-P., Rodriguez, E., Le Van Quyen, M., Lutz, A., Martinerie, J., & Varela, F. J. (2000). Studying single-trials of phase synchronous activity in the brain. *International Journal of Bifurcation and Chaos, 10* (10), 2429–2439.

Lachaux, J.-P., Lutz, A., Rudrauf, D., Cosmelli, D., Le Van Quyen, M., Martinerie, J., & Varela, F. (2002). Estimating the time-course of coherence between single-trial brain signals: An introduction to wavelet coherence. *Neurophysiologie Clinique, 32,* 157–174.

Lagerlund, T. D., Sharbrough, F. W., Busacker, N. E., & Cicora, K. M. (1995). Interelectrode coherences from nearest-neighbor and spherical harmonic expansion computation of laplacian scalp potential. *Electroencephalography and Clinical Neurophysiology, 95,* 178–188.

Le, J., & Gevins, A. (1993). Methods to reduce blur distortion from EEGs using a realistic head model. *IEEE Transactions on Biomedical Engineering, 40,* 517–528.

Llinás, R., & Ribary, U. (1993). Coherent 40-Hz oscillation characterizes dream state in humans. *Proceedings of the National Academy of Sciences USA, 90* (5), 2078–2081.

Lopes da Silva, F. (1991). Neural mechanisms underlying brain waves: From neural membranes to networks. *Electroencephalography and Clinical Neurophysiology, 79* (2), 81–93.

Makeig, S., Westerfield, M., Jung, T. P., Enghoff, S., Townsend, J., Courchesne, E., & Sejnowski, T. J. (2002). Dynamic brain sources of visual evoked responses. *Science, 295*, 690–694.

Mardia, K. V., & Jupp, P. E. (2000). *Directional statistics.* Chichester: John Wiley & Sons Ltd.

Müller, M. M., Junghöfer, M., Elbert, T., & Rockstroh, B. (1997). Visually induced gamma-band responses to coherent and incoherent motion: A replication study. *NeuroReport, 8*, 2575–2579.

Müller, M. M., Teder-Sälejärvi, W., & Hillyard, S. (1998). The time course of cortical facilitation during cued shifts of spatial attention. *Nature Neuroscience, 1*, 631–634.

Müller, M. M., Gruber, T., Keil, A., & Elbert, T. (2000). Modulation of induced gamma band activity in the human EEG by attention and visual processing. *International Journal of Psychophysiology, 38*, 283–299.

Neuper, C., & Pfurtscheller, G. (2001). Event-related dynamics of cortical rhythms: Frequency-specific features and functional correlates. *International Journal of Psychophysiology, 43*, 41–58.

Niedermeyer, E. (1997). Alpha rhythms as physiological and abnormal phenomena. *International Journal of Psychophysiology, 26* (1–3), 31–49.

Nunez, P. L., Silberstein, R. B., Cadusch, P. J., Wijesinghe, R. S., Westdorp, A. F., & Srinivasan, R. (1994). A theoretical and experimental study of high resolution EEG based on surface Laplacians and cortical imaging. *Electroencephalography and Clinical Neurophysiology, 90*, 40–57.

Nunez, P. L., Srinivasan, R., Westdorp, A. F., Wijesinghe, R. S., Tucker, D. M., Silberstein, R. B., & Cadusch, P. J. (1997). EEG coherency I: Statistics, reference electrode, volume conduction, Laplacians, cortical imaging, and interpolation at multiple scales. *Electroencephalography and Clinical Neurophysiology, 103*, 499–515.

Paluš, M. (1997). Detecting phase synchronization in noisy systems. *Physics Letters A, 235*, 341–351.

Pernier, J., Perrin, F., & Bertrand, O. (1988). Scalp current densities: Concept and properties. *Electroencephalography and Clinical Neurophysiology, 69*, 385–389.

Polich, J. (1997). EEG and ERP assessment of normal aging. *Electroencephalography and Clinical Neurophysiology, 104*, 224–256.

Quiroga, R. Q., & Garcia, H. (2003). Single-trial event-related potentials with wavelet denoising. *Clinical Neurophysiology, 114*, 376–390.

Rappelsberger, P., Pfurtscheller, G., & Filz, O. (1994). Calculation of event-related coherence—a new method to study short-lasting coupling between brain areas. *Brain Topography, 7*, 121–127.

Rodriguez, E., George, N., Lachaux, J.-P., Martinerie, J., Renault, B., & Varela, F. J. (1999). Perception's shadow: Long-distance synchronization of human brain activity. *Nature, 397*, 430–433.

Roelfsema, P. R., Engel, A. K., König, P., & Singer, W. (1997). Visuomotor integration is associated with zero time-lag synchronization among cortical areas. *Nature, 385*, 157–161.

Rosenblum, M., Pikovsky, A., & Kurths, J. (1996). Phase synchronization of chaotic oscillators. *Physical Review Letters, 76*, 1804–1807.

Rosenblum, M., Pikovsky, A., Kurths, J., Schaefer, C., & Tass, P. A. (2001). Phase synchronization: From theory to data analysis. In F. Moss & S. Gielen (Ed.), *Handbook of biological physics, volume 4* (pp. 279–231). Elsevier Science.

Salmelin, R., & Hari, R. (1994). Spatiotemporal characteristics of sensorimotor neuromagnetic rhythms related to thumb movement. *Neuroscience, 60*, 537–550.

Samar, V. J., Bopardikar, A., Rao, R., & Swartz, K. (1999). Wavelet analysis of neuroelectric waveforms. *Brain and Language, 66*, 7–60.

Sewards, T. V., & Sewards, M. A. (1999). Alpha-band oscillations in visual cortex: Part of the neural correlate of visual awareness? *International Journal of Psychophysiology, 33* (2), 177–179.

Schack, B., Chen, A. C. N., Mescha, S., & Witte, H. (1999). Instantaneous EEG coherence analysis during the Stroop task. *Clinical Neurophysiology, 110*, 1410–1426.

Schiff, S. J., Aldroubi, A., Unser, M., & Sato, S. (1994). Fast wavelet transformation of EEG. *Electroencephalography and Clinical Neurophysiology, 91* (6), 442–455.

Schreiber, T., & Schmitz, A. (2000). Surrogate time series. *Physica D, 142*, 346–382.

Srinivasan, R., Nunez, P. L., & Silberstein, R. B. (1998). Spatial filtering and neocortical dynamics: Estimates of EEG coherence. *IEEE Transactions on Biomedical Engineering, 45*, 814–826.

Steriade, M., McCormick, D. A., & Sejnowski, T. J. (1993). Thalamo-cortical oscillations in the sleeping and aroused brain. *Science, 262*, 679–685.

Steriade, M., Gloor, P., Llinás, R., Lopes da Silva, F., & Mesulam, M. (1990). Basic mechanisms of cerebral rhythmic activities. *Electroencephalography and Clinical Neurophysiology, 76* (6), 481–508.

Strüber, D., & Herrmann, C. S. (2002). MEG alpha activity decrease reflects destabilization of multistable percepts. *Cognitive Brain Research, 14* (3), 370–382.

Tallon, C., Bertrand, O., Bouchet, P., & Pernier, J. (1995). Gamma range activity evoked by coherent visual stimuli in humans. *European Journal of Neuroscience, 7*, 1285–1291.

Tallon-Baudry, C., Bertrand, O., & Fischer, C. (2001). Oscillatory synchrony between human extrastriate areas during visual short-term memory maintenance. *Journal of Neuroscience, 21*, 1–5.

Tallon-Baudry, C., & Bertrand, O. (1999). Oscillatory gamma activity in humans and its role in object representation. *Trends in Cognitive Sciences, 3*, 151–162.

Tallon-Baudry, C., Bertrand, O., Delpuech, C., & Pernier, J. (1996). Stimulus specificity of phase-locked and non-phase-locked 40 Hz visual responses in human. *Journal of Neuroscience, 16*, 4240–4249.

Tallon-Baudry, C., Bertrand, O., Delpuech, C., & Pernier, J. (1997). Oscillatory gamma-band (30–70 Hz) activity induced by a visual search task in humans. *Journal of Neuroscience, 17*, 722–734.

Tass, P., Rosenblum, M. G., Weule, J., Kueths, J., Pikovsky, A., Volkmann, J., Schnitzler, A., & Freund, H. J. (1998). Detection of n:m phase locking from noisy data: Application to magneto-encephalography. *Physical Review Letters, 81*, 3291–3294.

Tesche, C. D., & Karhu, J. (2000). Theta oscillations index human hippocampal activation during a working memory task. *Proceedings of the National Academy of Sciences USA, 97* (2), 919–924.

Theiler, J., Eubank, S., Longtin, A., Galdrikian, B., & Farmer, J. D. (1992). Testing for nonlinearity in time series: The method of surrogate data. *Physica D, 58*, 77–94.

Tiitinen, H., Sinkkonen, J., Reinikainen, K., Alho, K., Lavikainen, J., & Näätänen, R. (1993). Selective attention enhances the auditory 40-hz transient response in humans. *Nature, 364*, 59–60.

Varela, F., Lachaux, J.-P., Rodriguez, E., & Martinerie, J. (2001). The brainweb: Phase synchronization and large-scale integration. *Nature Reviews Neuroscience, 2*, 229–239.

von Stein, A., Rappelsberger, P., Sarnthein, J., & Petsche, H. (1999). Synchronization between temporal and parietal cortex during multimodal object processing in man. *Cerebral Cortex, 9* (2), 689–692.

Wang, K., Begleiter, H., & Pojesz, B. (1998). Spatial enhancement of event-related potentials using multiresolution analysis. *Brain Topography, 10* (3), 191–200.

Welch, P. D. (1967). The use of fast Fourier transform for the estimation of power spectra: A method based on time averaging over short, modified periodograms. *IEEE Transactions Audio Electroacoustic, AU-15*, 70–73.

Yordanova, J., Kolev, V., & Polich, J. (2001). P300 and alpha event-related desynchronization (ERD). *Psychophysiology, 38*, 143–152.

III Special Applications

12   ERPs in Developmental Populations

Tracy DeBoer, Lisa S. Scott, and Charles A. Nelson

A primary goal of developmental cognitive neuroscience is to elucidate the relation between brain development and cognitive development (see Nelson & Luciana, 2001). The study of this relation in children older than 5–6 years lends itself to many of the same tools used in the adult, such as functional magnetic resonance imaging (fMRI). However, in children younger than this, limitations in motor and linguistic abilities, coupled with abbreviated attention spans, make using such tools impractical. In contrast, event-related potentials (ERPs) provide one of the only methodological techniques in the armamentarium of cognitive neuroscientists that allow researchers to examine the relation between brain and behavior beginning at birth. ERPs are non-invasive and can be utilized across the entire lifespan, thereby permitting one to use the same methodological tool and dependent measure across a broad range of ages (although comparisons across large age spans may be challenging due to qualitative differences in the ERP response). Furthermore, due to the high temporal resolution of ERPs (on the order of milliseconds), researchers can index changes in the mental chronometry of a given system. Finally, ERPs do not require an overt behavioral or verbal response and therefore permit the study of phenomena that cannot be studied with behavioral methods (e.g., responses to the simultaneous presentation of multiple stimuli or stimuli presented so briefly so as to preclude a behavioral response). However, when a behavioral response is obtainable, ERPs can also provide an invaluable complement and an additional level of analysis to that behavioral measure by permitting one to glimpse (albeit imperfectly) the neural circuits underlying the behavior.[1]

Study Formation and Experimental Design

Hypotheses

Despite an increase in the use of ERPs with developmental populations, several obstacles remain that prevent testable hypotheses from appearing more often in the literature. First, the field has only begun to define ERP components of interest across development, and thus much discontinuity remains between age groups and across components of interest. Second, because relatively little is known about human brain development, it can be challenging to derive hypotheses based on the development of discrete neural circuits. Third, almost nothing is known about how physiologic activity in the developing brain propagates to the scalp surface, and thus, we do not know what the relation is between activity *in* the brain vs. *at* the scalp. With these caveats in mind, in this chapter we attempt to illustrate the kinds of questions that are particularly amenable to an electrophysiological investigation with developmental populations, but we also challenge researchers to perform the appropriate exploratory investigations so they can conduct more theoretically driven experiments with testable hypotheses.

Task Design

ERPs are, by definition, time-locked to the presentation of a stimulus. Therefore, constraints are constantly placed on the types of tasks amenable to ERP experiments, in both adult and developmental populations. However, due to the limited capacity of attention and restricted behavioral repertoire of infant and child populations, further considerations are necessary when designing experiments for these groups. Some developmental ERP tasks can be derived from ERP tasks used with adults and adjusted to take developmental differences into consideration (e.g., decreasing the number of independent variables or the complexity of the stimuli). However, as accommodations such as these are made it must be acknowledged that infants and children are not typically tested under the same conditions as adults (e.g., infants do not benefit from instructions) and therefore direct comparisons across large age differences are often difficult to interpret. Other age-appropriate ERP tasks can arise from modified versions of behavioral tasks known to tap certain cognitive functions of interest (e.g., speech discrimination tasks, habituation tasks, and recognition memory tasks). Finally, tasks used with other imaging techniques (such as those used in fMRI procedures) can be tailored to suit the constraints of developmental ERP research (e.g., the go/no-go tasks and serial reaction time tasks; see Davis et al., 2003).

Most developmental ERP studies conducted to date have used either the standard oddball paradigm or a combination of the oddball paradigm with an infant habituation paradigm. In the former, two or more stimuli are presented repeatedly, but with different frequencies. For example, in one study, 4- to 7-week-old infants were shown pictures of checkerboard patterns and geometric shapes. ERPs were recorded while one stimulus was repeated frequently (80% of the time) and the other stimulus was presented infrequently (20% of the time; Karrer & Monti, 1995). The combined oddball/habituation paradigm involves first familiarizing or habituating an infant to a stimulus (e.g., a face), and then presenting a series of stimuli, consisting of the now familiar stimulus and a novel stimulus (e.g., a new face) repeatedly with equal frequency (i.e., 50% of the time for each) while recording ERPs (e.g., Pascalis et al., 1998).

Important Considerations in Developmental Populations

Beyond paradigm considerations, one must also consider (1) age-related changes in the morphology and timing of ERP components of interest, and (2) changes in behavioral measures, including the availability, quality, and validity of these measures. We will discuss the above factors briefly in this section, but we will return to them throughout the chapter, as they are relevant to the remaining sections.

Developmental changes that are apparent in the morphology of the ERP waveform are often difficult to describe, and increasingly difficult to explain due to their complex and multifaceted nature. For instance, major developmental changes in synaptic density, myelination, and other physical maturational processes (e.g., changes in skull thickness and closing of the fontanel) may combine to influence amplitude and latency increases and decreases across different ages (Nelson & Luciana, 1998). Unexpectedly, ERPs of adults and newborns are similar to each other in amplitude, but very dissimilar compared to ERPs from older infants and young children (see figure 12.1 and plate 6 for illustration). Furthermore, in the first two years of life, reduced synaptic efficiency results in greater slow wave activity rather than peaked activity, the latter being more typical of adult ERPs. Thus, the infant ERP does not show as many well-defined peaked responses (especially in anterior components) when compared to adult responses. The characteristics of the peaked adult waveform typically begin to emerge when children reach 4 years of age and continue to develop well into adolescence (Friedman et al., 1984; Nelson & Luciana, 1998). In fact, because the distribution of activity across the scalp (i.e., topography) changes with age, we can infer that important changes are still taking place in the neural substrate generating the components of interest throughout development. Amplitudes also vary with task demands imposed on the participant. Presumably the easier the task, the less effort expended, and the less cortical activation required, ultimately resulting in smaller amplitudes (Nelson & Luciana, 1998). Finally, the general heuristic for changes that take place from early adulthood to later adulthood is that, overall, latencies of several ERP components appear longer and amplitudes appear smaller (see Kurtzberg et al., 1984; Nelson & Monk, 2001; and Taylor & Baldeweg, 2002 for further discussion).

A major change that also occurs with increasing age is the ability to "ground" the measure in behavior or correlate the brain's electrophysiological response with task performance. Infant ERP paradigms by necessity do not involve issuing instructions, nor do they require an overt behavioral response. However, most adult ERP paradigms include both instructions and a behavior response (even if only to ensure continued attention to the task). Therefore, because of the differences in testing conditions it is possible that, at some level, differences in ERP morphology are due to differences in task requirements.

The "passive" viewing paradigm (i.e., one in which no instructions are given) is useful for two reasons. First, developmental populations can be tested and their data

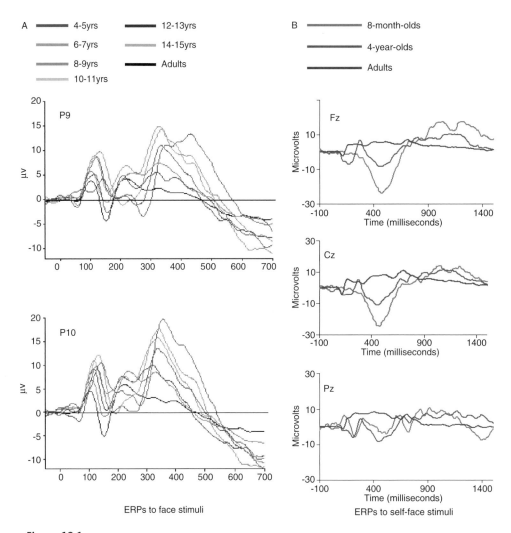

Figure 12.1

(*A*) Grand averaged ERPs from posterior, inferior temporal electrodes P9 (left parietal lobe) and P10 (right parietal lobe) in response to face stimuli for seven age groups. (*B*) Grand averaged ERPs from midline electrodes taken from a pilot study in which 8-month-olds, 4-year-olds, and adults passively viewed images of their own face in the context of a face recognition task. (*A* courtesy of Margot Taylor, Centre National Cervau et Cognition, Toulouse, France, and *B* courtesy of Lisa S. Scott, Institute of Child Development, University of Minnesota.) (See plate 6 for color version.)

compared to adults without modification to the paradigm. Second, passive paradigms may evoke basic perceptual components, without the added activity (or noise) that may be recorded when the subject is engaged in some task and/or a behavioral response is required. The drawback to using a passive task is that it is difficult to determine whether participants maintain attention throughout the task, or whether they are doing the task at all. Depending on the specific hypotheses, it may be important to be able to compare data sets across ages and use other means of monitoring attention (for example, video taping participants to ensure the infant was looking at the stimuli, and/or repeating trials in which it was obvious the participants were not attentive).

Although below the age of 4–5 years traditional button press responses cannot be used, there are some behavioral measures that researchers have used in developmental populations in conjunction with ERPs. The most informative behavioral measures are those that can be directly correlated with the electrophysiological response. For example, after recording ERPs in a visual oddball paradigm using two stimuli with different presentation frequencies, Karrer and Monti (1995) immediately presented the infant with four additional trials, and recorded visual fixations, analogous to a post-test after a traditional behavioral habituation paradigm. Specifically, they presented one of the two stimuli repeatedly until the infant looked away, followed by the presentation of the other stimulus until they looked away, and so on. Similarly, Snyder (2002) employed a design analogous to a habituation/dishabituation procedure that consists of recording ERPs during an initial exposure to a stimulus (the habituation phase), and then recording the duration of infants' visual fixations during a dishabituation phase. Snyder's study is unique in that it reflects a compromise between ERP methodology and stimulus exposure during a conventional infant controlled habituation procedure. During the familiarization phase, trials were continuously presented until the infant either became fussy, or looked away from the screen three times for at least 3 seconds each time. After the familiarization phase, infants were presented with serial presentations of familiar and novel stimuli and allowed one continuous look at each. Infant's visual preferences for test stimuli were computed as the proportion of fixation to the novel stimulus versus the total fixation time. Infants were subsequently divided into three groups: infants who showed a novelty preference at test (looked at the novel stimulus 55% or more of the time), those who showed a familiarity preference (looked at the novel stimulus 45% or less of the time), and those who did not show a preference. This method of combining ERPs with conventional behavioral measures permits researchers to examine directly the relation between preferential looking, which may be indicative of some aspect of attention or memory, and brain activity. A combination of techniques such as this provides information not accessible by either method alone.

Unfortunately, due to the highly constrained testing environment required by ERPs, it is not always feasible to record behavioral measures immediately following ERP collection. Therefore, some researchers have elected to record behavioral measures separately (e.g., after removing the electrodes when the infant is more attentive or better able to perform a required task). For example, Carver, Bauer, and Nelson (2000) combined behavioral performance on a deferred imitation task (which has been purported to tap explicit memory functions; see Bauer, 1995; Nelson, 1995) with electrophysiological responses. Before ERP recording, 9-month-old infants were behaviorally exposed to a unique sequence of events (e.g., the experimenter places a red cylinder into a wooden block, which is then pushed into the base of the apparatus, causing a green dinosaur puppet to pop up). After a one-week delay, the infant's ERP response to photographs of the now familiar event sequence and a novel event sequence were recorded. Four weeks later, the infants' delayed recall performance on the deferred imitation memory task was assessed. Infants were split into groups based on their behavioral performance: those who recalled the sequence and those who did not. Based on these groupings, Carver and colleagues (2000) examined the electrophysiological responses and found differentiation between the familiar and novel conditions for the infants who recalled after a one-month delay, but no such differentiation for the infants who did not display delayed recall.

In short, it is important that researchers continue to ground ERP measures in behavior. Such a combination will yield converging evidence and lead to more reliable results in predominately exploratory studies typical of the field at this time.

Breadth of Developmental ERP Research

Most developmental ERP studies to date have utilized only a single sensory modality to investigate any given cognitive process of interest. For example, recognition memory has typically been investigated using visual stimuli (Nelson, 1997, 1998), whereas language development has primarily utilized auditory stimuli (Cheour, Leppanen, & Kraus, 2000; Mills, Coffey-Corina, & Neville, 1993, 1997; Molfese, Narter, & Modglin, 2002; Molfese & Molfese, 2000). Few developmental ERP studies have used olfactory, gustatory, or tactile stimuli, although there are important exceptions. For example, Nelson, Henschel, and Collins, 1993, and Nelson et al., 2003, have employed a cross-modal task, in which infants are familiarized to a stimulus in the haptic modality and tested for recognition memory in the visual modality. However, it remains unknown whether the components observed in response to stimuli in one modality generalize to stimuli in another, nor is it apparent whether some pre-adult components are modality independent (such as the adult P300).

Over the past two decades, investigators have increasingly begun to use ERPs to examine early cognitive and linguistic development. Some specific abilities that researchers have studied include: attention (e.g., Richards, 2000, 2003; Taylor, Khan, & Malone, 1999), memory (Carver, Bauer, & Nelson, 2000; Nelson, 1995; Nelson & Monk, 2001), face and object processing (Courchesne, Ganz, & Norcia, 1981; de Haan,

Pascalis, & Johnson, 2002; de Haan & Nelson, 1997; Taylor et al., 1999), language (Holcomb, Coffey, & Neville, 1992; Mills & Neville, 1997; Molfese, Narter, & Modglin, 2002; Molfese & Molfese, 2000), and general cognitive development (for review, see Kurtzberg et al., 1984; Regan, 1989).

Developmental ERP Components

In the previous discussion of experimental design, we identified one of the major challenges presented by developmental ERP research as the limited information available on components of interest at various ages. We also commented on the complex changes that occur with increasing age in ERP morphology, amplitude, latency, and topography due to changes in physiology of the head, skull, and underlying brain tissue. In fact, although there are several well-documented infant ERP responses, studies of the development of these responses into more adultlike components remains limited (Nelson & Luciana, 1998). It is generally thought that by the age of 4 years, some semblance of the adult waveform can be discerned. However, relatively little work has been done in children 1.5–4 years of age, and changes in components during this time remain largely undocumented (Nelson & Luciana, 1998).

Extensive discussion of all ERP components found across development is beyond the scope of this *methodological* chapter. However, in the following section, we identify a few developmental ERP components and provide references for recent comprehensive reviews. However, due to space constraints, we will only elaborate on recognition memory components, which have been studied in infants and children in order to elucidate cognitive processes underlying memory development (i.e., the mid-latency negative component, positive slow wave, and negative slow wave activity) and the N170, a component reflecting face processing that has been studied from a developmental perspective from infancy to adulthood. This review of the face-processing component provides an excellent illustration of issues that arise when comparing ERP data across different age groups.

Researchers have identified several ERP components in infants, children, and adolescents (for review see: Nelson, 1994, 1995, 1996; Nelson & Luciana, 1998; Nelson & Monk, 2001; and Taylor & Baldeweg, 2002). These include components that are hypothesized to reflect sensory processing (e.g., the N1 component; Pang & Taylor, 2000; Polich & Luckritz, 1995; Taylor & Baldweg, 2002), obligatory attention (e.g., the negative component or Nc; Nelson, 1996), memory updating (e.g., positive slow wave activity, or PSW; Nelson, 1996), detection of expectant or discrepant events (e.g., the Pb component; Karrer & Ackles, 1990; and mismatch negativity or MMN; Cheour et al., 1998a; Cheour et al., 1998b; Cheour, Leppanen, & Kraus, 2000; Oades, 1997; Shafer, 2000), detection of novelty (e.g., negative slow wave, or NSW; Nelson, 1996), processing of linguistic stimuli, (e.g., the N400 component; Kutas & Hillyard, 1980; Mills, Coffey-Corina, & Neville, 1993; Neville, Mills, & Bellugi, 1994), and general

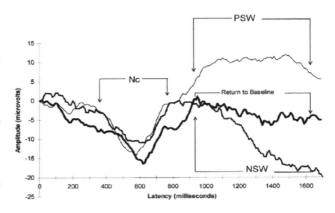

Figure 12.2
Schematic of different components observed in the infant event-related potential during a visual recognition memory task. (Reprinted with permission from M. de Haan and C. A. Nelson, 1997. Recognition of the mother's face by six-month-old infants: A neurobehavioral study. In *Child Development, 68*, 187–210.)

cognitive components commonly found in adults (e.g., the P300, P3a, or P3b; Regan, 1989).

Recognition Memory Components: An Elaboration   The negative component, or Nc, has been consistently observed in recognition memory paradigms (see figure 12.2). The Nc has a well-defined negative peak with maximum amplitude over central and frontal scalp leads (corresponding to Cz and Fz in the 10/20 classification system). The latency of this response generally declines from approximately 1000–1200 ms in the newborn to about 500 ms at 1 year (see Nelson, 1996 for a discussion). This negative peak can easily be discerned in both the single and averaged trial data and is presumed to reflect processes of attention (i.e., obligatory attention; Courchesne, 1977, 1978; Courchesne, Ganz, & Norcia, 1981; Karrer & Ackles, 1987, 1988; Karrer & Monti, 1995; Nelson & Collins, 1991, 1992). Whether this response is exogenous or endogenous in nature has not been determined, although it does share some similarities to the endogenous mismatch negativity in studies of auditory selective attention and is related to both the global and local probabilities of stimuli (Karrer & Ackles, 1990; Nelson & Luciana, 1998). Recently, Reynolds and Richards (2003) have used high-density recording, principle components analysis (PCA), and equivalent current dipole analysis to localize the cortical source of the Nc to several regions of the frontal cortex, including the anterior cingulate.

Following the Nc, there is typically one of three responses: a positive slow wave (PSW), negative slow wave (NSW), or return to baseline (see figure 12.2). Slow wave activity represents a deflection of the brain's electrical response to an event or stimulus, and is thought to reflect general or diffuse activation of neural systems that is characteristic of infant brain responses (de Haan & Nelson, 1997). A PSW is a positive shift late in the waveform that appears maximal at central and frontal scalp locations. It is thought to reflect the partial encoding of a stimulus that requires updating or periodic revision.

The NSW, on the other hand, is a negative shift in the waveform after the resolution of the Nc component that is only observed when novel stimuli are presented against a background of familiar or partially familiar stimuli. Therefore, the NSW is thought to reflect a comparative process, one that detects genuine novelty amidst relatively familiar surroundings (Nelson, 1994) or a disconfirmation of expectancy (Karrer & Ackles, 1990).

Finally, a return to baseline reflects a resolution of the waveform back to baseline indicating that the stimulus does not require memory updating. For example, de Haan and Nelson (1997) found a return to baseline response when 6-month-old infants viewed pictures of their mothers' faces (a fully encoded stimulus), but not when they viewed pictures of an unfamiliar woman's face.

The Face Processing Component: A Developmental Approach   A component that has received considerable attention from a developmental perspective is the N170 (see figure 12.1). In adults, studies using ERPs have found a negatively peaked component occurring approximately 170 ms after stimulus onset that differentiates faces and objects (for example, Jeffreys, 1989; Bentin et al., 1996; Carmel & Bentin, 2002) that is typically prominent over occipital and lateral leads (de Haan, Pascalis, & Johnson, 2002).

As an illustration of the complexities of investigating the development of a typical adult component, we will describe two compelling investigations that have attempted to find the developmental analog of this negative component. First, Taylor et al. (2001) investigated the neural changes associated with face and eye processing using ERPs in children 4–15 years old. Participants were presented with upright and inverted faces and eyes, to determine whether children were using featural versus configural information while processing faces. Findings revealed that the N170 undergoes developmental changes, including a decrease in peak latency and an increase in peak amplitude with increases in age. In addition, de Haan and colleagues (de Haan, Pascalis, & Johnson, 2002) studied both adults and 6-month-olds in a human and nonhuman primate face recognition ERP task in order to determine whether adults and infants show the same cortical specificity during face processing. This study was designed to answer questions regarding the basic nature of the face processing system as well as changes in specificity across development. Adults and infants were shown both non-human primate and human faces in upright and inverted orientations. In adults, all stimuli evoked an N170 over temporal and occipital leads. This N170 was larger in amplitude and longer in latency for upright monkey faces compared to upright human faces. Furthermore, inversion effects (i.e., increased amplitude and latency to inverted faces) were apparent in the human but not the monkey conditions. However, results also indicated that no component of the infant ERP showed the same specificity as the adult N170. Six-month-olds did show sensitivity to both inversion and species but it was distributed across two components in occipitotemporal leads. An early negative component (260–336 ms) was greater to human than monkey faces, and a later positive component (P400) was greater for upright compared to inverted faces. These findings suggest that adultlike patterns of face processing are not evident at 6 months of age. The authors suggest that these findings reflect a gradual specialization of cortical face processing systems. The above results illustrate that comparing components across age groups may be more difficult than originally thought, in that two or more developmental components may later combine into one mature adult component.

There are several factors to consider when identifying and interpreting components and tracking their changes across development. One challenge for future research is to create guidelines for choosing and labeling components that are revealed through new tasks and in previously unstudied age groups. When embarking on such an endeavor, one must keep in mind the variability both within and between participants and rely on subsequent replication before making strong conclusions. Furthermore, because of the relative lack of information on developmental components, it may be necessary for future research to extend initial study hypotheses and report additional components found post hoc. If this is the case, we encourage methods sections of developmental studies to clearly and consistently document paradigm parameters as well as component identification and analysis procedures in an attempt to find consistencies in component identification and selection across studies.

Data Collection Systems

Currently, there are several commercial systems available for purchase and use. These systems differ on features such as electrode and montage type, quantity, location, and placement. A major distinction among systems available to date is whether they are high- or low-density electrode montages. A low-density montage provides less coverage over the scalp (ranging from 1 to 32 electrodes), whereas high-density montages provide greater coverage across the scalp (ranging from 32 to 256 electrodes). The main advantages of high-density systems are increased opportunity for source localization, use of the average reference, and increased ability to detect subcortical electrical activity. When deciding whether to use a high- or low-density system in developmental populations there are several things to consider, such as: (1) where the data will be collected (e.g., in a MRI scanner that does not permit the presence of metal), (2) what hypotheses will guide data analysis (e.g., how important is spatial information), and (3) the proposed dependent measures for data analysis (e.g., amplitude differences at one electrode site or source localization procedures).

We have used two different methods for recording low-density ERPs in our developmental ERP lab. These methods differ in the number of electrodes and the method of placing the electrodes on the scalp. For both methods, the location of electrode placement follows the international 10–20 system of electrode placement commonly used in adults (Jasper, 1958). Each electrode is placed a percentage of the distance between the inion and nasion to ensure the ERPs are being recorded from approximately the same neural structures across all individuals regardless of age or head size. In addition, these low-density systems require slight scalp abrasion and the use of conductance cream in order to conduct the signal into the electrode on the scalp. Abrading the scalp may increase the risk of infection, and although it is not likely to occur, certain precautions are necessary (see Ferree et al., 2001; Putnam, Johnson, & Roth, 1992).

The first low-density approach is derived from methods with adults, in which researchers use a form of glue (collodion) to fix single electrodes filled with conductance cream to the scalp, and a solvent (acetone) to remove them. The advantage to this method is that the electrodes remain in the same place throughout the experiment. However, the disadvantage is that safety glasses, rubber gloves, and ventilation are recommended when using these products, as they may be irritating to the nose and throat. The modification we have used involves first slightly abrading the scalp with a cleansing solution such as NuPrep and holding single electrodes filled with conductance cream (EC2 cream) in place with adhesive backed foam pads, which in turn are held in place with Velcro headbands (see figure 12.3A). In studies with newborns, one can use disposable electrodes—which stick directly to the infant's scalp—instead of the single electrodes and foam (figure 12.3B). The advantage is that this procedure is typically no more aversive than putting on a hat. However, the disadvantage is that the foam pads can stick poorly to infants who have a great deal of hair or where the hair is braided, and thus have the potential to move around on the scalp unless one takes extra care. Typically 6–12 electrodes are used with this procedure, and it is most appropriate for infants under 12 months of age.

The second approach utilizes an electrode cap, made out of Spandex-like material that has electrodes sewn into it at standardized coordinates (this method is also commonly used with adults; see figure 12.3C). The advantage to this procedure is that one can position a greater number of electrodes on the scalp in relatively little time in comparison with the Velcro headband procedure and disposable electrodes. The scalp

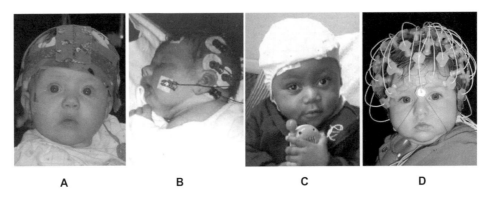

A   B   C   D

Figure 12.3
(A) Infant wearing 16 electrodes held in place with adhesive foam pads and Velcro headbands, (B) single disposable electrodes typically used in the newborn and NICU nurseries, (C) a 32-channel Electro-Cap, and (D) a 64-channel Electro Geodesic Sensor net.

is lightly abraded and conductance jelly inserted under each electrode site after the placement of the cap (this is typically done with a blunt tip syringe and cotton swab). This may be bothersome to some infants as it produces a sensation of a light scratching on the scalp. A chin or chest strap holds the cap in place. Although this strap does not entirely ensure that the cap will not shift on the head during the experiment, it does greatly reduce the risk of electrodes moving out of position. A disadvantage is that some infants' heads are asymmetrical and varied in size, making it difficult to ensure that the electrodes are fixed in the same location. In addition, the chin or chest strap used to hold the electrodes in place may bother some infants. Typically, electrode caps have 16–32 electrodes and can be used with infants as young as 9 months of age up through adulthood.

Recording high-density ERPs in developmental populations has been made possible by the Geodesic Sensor Net (GSN), which allows a very large number of electrodes (ranging from 64 to 256 electrodes) to be applied quickly to the surface of the scalp (Tucker, 1993). The GSN consists of an array of electrodes arranged in an elastic tension structure, which can be relatively quickly and easily slipped on and off the participants' head (see figure 12.3D). The arrangement of electrodes does not follow the international 10–20 system due to the fact that the tension structure conforms to the geometry of each individual's head, but ensures that the electrodes are all equidistant from one another, even on a variety of head shapes (which is a requirement for localization of underlying dipoles). One advantage of the GSN is its high-operating impedance level, which, when combined with amplifiers that allow high-input impedance, removes the need for scalp abrasion and conductance cream. The net is soaked in an electrolyte solution prior to application, which allows the signal to be conducted, recorded, and amplified by the high-input impedance amplifiers. A second advantage is the use of the average reference, which results in an unbiased estimate of noise across the scalp and thus unconfounds estimates of the amplitude and topography of components with the location of the reference electrode. A third advantage is that high-density montage arrays provide greater coverage of the scalp and thus are able to pick up activity in superficial cortical tissue (which, due to its proximity to the scalp, tends to produce smaller, more discrete patterns of activity). Finally, it takes a relatively short amount of time to apply the net in comparison to other procedures (Johnson et al., 2001).

There are a few disadvantages of high-density recordings worth mentioning as well. First, due to the fact that the electrodes are not fixed rigidly to the scalp, movement artifacts are common, and in some cases infants (6–12 months of age and older) may attempt to grab the net, frequently causing displacement and possible damage to the net (Johnson et al., 2001). A second disadvantage is that high-density systems are considerably more expensive than low-density systems, due to the increased cost of equipment and the need for several different net sizes to accommodate small differences in head size among participants. Nets are available in many different sizes, useful with newborns (64 or 128 electrodes), children up to 6 years of age (64 or 128 electrodes), and children age 6 years to adults (64, 128, or 256 electrodes). (For a complete review of recording high-density ERPs and strategies for analyzing high-density data with infants using the GNS, see Johnson et al., 2001.)

Thus far, comparisons of data collected from high- and low-density systems appear similar in quality (Carver et al., 1999; Johnson et al., 2001). The overall advantage of high-density montages is that they may allow for the use of the average reference, source separation and source localization, and due to greater spatial coverage of the scalp, high-density montages may be able to better pick up superficial cortical and subcortical activity. In contrast, low-density systems are more widespread in their use and are less expensive.

Participants

Ages
When selecting participants for a study, one should provide rationale for the selected age group. Common sources of rationale relate to (1) known changes occurring at the neurological or physiological level during some period in development, or (2) changes in behavior that are hypothesized to be related to changes in neurological substrates during a specific time in development. It is important, however, to keep in mind that the relation between ERPs and behavior is associative and not causal (Hood, 2001). Furthermore, as Hood (2001) argues, one should use caution when interpreting ERP data, because ERPs do not reflect the cause of the behavior, nor do they provide an

adequate explanation of the behavior. Areas may become activated simply as a consequence of connections with other more relevant areas. Nonetheless, once an age of interest has been selected for a given study, a specific age range must be set due to changes in ERPs that occur with increases in age. The previous discussion of the complex changes in ERPs should help with conceptualizing the fact that averaging over a wide age range may obscure developmental changes resulting from response variability (Taylor & Baldeweg, 2002). In fact, some recommend that in developmental studies, averages of group ERPs not be combined over more than 1- to 2-month intervals in infant studies, 1–2 years in childhood, and 2–3 years in adolescence (Taylor & Baldeweg, 2002; Picton et al., 2000). Our laboratory (based on knowledge of both brain and child development) typically recommends that averages for infants not be combined over more than 10 days in infants, 1 month in childhood, and 1 year in adolescence. Final decisions regarding age ranges of participant groups must be based on the specifics of each study, including considerations of task demands, task difficulty, and components of interest.

Screening

As in any research study, participants should be screened for several factors that might influence the dependent variable, although specific exclusion criteria may vary depending on the hypotheses, population, and age group of interest. For most populations, one should describe and/or document the following due to presumed or unknown influences these factors may have on the ERP response: age, gender (Hirayasu et al., 2000; Lavioe et al., 1998; Oliver-Rodriguez, Guan, & Johnston, 1999), sensory problems, medications, neurological and psychiatric disorders, and handedness (possibly including handedness of first degree relatives; see Oldfield, 1971, for an example of a handedness assessment). In addition, the following are relevant for developmental populations: pre- or postnatal difficulties, including prematurity (Lavioe et al., 1998; Stolarova et al., 2003), iron deficiency (deRegnier et al., 2000), head size (circumference, inion to nasion, and ear to ear measurements; Polich, Ladish, & Burns, 1990), memory span or intelligence assessment (Polich, Ladish, & Burns, 1990; Stauder, Van Der Molen, & Molenaar, 1998), time of day (especially in relation to feeding, see Geisler & Polich, 1990), and the main source of nutrition in early months of life (i.e., breast milk or formula). Finally, in late childhood and early adolescence it may also be important to document cognitive abilities (e.g., memory span), and pubertal status as studies have found that these factors may influence the ERP response (see Kaiser & Gruzelier, 1999; Polich, Ladish, & Burns, 1990).

Sample Size

A further consideration in developmental ERP studies is the number of participants required to obtain enough power to detect significant results. First, due to large variability in the ERP response (both between and within participants at younger ages), one must take care to ensure adequate power. Second, although collecting ERPs is considered a noninvasive procedure, preparation and participation in ERP studies does require a considerable amount of patience and cooperation on the part of the participant. In developmental populations this requirement is not easily realized. The behavioral and emotional state of young infants and children is extremely variable; many participants are unable to tolerate the preparation procedure or ERP recording and therefore do not produce utilizable data due to extreme fussiness or excessive movement artifacts. It is currently thought that it is this excessive movement (of the eyes and/or head) that accounts for much of the increased variability in developmental groups, although other sources of variability are suspected. Typical infant studies in our lab have enrollment numbers of 40 participants, with an expected 50–75% retention rate that is highly age dependent (e.g., 65% at 9 months, 50% at 12 months). However, we make every attempt to increase the amount of useable data from every session, such as using toys to distract the infant during electrode placement, having multiple testing partners who are experienced with children, and testing at a time of day that is best for the infant (see the section on data collection for more specific suggestions broken down by age group). However, due to high and variable rejection rates of developmental data, one must be mindful of differences that may arise due to the differential ability of infants and young children to successfully complete one condition versus another. Therefore, we strongly recommend that manuscript methods sections include complete descriptions of rejection criteria, including the number of participants indicated by the specific reasons for their exclusion.

Data Collection and Management

Recording

Due to developmental changes in skull thickness (including closure of fontanels in infancy) and variation in cell density, synaptic efficiency, and other physiological parameters, developmental groups require differences in the setup of the data acquisition system. Specifically, amplifier gain settings (i.e., resolution settings) must be altered in order to adequately resolve the ERP signal; sampling rates (i.e., the analog to digital conversion rate) may need to be adjusted in order to register signals of differing frequencies (with the minimum rate being twice the highest frequency of the signal to be measured); and filtering and scoring parameters need to be specified. For instance, in an experiment with 9-month-olds using a low-density Grass-Astromed amplifier, we commonly use a gain of 20,000 μV, a sampling rate of 200 Hz, a notch filter at 60 Hz, and headroom of ±250 μV. However, for the same study in adults, we would use a gain of 50,000 μV, a sampling rate of 200 Hz, a notch filter at 60 Hz, and headroom of ±100 μV. In short, headroom is a function of the range of values accepted by the A/D board

Table 12.1

Recommendations for event-related potential recording parameters in developmental populations

Age	Amplification Factor[a] (Gain)	Sampling Rate	Headroom	Scoring Parameters (A/D units)
0–2 months and 6 years and above	50,000	200 Hz	$\pm 100\ \mu V$	$\pm 100\ \mu V$
3 months to 6 years	20,000	200 Hz	$\pm 250\ \mu V$	± 100 to $\pm 225\ \mu V$[b]

[a]High-density systems, such as the EGI system, have high input impedance amplifiers and gain settings may vary.

[b]For example, using the following equations: Minimum A/D units: $0 + (\text{headroom}/2) - X\ \mu V/\text{precision})$ and Maximum A/D units: $4096 - (\text{headroom}/2) - X\ \mu V/\text{precision})$. If headroom is $\pm 250\ \mu V$, the gain is 20,000, and data that exceeds $\pm 100\ \mu V$ needs to be rejected, the calculation (using a 16-bit data acquisition board) is

Min A/D units: $0 + (250 - 100)\ \mu V/(500/4096)) = \sim 1229$,

Max A/D units: $4096 - (250 - 100)\ \mu V/(500/4096)) = \sim 2867$.

and the gain. For adults, data are typically collected with a $\pm 100\ \mu V$ headroom; this usually does not need to be reduced (or "scored down") any further off line because normal adult brain activity falls within these bounds. However, for infants, due to the large variability and increased amount of movement artifacts, researchers use a wider headroom range for data collection. This range is then reduced off line, in order to remove large artifact signals. Although there is still debate about the range of amplitude of typical infant and child brain activity, current consensus is somewhere between ± 100 to $150\ \mu V$. Table 12.1 provides guidelines from our laboratory. However, these values may differ for various recording systems. Furthermore, these settings may be changed depending on how the data are to be used. For example, if directly comparing 6- and 9-month-olds, it would be appropriate to have the same recording specifications for both ages.

Testing Session Specifics

There are several factors in developmental ERP testing sessions that differ from adult ERP testing sessions. For groups of all ages, researchers should consider the session length (including preparation) and the number of trials attempted and expected to be completed. In our laboratory, we have found the following recommendations useful regardless of the age of the participant group; in the sections following, we make additional recommendations that apply to specific age groups. First, experience with infants and children is desirable due to the fact that the procedure is often a very novel experience to infants and children and it is important to make the participants and their caregivers comfortable. Second, a welcoming preparation room with many toys and "distracter" items will also help both the child and the caregiver feel comfortable in the unfamiliar surroundings during the introduction to the procedure and preparation. In the actual testing room we recommend placing a screen around the area where the infant or child is sitting and removing any distracting items from the room, in order to keep their attention focused on the computer screen. This will help minimize movement artifacts. Finally, we recommend, for all age groups, that the experimenter(s) have some means, either during data collection or during data analysis, to ensure that data are accepted only when the infants are motionless and attending to the stimuli. For example, experimenters could monitor infants' looking during the task and have access to both a repeat button and a pause button. This will reduce artifacts due to either movement or eye blinks and will allow the experimenter to take short breaks from testing if the infant becomes fussy.

Newborns   Data collection with newborn infants involves "passive" viewing or listening paradigms. During auditory tasks newborns are typically in an active state of sleep or awake, and artifacts are uncommon due to the newborn's limited range of movement. In fact, most newborn infants are able to complete 50–200 trials, as the experiment can usually be paused to accommodate changes in the newborn's state (e.g., if the newborn becomes fussy). One important consideration when studying newborns is the portability of the ERP collection system. Often it is desirable to record ERPs within a day of birth, which requires that these studies take place in a hospital setting, preferably in a different hospital room so that disturbance to baby and mother is minimal.

Infants   Data collection in infants also typically involves passive viewing or listening paradigms. For the most part, infants are easily distracted during preparation by playing with a second experimenter, or engaging with toys. Depending on the age and locomotor abilities of the child, we recommend using a highchair or self-contained walker to keep the infant from crawling around the room during preparation. During ERP recording, it is preferable if infants remain in a highchair or car seat in front of the computer screen presenting stimuli, with the caregiver seated a little behind and to the side. It is important to minimize the amount the infant turns to look at his/her caregiver. In some cases, infants may be more comfortable sitting on their caregiver's lap during stimulus presentation and ERP recording, but this typically increases movement artifact. If the infant sits on the caregiver's lap, we recommend instructing the caregiver to let the infant move around only as much as necessary, but request that the caregiver not bounce the infant on his/her knee, as such movement creates artifacts in the data. Furthermore, in looking paradigms (such as habituation paradigms) we suggest that the parent be blindfolded to reduce possible biases.

Often during ERP recording, infants become inattentive, restless, or fussy. Therefore, in visual experiments an experimenter usually sits next to the infant and directs infants' attention to the stimuli by tapping or pointing at the screen. (Note: To decrease potential biases in the data due to artifacts that result from consistent movements to only one side, the side on which the experimenter sits should be counterbalanced or randomized.) Additionally, the experimenter who is directing the infants' attention to the stimuli should be naive to stimuli or conditions of interest in order to reduce possible biases.

In auditory ERP studies, it is also important to achieve eye fixation and reduce movement in order to minimize artifacts. In such cases, providing an interesting screen saver or object (e.g., bubbles) for the infant to watch can be quite useful.

One can either present visual stimuli at a constant rate, with the option to repeat a trial or pause the experiment if the infant is not attending to the stimuli, or the experimenter can control stimulus presentation and only present stimuli when the infant is attending. One experimenter may need to control the stimulus presentation and determine when the infant is attending to the stimulus, while the other experimenter directs the infant's attention. If necessary, the infant may have a pacifier, bottle, dry cereal, cookie, or teether, although there is some concern that sucking on such objects may result in movement artifacts and thus should be well documented and examined to determine any influence such items have on the data (cf. Picton et al., 2000; Johnson et al., 2001).

Younger Children (Ages 2–6 Years) Many of the same concerns that we addressed with infants regarding stimulus presentation and artifacts remain when testing young children. In addition, our laboratory has found it helps to use a theme that makes the experience more interesting and/or familiar (such as referring to the electrode cap as a "toy hat," "astronaut hat," or letting the child put a different cap on a stuffed animal or doll). In addition, if using single adhesive electrodes to record eye movements or for reference electrodes, the experimenter may give stickers to the children to allow some comparison with familiar items. Children may also perform more attentively if the experimenter sits next to them during ERP recording providing words of encouragement at random intervals (e.g., "Great job!" or "Just a few more pictures!").

Older Children (Ages 6–12 Years) Similar concerns addressed with infants and young children regarding stimulus presentation, artifacts, and testing environment remain when testing older children. Additionally, at older ages, a behavioral response (e.g., button press or verbal response) may be desirable. We recommend using a button press with only one or two buttons with older children, as we have found that requiring more than this increases movement artifacts as the children tend to look at their fingers when making responses. In addition, there needs to be enough time between trials for responses due to children's slower reaction times. Finally, one should obtain informed assent from children ages 8 years and above, in addition to obtaining informed consent from their caregiver. When explaining the procedure and obtaining informed assent, one should use caution in order to ensure that both the details of the procedure and the reason for doing the experiment are clear to the child. Furthermore, it should be clear to the child that they can ask questions or withdraw from the experiment at any time if they do not wish to participate.

Adolescents   Although testing adolescents is very similar to testing adults and many of the issues discussed for younger age groups do not apply, one recommendation is that the pubertal status of adolescents be determined due to unknown effects that hormonal changes during this period may have on the central nervous system and, therefore, the ERP response. For example, Kaiser and Gruzelier (1999) reported P3 latency differences in late versus early maturing females at posterior midline electrode sites. It is important to note, however, that this investigation was based on adults' retrospective reports regarding pubertal maturation; therefore, it is not possible to determine what factors other than pubertal timing may have contributed to the pattern of findings.

   In sum, there are several ways to create a more comfortable atmosphere for developmental ERP participants and their caregivers both during preparation and ERP recording. We encourage researchers to try several of the suggestions mentioned above and create new strategies that are appropriate for different types of studies. However, we conclude this section by acknowledging that there is a trade off between entering in exogenous factors that may influence data (e.g., pacifiers, short breaks, etc.) and keeping participants comfortable and happy in order to acquire useable data.

Reference Montages

The appropriate type of recording reference depends primarily on the inter-electrode distance. Typically, low-density montages (32 electrodes or fewer) use a common bipolar reference. The difference in amplitude between the scalp electrode of interest and a reference electrode that is equidistant from all other electrodes (commonly the vertex or Cz in the 10–20 system) is recorded during data collection, and then the data are re-referenced off line to a mathematically linked reference recorded separately from two single sources (e.g., the ear lobes or mastoids). With high-density montages such as the EGI system (64, 128, 256 electrodes), researchers typically use an average reference, calculated by subtracting the mean of all electrodes from each channel. An important note here is that it is not the density that determines the type of reference per se, but instead the inter-electrode distance. Experimenters can use an average reference when the inter-electrode distance is less than 2–3 cm. Junghöfer and colleagues (1997) suggest that the optimal number of electrodes on an adult head is approximately 256, and on the infant head about 128 (although 64, and possibly 32, electrodes can yield a sampling density of less than 3 cm in infants depending on the age of the infant and size of the infant's head; Junghöfer et al., 1997, cited in Johnson et al., 2001).

In our experience, the best way to record a linked reference is by affixing electrodes to an adhesive foam pad and placing them behind the infant's or child's ears on the mastoid bone. However, this is problematic if the infant has a great deal of hair; the adhesive pad may stick to the hair and not remain in place. Ear clips are also available that clip to the infant's ear lobes, but our lab has found that these do not consistently remain on the infant's ears and have to be replaced frequently during the recording session. In contrast, an average reference is recorded from one of the electrodes on the scalp (usually the vertex) and therefore does not present any unique problems except ensuring that this essential electrode has a low impedance connection with the scalp.

Data Reduction

Artifact Rejection   Artifacts refer to unwanted noise in the ERP signal that can result from many sources. The largest source of artifact in infant ERPs is movement artifact unrelated to EMG (i.e., high-amplitude or off-scale activity as opposed to high-frequency activity of electromyogram, or EMG). However, artifacts can also be caused by EMG (e.g., head or body movements) and eye movements (e.g., blinking). In the previous section, we made several suggestions as to how to reduce artifacts and ensure that the infant attends to the stimuli. Far more challenging are artifacts resulting from eye movements, which may disproportionately contaminate anterior recording electrodes. These artifacts may result in the misattribution of the component source to the frontal region of the brain, when it rightly belongs in the eyes and should be excluded from data analysis (Nelson, 1994). Fortunately, infant ERPs tend to be much larger than adult ERPs (most likely due to physiological differences such as thinner skulls and less dense cell packing in brain tissue). As a result, developmental researchers have found that it takes considerably more eye activity to contaminate the ERP signal in infants compared to adults (see Nelson, 1994 for further discussion). However, to ensure against contamination due to electro-oculogram (EOG) activity, we recommend recording eye movements, using computer algorithms and visual inspection of the data to identify and delete corrupted trials (see Nelson, 1994, for details).

Specifically, our lab uses a bipolar recording for the EOG recording (i.e., referencing the upper eye to the lower eye), which provides us with a measure of the eye activity itself. Typically, the recording configuration consists of two electrodes placed on the supra and inferior orbital ridges of the eye. This configuration allows for detecting blinks and, with somewhat less precision, horizontal eye movements (e.g., saccades).

In an ideal situation, recording both vertical and horizontal eye movements is preferable, but from a practical perspective, if participants are not able to tolerate multiple electrodes near the eye, vertical eye movements are considered more essential and should be recorded. If the study involves presenting stimuli in the periphery, it is necessary to record both vertical and horizontal eye movements. Although it is becoming increasingly common with adult participants to use mathematical routines for identifying and subtracting artifacts due to eye movements to preserve the trial for averaging and analysis, this technique should only be used when it is ensured that the infant's eyes were not moving during stimulus presentation. Moreover, given differences in head size and shape between infants and adults, different propagation factors may dictate the utilization of different algorithms for subtracting EOG artifacts. In practice, our lab has adopted the following procedures for dealing with EOG activity. If the EOG activity exceeds 250 μV, we reject the entire trial. If EOG activity is below 250 μV *and* the infant's eyes were fixated during the stimulus presentation, we apply a blink correction algorithm (Gratton, Coles, & Donchin, 1983). After editing the data for EOG artifacts, we visually inspect each individual participant's data; if it appears that eye movements were occurring consistently and appear to distort the ERP signal, especially at the anterior electrode sites, we reject those trials from the average and subsequent analyses.

With older children, blink activity remains a problem, and although they may be able to follow instructions, we do not recommend giving instructions regarding eye movements (i.e., blinking). However, if instructions become necessary, we recommend that participants be instructed *when* to blink, as opposed to when *not* to blink, and that these instructions be given in a similar manner across all conditions to all participants as they may alter the ERP response by adding an additional component to the task (Ochoa & Polich, 2000).

When editing data for artifacts, one can detect many benign sources of activity (e.g., head movements, eye movements, blinks, and so on). In addition, sources of abnormal activity, such as seizure activity, may also become apparent during data collection or data analysis. A final recommendation is that researchers be generally familiar with the appearance of seizure activity and establish procedures for reporting it if and when it is suspected (either during or after data collection). Although this is very rare, due to the young age of some participants, many seizure disorders may not yet be detected (situations such as this are similar to incidental findings of structural abnormalities in the brains of normal or typical participants in fMRI studies and should be handled in a similar manner). Notifying the parents of such a possible concern should be done with great care and accompanied with a referral to a competent physician.

Averaging Another issue pertinent to developmental ERP data concerns the large variability in waveforms (both between and within subjects). Indeed, Nelson and colleagues report more between-subject variability in infants than in adults and children tested under the same conditions (Nelson, 1994). Although part of this variability is the result of increases in artifacts (as discussed above), there is a great deal of variability between subjects as a function of the total number of trials contributed by each infant during the ERP session (Snyder, Webb, & Nelson, 2002). Infants vary widely in the number of trials they complete in an ERP session, with some completing as few as 20 trials and others completing over 100 trials. Importantly, between-subject differences that arise from differences in the number of completed trials have been associated with both amplitude and latency differences in certain components (e.g., the Nc component in 6-month-olds; see Snyder, Webb, & Nelson, 2002).

In addition to the differences that lead to increased between-subject variability, there is often a great deal of within-subject variability in developmental ERP data. In fact, some have reported variability in the infant's brain response to the same stimulus over time. Differences in topography (of both the Nc and slow wave activity) have been detected in the same subject's data depending on whether the first half or the second half of their data from one testing session was included in their final data set. These differences may depend on the infant's familiarity with the stimulus (Snyder, Webb, & Nelson, 2002), yet they also may arise from state changes in the infant during data collection (e.g., changes in sleepiness, fussiness, or comfort level).

Such individual differences are important and can be analyzed separately to answer a different line of questions. However, these differences can result in an extraordinary amount of variability in group data sets. In fact, it is not uncommon to fail to find statistical differences between two experimental conditions that visually appear to be vastly different from one another. These findings may, of course, reflect the actual equivalence of two experimental conditions. However, null findings can also be due to insufficient power to detect differences due to large between and within subject variability. Although methods for analyzing such variability exist (e.g., analyzing variances instead of means) these methods are not common in the literature due to the fact they are mathematically complex and not easily implemented or interpretable (Nelson, 1994; Taylor & Baldeweg, 2002). Therefore, our solution to date has been to collect as many artifact free trials as possible from a large number of infants and to be conservative in reporting our findings (Nelson, 1994). Although it varies from study to study, our current heuristic is to require that an infant contribute *at least* 10–20 artifact-free trials to their individual average and at least 10–15 infants contribute data for each experimental condition. Without these or more stringent criteria, the signal-to-noise ratio is often compromised and significant results remain elusive despite genuine differences between experimental conditions (i.e., a type II error). Therefore, we recommend that investigators report estimates of effect size and conduct power analyses to determine the number of participants required to obtain significant effects and caution the interpretation of null findings with small sample sizes.

Statistical Analysis

In the following sections we comment on the utilization of different techniques used to statistically analyze developmental data, including ANOVA and MANOVA, hierarchical linear modeling (HLM), independent components analysis (ICA), and principle components analysis (PCA). For a full discussion, we refer the reader to other chapters in this book on these selected topics, as our discussion will highlight concepts that are especially relevant when working with developmental data.

In adult ERP studies, the typical dependent or response variables include average or peak amplitude, area below or above the curve, and latency to peak measurements. The independent or predictor variables include condition or task factors. Researchers typically use average amplitude measurements and area measures with components that do not exhibit a distinctly peaked component. For example, some investigators have used average amplitude to analyze the N400 component (e.g., Eimer, 2000; Bentin & Deouell, 2000). For data occurring in longer latency windows, such as slow wave activity, researchers typically use area measurements. Area measurements tend to be less sensitive to noise but may also underestimate differences among participants, conditions, and electrodes (van Boxtel, 1998). For clearly defined components, such as the N170 or the P300, researchers often use peak amplitude and corresponding latency measures with similar criteria as those used in adult data (Carmel & Bentin, 2002; Donchin et al., 1983).

Statistical Tests

Currently, statistical analyses that use the appropriate dependent variable mentioned above are similar if not the same as those analyses conducted with adult ERP data. Picton and colleagues (2000), as well as van Boxtel (1998), provide guidelines for statistical analyses with ERP data that we summarize briefly. The experimenter should use statistical analyses that are appropriate to both the nature of the data and the goal of the study. Typically, one uses repeated measures ANOVA models to test hypotheses with ERP data (see chapter 4 of this volume). As with any ANOVA, repeated measures ANOVAs test the equality of means. This type of analysis is used when all members of a random sample are measured under a number of different conditions. As the sample is exposed to each condition, the measurement of the dependent variable is repeated (i.e., amplitude or latency at different leads). Using ANOVA techniques is not appropriate in this case because it fails to model the correlation between the repeated measures (the psychophysiological data often violate the ANOVA assumption of independence). To compensate for violations, one can reduce the degrees of freedom by calculating epsilon, as described by Greenhouse and Geisser (1959) or Huynh and Feldt (1970).

One can also use MANOVA analyses to analyze ERP data. As long as the sample size exceeds the number of repeated measures by "a few," MANOVA analyses will range from being slightly less powerful than the adjusted method (described above) to infinitely more powerful (Davidson, 1972). Davidson (1972) suggests that the MANOVA approach is the best in cases when one expects small but reliable effects. He also suggests that when using MANOVA, one should choose a sample size that exceeds the number of repeated measurements by 20 or more. Thus, the only case when one should use adjusted ANOVA tests is when the sample size becomes as small as the number of repeated measurements in the design. These typical statistical methods used with ERP data in adults (ANOVA, MANOVA, etc.) that can also be utilized for the statistical analysis of developmental ERP data have several assumptions. For instance, (1) there cannot be any missing data (cases are deleted listwise), (2) all subjects must be measured at the same equally spaced time points (e.g., using the same leads across all subjects), (3) the response variable must be normally distributed, and (4) there is homogeneity of variance (either across time or across measurements). Violations in the above assumptions that, unfortunately, are often common in developmental ERP data, result in deletion of cases and an unbalanced design. However, recent statistical advances such as the use of hierarchical linear modeling (HLM) to analyze longitudinal and repeated measure data sets may be especially relevant for developmental ERP data due to the fact that it is not constrained by these assumptions. For example, HLM can accommodate unbalanced designs or data sets by estimating missing data. This accommodation may allow researchers to include more data that ultimately results in an increase in the retention rate. HLM can be used to include data from participants who may have unusable or artifact contaminated data at specific electrode locations (e.g., subjects with data that was selectively contaminated at anterior electrode sites by eye artifacts). Furthermore, infants will often only finish one of two experimental conditions (e.g., due to fussiness). The use of HLM may allow one to keep data from the first condition for subsequent data analysis, as opposed to deleting all of this participant's data.

Source Separation and Localization Techniques

An increase in the number of electrodes and a concomitant decrease in inter-electrode distances results in increased spatial resolution in high-density recording methods (see chapter 8 of this volume). Conventional methods of analyzing ERP data do not take advantage of this added spatial information; thus, several investigators have used source separation and localization techniques to statistically identify source generators in the brain (for further illustration, see Johnson et al., 2001; Reynolds & Richards, 2003; and Richards, 2000).

A well-known challenge in ERP research is localizing activity that is volume conducted to the scalp surface. This problem, known as the inverse problem, refers to the relative difficulty we have calculating the distribution of electrical current in the brain from surface measurements (see chapter 7 of this volume). Electrical recordings taken from the scalp reflect a mixture of the activity of a number of underlying neural sources (dipoles) in the brain. Source separation consists of identifying sources that account for the largest portion of variance in the data. One method of source separation is independent component analysis (ICA), which decomposes spatiotemporal data into separate, or independent, components. One can think of ICA as an extension of a more commonly applied method, principal component analysis (PCA), which uses factor analysis to identify the components that account for the largest amount of variance in the data, then the next largest and so on. Compared to ICA, which is not restricted to normally distributed components, PCA yields statistically independent components if they are normally distributed (Johnson et al., 2001). ICA assumes that electrical activity recorded at scalp electrode sites represents a linear combination of the concurrent electrical activity evoked by networks of neurons within the brain. It is assumed that these networks are spatially fixed and operate independently in time. However, the "sources" of ICA components may be one or more distributed brain networks rather than modularly active brain regions. Source localization procedures assume that brain networks (or dipoles) are physically isolated from one another, whereas ICA procedures only assume that brain networks act independently. Therefore, ICA may be useful as a preprocessing step prior to attempting source localization (Makeig et al., 1996). However, this does not solve the problem of source localization. Johnson and colleagues (2001) suggest that ICA may be useful in reducing intertrial variability in analyses of infant ERP data. They state that ICA may be able to extract components from more noisy data (common in infant data) that are similar to those extracted from a data set that has been previously corrected for artifacts. In sum, for developmental ERP data, ICA could provide a method for examining both intersubject and intertrial variability.

Source localization is a different process than source separation. Source localization attempts to identify the location, orientation, and magnitude of dipoles in the brain that may be responsible for specific ERP components (Nunez, 1990). The software package Brain Electrical Source Analysis (BESA) identifies candidate dipoles in the brain by analyzing the distribution of electrical activity recorded at the scalp (Scherg & Berg, 1996). This activity is applied to simplified models of the head in order to determine neural sources. Johnson and colleagues (2001) voice several concerns regarding the use of source localization methods in infants. First, skull thickness, density, and fontanel closure are different in adults relative to infants. Thus, localization techniques used with adults may not be applicable to all developmental populations. Second, the spherical head model used in source localization may be less appropriate for developmental populations, as factors such as skull thickness and head circumference may be more variable in infant compared to adult populations. To date, there are currently no software packages (such as BESA) that attempt to compensate for these differences. Developmentally appropriate head models may increase the feasibility of source localization in developmental populations. Although high-density ERP techniques appear to provide researchers will the ability to estimate sources of neural activity, source localization should only be combined with strong theoretical foundations concerning anatomical localization (e.g., Richards, 2003). In fact, Hood argues that although relatively specific areas may "light up" under some conditions, such localization is of limited value on its own as explanation, and provocatively claims that "in most cases it [source localization] simply confirms the experimenters expectation that there is event-related activity occurring in the brain" (Hood, 2001, p. 215).

Converging Measures

A general consensus in psychology is that the most reliable test of a theory is convergent evidence. It is not surprising, then, that many have begun to argue that ERPs should be used in conjunction with other imaging techniques, such as fMRI, and behavioral measures, such as reaction time. The combination of these techniques and measures provides complementary information that may strengthen data interpretations (see chapter 15 of this volume).

Specifically, due to the excellent spatial resolution of fMRI and superior temporal resolution of ERPs, the combination of these two techniques is well suited to provide spatiotemporal information superior to either method alone (de Haan & Thomas, 2002). For example, research on face processing, face detection, and recognition of facial expressions of emotion has combined ERP and fMRI research, and similar collaborative innovations are encouraged in other areas (for further discussion see de Haan & Thomas, 2002).

ERPs and Special Populations

Recently several researchers have begun to use ERPs as a tool to investigate deficits and impairments across a wide range of developmental disorders, including autism spectrum disorder (Dawson et al., 2002a, 2002b), attention deficit hyperactivity disorder (Jonkman et al., 2000), language disorders (Molfese, Molfese, & Modglin, 2001), individuals who have experienced maltreatment (Pollak et al., 2001), individuals who are at high risk for alcoholism (Hill et al., 1999), or individuals who, due to pre- or perinatal complications, are at risk for neurobehavioral sequelae (deRegnier, Georgieff, & Nelson, 1997; deRegnier et al., 2000; Nelson et al., 2000; for review of examples of atypical development, see Nelson & Luciana, 1998). For example, Dawson et al. (2002a) used high-density ERPs to examine whether children with autism spectrum disorder (ASD) have impairments in face recognition abilities that originate at the cortical level. Relative to a typically developing group of children and a group of children with developmental delays, children with ASD failed to show differences in ERPs to familiar (i.e., their mother's face) versus unfamiliar faces, but did show differentiation to familiar versus unfamiliar toys. These results imply that children with autism may have deficits in face processing cortical circuitry but concurrent sparing of object processing circuitry.

Indeed, combined with typical behavioral assessment and diagnostic tools, ERPs may prove useful in understanding developmental disorders, as well as for prevention and intervention programs (Otto et al., 1984). Elucidation of the cause, nature, and treatment of childhood disorders may require an integration of approaches and empirical techniques informed by multilevel analyses from brain to behavior. Although the application of ERP techniques to special populations for clinical purposes is encouraging, researchers must exert caution when looking at individual and group data. Results are often based on averaged responses from groups of individuals, and until single-trial analyses are possible in individual participants, such research is limited to general statements regarding groups of individuals who have experienced a set of common circumstances or exhibit similar symptoms.

Future Directions

There are several areas of developmental ERP research in need of improvement. First, more headway in grounding developmental ERP research in behavior is needed. Researchers need to use new behavioral measures in conjunction with ERP measures, and need to design new paradigms that facilitate a convergence of behavioral and electrophysiological data. Second, future research should aim to explore the development of ERP components. We can combine such knowledge with our increasing knowledge of the development of the brain in order to refine data collection parameters. This will allow ERP recordings to accurately capture the dynamic development of the brain. Third, we should apply statistical methods that can accommodate missing data to developmental data sets. This strategy will help ensure that valuable information is not lost due to insufficient statistical techniques. In addition, experimenters should alter algorithms used to identify artifacts in adult ERP data analysis to accommodate the wide variability in infant data. This will ensure that similar techniques will be useful across age groups. Finally, if researchers continue to use source localization techniques, they need to develop parameters suitable for infant and child data and establish them in available software.

In conclusion, the challenges of developmental research include issues ranging from designing studies that are sufficiently interesting in order to recruit and sustain infants' attention, to successfully placing the desired number of electrodes on infants' heads, to the careful reduction of variability in data and rejection of artifact contaminated data. However, the ultimate challenge in conducting developmental ERP research is to take what we know from other areas of research, which utilize different methodologies, and combine this information with electrophysiological data in innovative ways to produce converging evidence in support of theoretical claims. The use of consistent and appropriate methods will, we hope, contribute to this goal. Furthermore, we hope that methods for developmental ERP research will continue to be refined. We underscore the importance of a collaborative approach that will prove to be the most powerful tool in examining complex developmental changes in the brain from infancy forward.

Acknowledgments

The authors would like to thank the members of the Developmental Cognitive Neuroscience and the Cognition in the Transition labs at the University of Minnesota for their comments on the chapter. Support for the writing of this chapter was made possible by grants to the third author from the NIH (NS329976), and to the second author from a training grant from the National Institute of Child Health & Human Development to the Center for Cognitive Sciences at the University of Minnesota (5T32 HD07151).

Note

1. The field of developmental electrophysiology is continually evolving; subsequently, developmental electrophysiological research remains a broad area. Currently, the term *developmental* is used not only to refer to authentic change overtime (e.g., changes in components, changes in brain structures, or changes in children's behavior) but also is used to refer to research that, ultimately, will contribute to knowledge regarding such change. Therefore, in this chapter, we will use "developmental" to refer to both circumstances (e.g., studying the development of actual entities, such as components, and the utilization of ERP components in developmental [i.e., child] populations to better understand development more generally).

References

Bauer, P. J. (1995). Recalling past events: From infancy to early childhood. *Annals of Child Development, 11*, 25–71.

Bentin, S., Allison, T., Puce, A., Perez, E., & McCarthy, G. (1996). Electrophysiological studies of face perception in humans. *Journal of Cognitive Neuroscience, 8*, 551–565.

Bentin, S., & Deouell, L. Y. (2000). Structural encoding and identification in face processing: ERP evidence for separate mechanisms. *Cognitive Neuropsychology, 17*, 35–54.

Carmel, D., & Bentin, S. (2002). Domain specificity versus expertise: Factors influencing distinct processing of faces. *Cognition, 83*, 1–29.

Carver, L. J., Bauer, P. J., & Nelson, C. A. (2000). Associations between infant brain activity and recall memory. *Developmental Science, 3*, 234–246.

Carver, L. J., Wewerka, S. S., Gary, J. W., Panagiotides, H., Tribby-Walbridge, S. R., Rinaldi, J. A., & Werner, E. B. (1999). Neural correlates of recognition memory during the second year of life. Poster presented at the Biennial Meeting of the Society for Research in Child Development, Albuquerque, NM.

Cheour, M., Alho, K., Ceponiene, R., Reinikainen, K., Sainio, K., Pohjavuori, M., Aaltonen, O., & Naeaetaenen, R. (1998a). Maturation of mismatch negativity in infants. *International Journal of Psychophysiology, 29,* 217–226.

Cheour, M., Ceponiene, R., Lehtokoski, A., Luuk, A., Allik, J., Alho, K., & Naatanen, R. (1998b). Development of language-specific phoneme representations in the infant brain. *Nature Neuroscience, 1,* 351–353.

Cheour, M., Leppanen, P. H. T., & Kraus, N. (2000). Mismatch negativity as a tool for investigating auditory discrimination and sensory memory in infants and children. *Clinical Neurophysiology, 111,* 4–16.

Courchesne, E. (1977). Event-related potentials: A comparison between children and adults. *Science, 197,* 589–592.

Courchesne, E. (1978). Neurophysiological correlates of cognitive development: Changes in long-latency event-related potentials from childhood to adulthood. *Electroencephalography and Clinical Neurophysiology, 45,* 468–482.

Courchesne, E., Ganz, L., & Norcia, A. M. (1981). Event-related brain potentials to human faces in infants. *Child Development, 52,* 804–811.

Davidson, M. L. (1972). Univariate versus multivariate tests in repeated-measures experiments. *Psychological Bulletin, 77,* 446–452.

Davis, E. P., Bruce, J., Snyder, K., & Nelson, C. A. (2003). The X-trials: Neural correlates of an inhibitory control task in children and adults. *Journal of Cognitive Neuroscience, 77,* 432–443.

Dawson, G., Carver, L., Meltzoff, A., Panagiotides, H., McPartland, J., & Webb, S. J. (2002a). Neural correlates of face and object recognition in young children with autism spectrum disorder, developmental delay and typical development. *Child Development, 73,* 700–717.

Dawson, G., Webb, S., Schellenberg, G. D., Dager, S., Friedman, S., Aylward, E., & Richards, T. (2002b). Defining the broader phenotype of autism: Genetic, brain, and behavioral perspectives. *Development & Psychopathology, 14,* 581–611.

de Haan, M., & Nelson, C. A. (1997). Recognition of the mother's face by 6-month-old infants: A neurobehavioral study. *Child Development, 68,* 187–210.

de Haan, M., Pascalis, O., & Johnson, M. H. (2002). Specialization of neural mechanisms underlying face recognition in human infants. *Journal of Cognitive Neuroscience, 12,* 199–209.

de Haan, M., & Thomas, K. M. (2002). Application of ERP and fMRI techniques to developmental science. *Developmental Science, 5,* 335–343.

deRegnier, R.-A. O., Georgieff, M. K., & Nelson, C. A. (1997). Cognitive event-related potentials in four-month-old infants at risk for neurodevelopmental impairments. *Developmental Psychobiology, 30*, 11–28.

deRegnier, R.-A., Nelson, C. A., Thomas, K., Wewerka, S., & Georgieff, M. K. (2000). Neurophysiologic evaluation of auditory recognition memory in healthy newborn infants and infants of diabetic mothers. *Journal of Pediatrics, 137*, 777–784.

Donchin, E., McCarthy, G., Kutas, M., & Ritter, W. (1983). Event-related brain potentials in the study of consciousness. In R. J. Davidson, G. E. Schwartz, & D. Shapiro (Eds.), *Consciousness and self-regulation Vol. 3*, (pp. 81–121). New York: Plenum.

Eimer, M. (2000). Effects of face inversion on the structural encoding and recognition of faces: Evidence from event-related brain potentials. *Cognitive Brain Research, 10*, 145–158.

Ferree, T. C., Luu, P., Russell, G. S., & Tucker, D. M. (2001). Scalp electrode impedance, infection risk, and EEG data quality. *Clinical Neurophysiology, 112*, 536–544.

Friedman, D., Brown, C. III., Cornblatt, B., Vaughan, H. G., & Erlenmeyer-Kimling, L. (1984). Changes in the late task-related brain potentials during adolescence. *Annals of the New York Academy of Sciences, 425*, 344–352.

Geisler, M. W., & Polich, J. (1990). P300 and time of day: Circadian rhythms, food intake, and body temperature. *Biological Psychology, 31*, 117–136.

Gratton, G., Coles, M. G. H., & Donchin, E. (1983). A new method of off-line removal of ocular artifact. *Electroencephalography and Clinical Neurophysiology, 55*, 468–484.

Greenhouse, S. W., & Geisser, S. (1959). On methods in the analysis of profile data. *Psychometrika, 24*, 95–112.

Hill, S. Y., Shen, S., Locke, J., Steinhauer, S. R., Konicky, C., Lowers, L., & Connolly, J. (1999). Developmental delay in P300 production in children at high risk for developing alcohol-related disorders. *Biological Psychiatry, 46*, 970–981.

Hirayasu, Y., Samura, M., Ohta, H., & Ogura, C. (2000). Sex effects on rate of change of P300 latency with age. *Clinical Neurophysiology, 111*, 187–194.

Holcomb, P. J., Coffey, S. A., & Neville, H. J. (1992). Visual and auditory sentence processing: A developmental analysis using event-related brain potentials. *Developmental Neuropsychology, 8*, 203–241.

Hood, B. M. (2001). Combined electrophysiological and behavioral measurement in developmental cognitive neuroscience: Some cautionary notes. *Infancy, 2*, 213–217.

Huynh, H., & Feldt, L. S. (1970). Conditions under which mean square ratios in repeated measures designs have exact F-distributions. *Journal of the American Statistical Association, 65*, 1582–1589.

Jasper, H. H. (1958). The ten-twenty electrode system of the international federation. *Electroencephalography Clinical Neurophysiology, 10*, 371–375.

Jeffreys, D. A. (1989). A face-responsive potential recorded from the human scalp. *Experimental Brain Research, 78*, 193–202.

Johnson, M. H., de Haan, M., Oliver, A., Smith, W., Hatzakis, H., Tucker, L. A., & Cisbra, G. (2001). Recording and analyzing high-density event-related potentials with infants using the geodesic sensor net. *Developmental Neuropsychology, 19*, 295–323.

Jonkman, L. M., Kemner, C., Verbaten, M. N., Van Engeland, H., Camfferman, G., Buitelaar, J. K., & Koelega, H. S. (2000). Attentional capacity, a probe ERP study: Differences between children with attention-deficit hyperactivity disorder and normal control children and effects of methylphenidate. *Psychophysiology, 37*, 334–346.

Junghöfer, M., Elbert, T., Leiderer, P., Berg, P., & Rockstroh, B. (1997). Mapping EEG-potentials on the surface of the brain: A strategy for uncovering cortical sources. *Brain Topography, 9*, 203–217.

Kaiser, J., & Gruzelier, J. H. (1999). Effects of pubertal timing on EEG coherence and P3 latency. *International Journal of Psychophysiology, 34*, 225–236.

Karrer, R., & Ackles, P. K. (1987). Visual event-related potentials of infants during a modified oddball procedure. In R. Johnson, Jr., J. W. Rohrbaugh, & R. Parasuraman (Eds.), *Current trends in event-related potential research. Vol. 40 Electroencephalography and clinical neurophysiology supplement* (pp. 603–608). Amsterdam: Elsevier.

Karrer, R., & Ackles, P. K. (1988). Brain organization and perceptual/cognitive development in normal and Down syndrome infants: A research program. In P. M. Vietze & H. G. Vaughan, Jr. (Eds.), *Early identification of infants with developmental disabilities* (pp. 210–234). New York: Guilford Press.

Karrer, R., & Ackles, P. K. (1990). ERP evidence for expectancy in six-month-old infants. In C. H. M. Brunia, A. W. K. Gillard, & A. Kolk (Eds.), *Psychophysiological brain research, Vol. 2* (pp. 157–160). Tilburg: Tilburg University Press.

Karrer, R., & Monti, L. A. (1995). Event-related potentials of 4–7-week-old infants in a visual recognition memory task. *Electroencephalography and Clinical Neurology, 94*, 414–424.

Kurtzberg, D., Vaughan, H. G. Jr., Courchesne, E., Friedman, D., Harter, M. R., & Putnam, L. E. (1984). Developmental aspects of event-related potentials. *Annals of the New York Academy of Sciences, 425*, 300–318.

Kutas, M., & Hillyard, S. A. (1980). Reading senseless sentences: Brain potentials reflect semantic incongruity. *Science, 207*, 203–205.

Lavioe, M. E., Robaey, P., Stauder, J. E. A., Glorieux, J., & Lefebvre, F. (1998). Extreme prematurity in healthy 5-year-old children: A re-analysis of sex effects on event-related brain activity. *Psychophyisology, 35*, 679–689.

Makeig, S., Bell, A. J., Jung, T.-P., & Sejnowski, T. J. (1996). Independent component analysis of electroencephalographic data. *Advances in Neural Information Processing Systems, 8*, 145–151.

Mills, D. L., Coffey-Corina, S. A., & Neville, H. J. (1993). Language acquisition and cerebral specialization in 20-month-old infants. *Journal of Cognitive Neuroscience, 5*, 317–334.

Mills, D. L., Coffey-Corina, S., & Neville, H. J. (1997). Language comprehension and cerebral specialization from 13 to 20 months. *Developmental Neuropsychology, 13*, 397–445.

Mills, D., & Neville, H. J. (1997). Electrophysiological studies of language and language impairment. In I. Rappin & R. Nass (Eds.), Special issue: EEG, ERP, and MEG in children with developmental and acquired language disorders. *Seminars in Pediatric Neurology, 4*, 125–134.

Molfese, D. L., & Molfese, V. J. (2000). The continuum of language development during infancy and early childhood: Electrophysiological correlates. In C. Rovee-Collier, L. P. Lipsitt, & H. Hayne (Eds.), *Progress in infancy research, Vol. 1* (pp. 251–287). Mahwah, NJ: Lawrence Erlbaum Associates, Inc.

Molfese, D. L., Molfese, V. L., & Espy, K. A. (1999). The predictive use of event-related potentials in language development and the treatment of language disorders. *Developmental Neuropsychology, 16*, 373–377.

Molfese, V. J., Molfese, D. L., & Modgline, A. A. (2001). Newborn and preschool predictors of second-grade reading scores: An evaluation of categorical and continuous scores. *Journal of Learning Disabilities, 34*, 545–554.

Molfese, D. L., Narter, D. B., & Modglin, A. (2002). The relation between language development and brain activity. In Dennis L. Molfese & Victoria J. Molfese (Eds.), *Developmental variations in learning: Applications to social, executive function, language, and reading skills* (pp. 187–224). Mahwah, NJ: Lawrence Erlbaum Associates, Inc.

Nelson, C. A. (1994). Neural correlates of recognition memory in the first postnatal year of life. In G. Dawson & K. Fischer (Eds.), *Human behavior and the developing brain* (pp. 269–313). New York: Guilford Press.

Nelson, C. A. (1995). The ontogeny of human memory: A cognitive neuroscience perspective. *Developmental Psychology, 31*, 723–738.

Nelson, C. A. (1996). Electrophysiological correlates of memory development in the first year of life. In H. W. Reese & M. D. Franzen (Eds.), *Thirteenth West Virginia University conference on life span developmental psychology: Biological and neuropsychological mechanisms* (pp. 95–131). Mahwah, NJ: Lawrence Erlbaum.

Nelson, C. A. (1997). The neurobiological basis of early memory development. In N. Cowan (Ed.), *The Development of Memory in Childhood* (pp. 41–82). Hove, East Sussex: Psychology Press.

Nelson, C. A. (1998). The nature of early memory. *Preventive Medicine, 27*, 172–179.

Nelson, C. A., & Collins, P. F. (1991). Event-related potential and looking time analysis of infants' responses to familiar and novel events: Implications for visual recognition memory. *Developmental Psychology, 27*, 50–58.

Nelson, C. A., & Collins, P. F. (1992). Neural and behavioral correlates of recognition memory in 4- and 8-month-old infants. *Brain and Cognition, 19,* 105–121.

Nelson, C. A., Henschel, M., & Collins, P. F. (1993). Neural correlates of cross-modal recognition memory by 8-month-old infants. *Developmental Psychology, 29,* 411–420.

Nelson, C. A., & Luciana, M. (1998). Electrophysiological studies II: Evoked potentials and event-related potentials. In C. E. Coffey & R. A. Brumback (Eds.), *Textbook of pediatric neuropsychiatry* (pp. 331–356). Washington, D.C.: American Psychiatric Press.

Nelson, C. A., & Luciana, M. (2001). *Handbook of developmental cognitive neuroscience.* Cambridge, MA: MIT Press.

Nelson, C. A., & Monk, C. (2001). The use of event-related potentials in the study of cognitive development. In C. A. Nelson & M. Luciana (Eds.), *Handbook of developmental cognitive neuroscience* (pp. 125–136). Cambridge, MA: MIT Press.

Nelson, C. A., Wewerka, S., Borscheid, A. J., deRegnier, R.-A., & Georgieff, M. K. (2003). Electrophysiologic evidence of impaired cross-modal recognition memory in 8-month-old infants of diabetic mothers. *Journal of Pediatrics, 142,* 575–582.

Nelson, C. A., Wewerka, S., Thomas, K. M., Tribby-Walbridge, S., deRegnier, R.-A., & Georgieff, M. (2000). Neurocognitive sequelae of infants of diabetic mothers. *Behavioral Neuroscience, 114,* 950–956.

Nunez, P. L. (1990). Physical principles and neurophysiological mechanisms underlying event-related potentials. In J. W. Rohrbach, R. Parasuraman, & R. Johnson, Jr., (Eds.), *Event-related potentials: Basic issues and applications* (pp. 19–36). New York: Oxford University Press.

Oades, R. D. (1997). Development and topography of auditory event-related potentials (ERPs): Mismatch and processing negativity in individuals 8–22 years of age. *Psychophysiology, 34,* 677–693.

Ochoa, C. J., & Polich, J. (2000). P300 and blink instructions. *Clinical Neurophysiology, 11,* 93–98.

Oldfield, R. C. (1971). The assessment and analysis of handedness: The Edinburgh inventory. *Neuropsychologia, 9,* 97–113.

Oliver-Rodriguez, J. C., Guan, Z., & Johnston, V. S. (1999). Gender differences in late positive components evoked by human faces. *Psychophysiology, 36,* 176–185.

Otto, D., Karrer, R., Halliday, R., Horst, R. L., Klorman, R., Squires, N., Thatcher, R. W., Fenelson, B., & Lelord, G. (1984). Developmental aspects of event-related potentials: Aberrant development. *Annals of the New York Academy of Sciences, 425,* 319–337.

Pang, E. W., & Taylor, M. J. (2000). Tracking the development of the N1 from age 3 to adulthood: An examination of speech and non-speech stimuli. *Clinical Neurophysiology, 111,* 388–397.

Pascalis, O., de Haan, M., Nelson, C. A., & de Schonen, S. (1998). Long-term recognition memory assessed by visual paired comparison in 3- and 6-month-old infants. *Journal of Experimental Psychology: Learning, Memory, and Cognition, 24*, 1–12.

Picton, T. W., Bentin, S., Berg, P., Donchin, E., Hillyard, S. A., Johnson, R. Jr., Miller, G. A., Ritter, W., Ruchkin, D. S., Rugg, M. D., & Taylor, M. J. (2000). Guidelines for using human event-related potentials to study cognition: Recording standards and publication criteria. *Psychophysiology, 37*, 127–152.

Polich, J., Ladish, C., & Burns, T. (1990). Normal variation of P300 in children: Age, memory span, and head size. *International Journal of Psychophysiology, 9*, 237–248.

Polich, J., & Luckritz, J. Y. (1995). EEG and ERPs in young and elderly subjects. *Electroencephalography and Clinical Neurophysiology Supplement, 44*, 358–368.

Pollak, S. D., Klorman, R., Thattcher, J. E., & Cicchetti, D. (2001). P3b reflects maltreated children's reactions to facial displays of emotion. *Psychophysiology, 38*, 267–274.

Putnam, L. E., Johnson, R. Jr., & Roth, W. T. (1992). Guidelines for reducing the risk of disease transmission in the psychophysiology laboratory. SPR Ad Hoc Committee on the Prevention of Disease Transmission. *Psychophysiology, 29*, 127–141.

Regan, D. (1989). *Human brain electrophysiology: Evoked potentials and evoked magnetic fields in science and medicine.* New York: Elsevier.

Reynolds, G., & Richards, J. (2003). The impact of familiarization on electrophysiological correlates of recognition memory in infants. Poster presented the Annual Meeting of the Cognitive Neuroscience Society, New York City, NY.

Richards, John E. (2000). Localizing the development of covert attention in infants with scalp event-related potentials. *Developmental Psychology, 36*, 91–108.

Richards, J. E. (2003). Attention affects the recognition of briefly presented visual stimuli in infants: An ERP study. *Developmental Science, 6*, 312–328.

Scherg, M., & Berg, P. (1996). BESA-Brain Electromagnetic Source Analuss User Manual (Version 2.2). Munchen, Germany: MEGIS Software GmbH.

Shafer, V. L. (2000). Maturation of mismatch negativity in school-age children. *Ear & Hearing, 21*, 242–251.

Snyder, K. A. (2002). Neurophysiological correlates of habituation and novelty preferences in human infants. Presented at the International Conference on Infant Studies, Toronto, Canada.

Snyder, K., Webb, S. J., & Nelson, C. A. (2002). Theoretical and methodological implications of variability in infant brain response during a recognition memory paradigm. *Infant Behavior and Development, 25*, 466–494.

Stauder, J. E. A., Van Der Molen, M. W., & Molenaar, P. C. M. (1998). Changing relations between intelligence and brain activity in late childhood: A longitudinal event-related potential study. *Brain & Cognition, 37*, 119–122.

Stolarova, M., Whitney, H., Webb, S., deRegnier, R.-A., Georgieff, M., & Nelson, C. A. (2003). Electrophysiological brain responses of six-month-old low-risk premature infants during a visual priming task. *Infancy, 4*, 437–450.

Taylor, M. J., & Baldeweg, T. (2002). Application of EEG, ERP and intracranial recordings to the investigation of cognitive functions in children. *Developmental Science, 5*, 318–334.

Taylor, M. J., Edmonds, G. E., McCarthy, G., & Allison, T. (2001). Eyes first! Eye processing develops before face processing in children. *NeuroReport, 12*, 1671–1676.

Taylor, M. J., Khan, S. C., & Malone, M. A. (1999). Parallel and serial attentional processes: A developmental ERP study. *Developmental Neuropsychology, 15*, 351–358.

Taylor, M. J., McCarthy, G., Saliba, E., Degiovanni, E. (1999). ERP evidence of developmental changes in processing of faces. *Clinical Neurophysiology, 110*, 910–915.

Tucker, D. (1993). Spatial sampling of head electrical fields: The geodesic sensor net. *Electroencephaolgraphy and Clinical Neurophysiology, 87*, 154–163.

van Boxtel, G. (1998). Computational and statistical methods for analyzing event related potential data. *Behavior Research Methods, Instruments and Computers, 30*, 87–102.

13   ERPs in Neuropsychological Populations

Diane Swick

The field of neuropsychology has a lengthy history within the science of brain-behavior relationships. Researchers have made important discoveries about the anatomical regions involved in particular cognitive functions from observations of the behavioral deficits exhibited by neurological patients (Bouillard, 1825; Broca, 1861; Harlow, 1868; Dejerine, 1892). This line of research has led to a number of critical observations about the brain regions necessary for normal cognitive functions, such as speech, emotional control, and reading. Traditional neuropsychology entered the era of contemporary cognitive neuroscience with the development of computed tomography (CT) and magnetic resonance imaging (MRI) methods that provide accurate images of the living human brain. The evolution of structural mapping techniques, including three-dimensional reconstruction methods (Damasio & Frank, 1992; Frank, Damasio, & Grabowski, 1997), diffusion-tensor imaging (Conturo et al., 1999), and voxel-based lesion-symptom mapping (Bates et al., 2003) have further refined our ability to quantify and localize brain injuries due to stroke, head injury, and surgical intervention. This chapter will describe how event-related potential (ERP) recordings in neurological patients can enrich our understanding of neuropsychological issues and, in turn, how precise structural lesion information can assist in localizing the neural generators of various ERP components.

In contrast to their spectacular temporal resolution, the spatial resolution of scalp-recorded ERPs is relatively poor. A number of techniques have improved localization accuracy and increased our knowledge of the underlying anatomical substrates, but each has its own set of advantages and disadvantages (see chapters 7, 8, and 15 of this volume). Determining the neural structures involved in generating scalp-recorded ERP components from their absence or alteration in patients with focal brain lesions has yielded suggestive evidence, although one must take interpretative issues into account. If a lesion abolishes an ERP component, it may not necessarily be because the neural substrate itself has been destroyed, but rather because of damaged input to the generators. One must take physical changes in the brain and skull (in neurosurgical patients) into account. For instance, loss of tissue can alter the configuration of the generators, thereby changing scalp topography. The removal of skull in patients undergoing resection of tumors or epileptogenic foci presumably alters intracranial conductivity and surface ERP topography postsurgically (Vaughan, 1987). Likewise, it can be difficult to determine whether an intracranial potential recorded directly from a particular brain structure contributes to a potential recorded concurrently on the scalp. Indeed, late positive potentials resembling the P300 have been recorded from the medial temporal lobes (MTL) during oddball tasks, for example (Halgren et al., 1980; McCarthy et al., 1989), but MTL lesions do not alter scalp-recorded P300 in a manner consistent with an MTL primary generator (Stapleton, Halgren, & Moreno, 1987; Johnson, 1988).

This is likely due to the "closed field" source configuration of the hippocampus (Kutas & Dale, 1997). The study by Fernandez and colleagues (1999) further illustrates this. Depth electrodes were placed in MTL structures for surgical monitoring of seizure activity in epilepsy patients (see chapter 14 of this volume). ERPs were recorded while the patients were engaged in a word list learning task. In the anterior parahippocampal gyrus, a large negative potential peaked at 440 ms. This anterior MTL-N400 was larger for words that were later remembered than for those that were forgotten (the subsequent memory effect, or Dm, difference related to memory encoding; Paller, Kutas, & Mayes, 1987). In the hippocampus proper, a large positivity from 500–2,000 ms distinguished between subsequently remembered and forgotten words. This Dm effect was recorded within, but not immediately outside, the hippocampus. Fernandez et al. (1999) point out that the organization of hippocampal neurons results in a radially symmetric, closed field that is isopotentially zero outside the hippocampus. Therefore, this hippocampal potential does not contribute directly to Dm effects recorded from the scalp. However, the hippocampus is most plausibly part of a circuit that does participate in memory-related ERP effects recorded from surface electrodes. The reduction of memory effects in patients with MTL lesions offers supportive evidence (Smith & Halgren, 1989; Rugg et al., 1991; Johnson, 1995).

Preliminary ERP data from two sudden cardiac arrest survivors (figure 13.1) also endorse the view that damage to the hippocampus affects ERPs recorded during recognition memory (Swick, Knight, Kixmiller, & Sauvé, unpublished observations). Individuals who are resuscitated after anoxic events of this type often show persistent memory deficits (Sauvé et al., 1996). Both MRI (Reed & Squire, 1997) and postmortem neuropathological analyses (Zola-Morgan, Squire, & Amaral, 1986; Rempel-Clower et al., 1996) have demonstrated that anoxia is associated with loss of neurons in the CA1 field of the hippocampus; this lesion is sufficient to cause moderate to severe anterograde amnesia. Even though hippocampal potentials do not propagate to the scalp, the two patients in our study showed a reduction of the ERP old/new effect (figure 13.1) after probable cell loss in this structure.

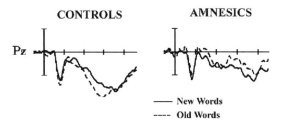

Figure 13.1
Grand averaged ERPs to new words and correctly recognized old words in a continuous recognition memory task. Older control subjects showed greater positivity from 400 to 600 ms at a fairly short retention interval. The two amnesic patients were impaired at recognition accuracy and did not show the old/new effect. Stimulus onset is indicated by the vertical calibration bar, which is ± 5 µV. Negative is up, and tick marks are 200 ms.

A related issue concerns the indirect and compensatory effects of lesions. Recovery of function after brain damage can change the neural circuits recruited for a specific cognitive task. Damage to a particular brain area may disrupt connections to remote regions, thereby influencing function in distant sites. However, the observation of changes remote from the site of lesion can reveal information about connectivity and modulatory interactions. For instance, lesions of dorsolateral prefrontal cortex (PFC) can influence visual processing in extrastriate temporal-occipital areas by reducing the amplitude of the visual N1 (N170) and N2 components (Swick & Knight, 1998; Barceló, Suwazono, & Knight, 2000). In the experiment by Barceló and colleagues (2000), the ipsilesional ERP abnormalities were associated with visual target detection deficits in the contralesional hemifield. These changes could be due to the loss of a gain-enhancing signal from the PFC to the extrastriate generators of these components. This interpretation is in accord with the biased competition model of visual attention, which postulates that PFC neurons provide top-down biasing signals to visual cortical regions coding for the attributes relevant for the task at hand (Desimone & Duncan, 1995; Miller & Cohen, 2001). Another example of remote modulatory influences on ERPs was provided by a monkey model of the P300, in which lesions of the noradrenergic nucleus locus coeruleus produce a reduction of P300 amplitude (Pineda, Foote, & Neville, 1989). Damage to this brainstem nucleus deprives the cortical generators of norepinephrine, a transmitter that boosts the signal-to-noise ratio of postsynaptic neurons, and diminishes the magnitude of P300 responses to auditory oddball stimuli.

An important advantage of the lesion method is determining the *necessity* of a particular brain region for a particular cognitive function. Multiple cortical and limbic sites generate large potentials during simple sensory discriminations (Halgren et al.,

1995), for example, but many of these areas may be unnecessary for task performance. Thus, ERP studies in neurological patients can constrain the list of plausible sources for a given component.

Practical Considerations

When working with patient populations, there are a number of things to consider about experimental design, recording parameters, and session length. Many of these issues also apply to studies of elderly control subjects and psychiatric populations. Of paramount importance is the comfort of your experimental participants. It is wise to keep the recording session as brief as possible, including electrode application time. High-density electrode mapping studies may not be indicated in many patient groups, so the use of fewer electrodes is most acceptable. Experimental blocks should be short (~5 min) whenever possible to allow for frequent rest periods. Another consideration is that the number of trials in your experiment must allow for a higher artifact rejection rate than in studies of college students. Blink correction algorithms (Gratton et al., 1983; Berg & Scherg, 1994; Dale, 1994; see chapter 6 of this volume) are most helpful in recovering data from individuals who blink a lot. One must also consider the lesion etiology and the time since brain injury. If short, edema and diaschisis may not have resolved, which can complicate the interpretation of results. ERP studies with reasonably uniform groups of similar patients are preferred, but the single-case study can be a viable approach if one proceeds with caution (Swick & Turken, 2002; D'Arcy et al., 2003). Finally, be sensitive to the patients' deficits and provide words of encouragement throughout the experiment.

Researchers have generally taken two major approaches to ERP experimentation in neurological patients: (1) a focal lesion/localization approach, and (2) a syndrome-based approach. The first tactic is primarily concerned with inferring the neural sources of scalp-recorded ERPs by their presence, absence, or alteration in patients with focal brain lesions. Consideration of studies using this approach can provide critical insight into how abnormal ERP patterns in neuropsychological populations are interpreted. The second methodology is aimed at providing neurophysiological measures that can serve as a complement to behavioral testing in patients with clinical problems such as traumatic brain injury, visuospatial neglect, and aphasia. The syndrome-based approach can also address theoretical issues concerning the underlying cognitive deficits in a specific patient group (Hagoort & Kutas, 1995).

Approach 1—Localization

The major components discussed here are the mismatch negativity (MMN), the P300 and other late positive components (LPCs), the N400, and the error-related negativity

(ERN). The MMN is a measure of auditory sensory memory elicited by deviant stimuli embedded in sequences of standard stimuli (Näätänen, 1990), sometimes called the N2a. It precedes the P300 complex and is observed in conditions similar to the novelty P300 (P3a). Overt attention and active task performance are not required (MMN can be recorded while participants are reading a book, for example), so this component is thought to be relatively automatic. The P300 consists of multiple subcomponents. The P3b shows a maximal amplitude at central-parietal scalp sites and peaks about 300 to 600 ms after the detection of infrequent targets embedded in a series of background stimuli (the "oddball" paradigm, Squires, Squires, & Hillyard, 1975). A variety of cognitive processes have been associated with P300, including context-updating, stimulus categorization, cognitive closure, and template matching (Donchin & Coles, 1988; Verleger, 1988). The earlier latency P3a, largest at frontocentral sites, is elicited by rare, task irrelevant stimuli and has been associated with orienting, arousal, and the novelty response (Squires, Squires, & Hillyard, 1975). Related to the P300 are late positive components (LPCs) that have been recorded in explicit memory tasks (Friedman, 1990) and in implicit paradigms such as the incidental repetition of words in lists, sentences, and text (Karayandis et al., 1991; Van Petten et al., 1991; Besson, Kutas, & Van Petten, 1992). The N400 is a mainstay of language processing tasks (see Kutas & Van Petten, 1994 for review). Kutas and Hillyard (1980) first described it as being elicited by violations of semantic expectancies at the end of sentences. Subsequent research has proven it to be an exquisite indicator of how easily a word is integrated into its semantic context. We will discuss the N400 in relation to memory-related effects and ERP observations of patients with language disorders. The error-related negativity (ERN or Ne) is detected in waveforms that are time-locked to the occurrence of erroneous responses in speeded reaction time tasks (Falkenstein et al., 1990; Gehring et al., 1993). The ERN is considered to be an index of performance monitoring (Falkenstein et al., 2000).

Mismatch Negativity (MMN)

Patient studies of the MMN indicate that temporoparietal cortex and dorsolateral PFC both contribute to this measure of auditory sensory memory (Alho et al., 1994; Alain, Woods, & Knight, 1998). In the study by Alho and colleagues (1994), ERPs to non-attended auditory stimuli (1000 Hz standard tones and 1300 Hz infrequent tones) were recorded while subjects performed a visual reaction time task. Patients with lesions of dorsolateral PFC showed a reduction in the MMN elicited by deviant tones. A subsequent experiment evaluated three groups of patients with damage to posterior association cortex (temporoparietal junction), the hippocampus and adjacent MTL regions, or dorsolateral PFC (Alain, Woods, & Knight, 1998). The MMN was recorded in response to deviant tones and to pattern deviations during performance of a difficult visual discrimination task (figure 13.2). In a separate session, subjects performed an auditory

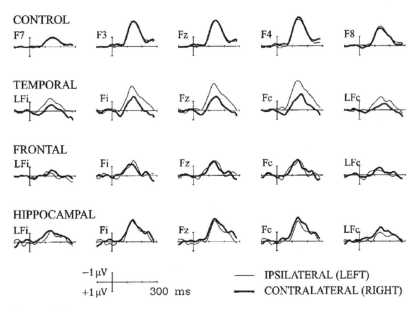

Figure 13.2
The mismatch negativity (MMN) in controls and three patient groups. The MMN shown here was obtained by subtracting the ERPs to auditory deviant stimuli from the ERPs to standard tones. Electrodes have been transposed in patients with right hemisphere lesions, so that those on the left of the figure are ipsilateral to the lesion. Electrodes are labeled accordingly (*i* is ipsilateral to the lesion, *c* is contralateral). Stimulus onset is indicated by the vertical bar and negativity is plotted upward. (Taken from figure 6 of Alain et al., 1998.)

discrimination task to assess their abilities to detect the frequency and pattern deviants presented in the ERP study. Patients with temporoparietal lesions had impaired auditory discrimination and reduced MMN amplitudes for stimuli presented in the ear contralateral to the lesioned hemisphere, suggesting that auditory sensory memories are predominantly stored in cortex contralateral to the stimulated ear. In contrast, unilateral frontal lesions impaired performance and reduced MMNs for stimuli presented in either ear, implying that dorsolateral prefrontal cortex influences sensory memory storage in bilateral auditory cortices. Hippocampal lesions did not affect MMN amplitudes or behavioral performance. These results suggest that prefrontal-temporal projections are critical for the transient storage of auditory stimuli (Alho et al., 1994; Alain, Woods, & Knight, 1998).

P300

The most widely studied component using the lesion technique is the P300. A number of studies have focused on the generators of the P300 recorded in simple target detection tasks. This research has shown that the P3a subcomponent, an index of phasic attention to novel events, is dependent on a prefrontal-hippocampal network (Knight, 1984, 1996), whereas temporoparietal junction is a crucial generator of the P3b subcomponent (Knight et al., 1989). We give only a brief overview here (for more extensive reviews, see Swick, Kutas, & Neville, 1994; Knight & Scabini, 1998; Soltani & Knight, 2000).

In patients with unilateral lesions of dorsolateral PFC, P3a responses to novel auditory stimuli were reduced at frontocentral sites and instead exhibited a more parietal distribution (Knight, 1984). These patients showed normal, parietally distributed P3bs to auditory targets. Likewise, the somatosensory P3a to tactile novels and shocks was decreased by PFC lesions, particularly at frontal sites (Yamaguchi & Knight, 1991), with P3b to tactile targets showing only slight reductions. The P3b to auditory targets was abolished and P3a to novels was substantially reduced at central and parietal sites in patients with lesions of the temporoparietal junction (Knight et al., 1989), with similar results in the somatosensory modality (Yamaguchi & Knight, 1991). Patients with lesions restricted to more superior regions of parietal cortex exhibited normal P3a and P3b potentials.

In oddball paradigms, the modality-specific N200 precedes P3a and P3b (Squires, Squires, & Hillyard, 1975). Lesions of lateral parietal cortex significantly reduced N200 to target and novel stimuli in both auditory (Knight et al., 1989) and somatosensory (Yamaguchi & Knight, 1991) modalities. Lesions of the temporoparietal junction, conversely, did not affect N200 amplitude in either modality. Additionally, PFC lesions reduced the amplitude of somatosensory N200 to novels and targets (Yamaguchi & Knight, 1991) and auditory N200 to novels only (Knight, 1984). The dissociation between N200 and P300 observed in these studies suggests that they have different neural sources.

Studies of patients with MTL damage have demonstrated that the late positive component observed during recognition memory and the oddball P300 also have dissociable neural generators. Surgical excision of the left anterior temporal lobe abolished the LPC to repeated words but not the P300 to rare tones (Smith & Halgren, 1989). Amnesic patients with bilateral hippocampal lesions showed normal scalp-recorded P3b responses to auditory and visual target stimuli (Polich & Squire, 1993). By contrast, similar amnesic patients showed a decrement in the memory-related LPC (figure 13.1). Patients with more extensive bilateral MTL damage (due to encephalitis) showed reductions in auditory P3b amplitude at lateral frontal and anterior temporal sites but not at midline, posterior temporal, lateral parietal, or occipital electrodes (Onofrj et al., 1992). In addition to providing another demonstration that intact MTLs are not necessary for generating P300 at Cz and Pz, this finding suggests that the MTL contributes to the positivity recorded at other scalp sites and strongly implies multiple P300 sources.

(a)

FRONTALS

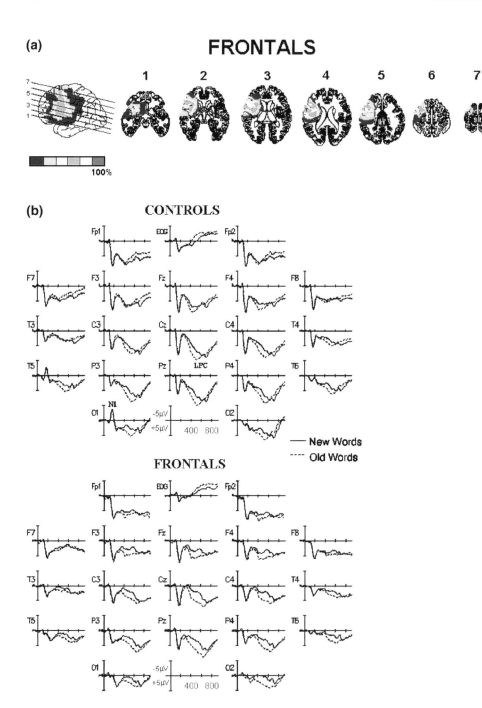

(b)

CONTROLS

FRONTALS

— New Words
---- Old Words

N400/Late Positive Component—ERP Old/New Effect

ERP studies of memory retrieval have focused on the word repetition effect (or "old/new effect"), in which previously studied words elicit larger positive potentials than new words, beginning at 300–500 ms poststimulus and lasting for several hundred ms (reviewed in Friedman & Johnson, 2000; Rugg & Allan, 2000). The first ERP component that comprises the old/new response is the N400. Because its amplitude is modulated by the extent to which a word is related to its prior context, the N400 is sensitive to repetition. The second element of the old/new effect, the LPC, peaks at about 600 ms. Use of the "remember/know" paradigm, based on dual-process models of recognition memory (Tulving, 1985), has shown the LPC to be a sensitive measure of recollective experience. During old/new recognition judgments, old words that are associated with conscious recollection ("remember") evoke larger positive shifts than items associated with only a general feeling of familiarity (or "know," Smith, 1993; Düzel et al., 1997). The ERP old/new effect shows a voltage distribution that is maximum over central-parietal and posterior temporal scalp electrodes (sometimes with a left greater than right hemisphere asymmetry), and that is typically smaller over frontal electrodes.

As previously mentioned, anterior temporal lobectomy reduces the amplitude of the scalp-recorded repetition effect during recognition (Smith & Halgren, 1989; Johnson, 1995), but the consequences of other lesions on this ERP response are relatively less known. For the last 10 years, PET and fMRI studies have implicated the PFC in episodic encoding and retrieval tasks (Buckner, 2000), although it is still debated if this activity is a direct reflection of mnemonic processes, cognitive "effort," or postretrieval monitoring. Because of their superior temporal resolution, ERPs are a good choice to help clarify this debate, and testing patients with focal PFC damage can determine whether this region generates the ERP old/new effect.

ERPs and behavioral performance were examined in 11 patients with frontal lesions (10 left, 1 right hemisphere) centered in areas 9 and 46 of dorsolateral PFC (figure

◀ **Figure 13.3**

(*a*) Averaged lesion reconstructions for the group of 11 frontal patients illustrate dorsolateral PFC damage with variable extent into ventrolateral prefrontal cortex, the anterior temporal tip, and insular cortex. Lesions were estimated from CT or MRI scans and transcribed onto sequential axial templates. All lesions are projected onto the left hemisphere. The scale indicates the percentage of patients with damage in the corresponding areas. Lines through the lateral view show the level of the axial cuts from ventral (1) to dorsal (7). (Adapted from figure 2 of Swick & Knight, 1999.) (See plate 7 for color version.) (*b*) Grand average ERPs recorded from controls (*top*) and frontal patients (*bottom*) in the recognition memory task. Old words were collapsed across the three lags. The N170 (N1) and late positive component (LPC) are labeled. (Taken from figure 5 of Swick & Knight, 1999.)

13.3a and plate 7; Swick & Knight, 1999). Verbal stimuli repeated after one of three delays in a continuous recognition paradigm. In the analysis of correctly recognized old items (hit rates), all subjects were most accurate for immediately repeated stimuli, and accuracy declined as lag increased. The hit rates of patients did not differ from controls. However, analysis of false alarms revealed that patients with frontal lesions were more likely to respond incorrectly to new stimuli. This pattern of results suggests that their deficit may be a strategic or attentional one, rather than purely mnemonic in nature.

In support of this view, the PFC group showed an intact ERP repetition effect (figure 13.3b), which would not have been predicted if the patients had engaged in an undue number of "lucky guesses" for old stimuli, which would have diluted the size of the ERP response. Correctly remembered words elicited more positive-going ERPs than new words in both groups: from 400 to 600 ms in controls and 400 to 700 ms in the patients. However, the patients did show amplitude reductions in their ERPs to new words from 500 to 600 ms, suggesting an impairment in detecting and responding to novel stimuli, in accord with their higher false alarm rates and diminished P3a novelty responses (Knight, 1984).

Because the onset of the old/new effect occurs several hundred ms prior to RTs for correctly recognized words, left PFC is not necessary for the ERP modulation associated with successful recognition. Other neural sources, some in the MTL, are still able to modulate this electrical response in the frontal patients. Its scalp distribution and recent neuroimaging evidence have led to the speculation that the old/new effect is actually generated in left parietal cortex (Rugg, Otten, & Henson, 2002). Thus, it would be interesting to examine whether the old/new effect is diminished in patients with left parietal lesions.

In contrast to the lack of PFC involvement in generating ERP effects during word recognition, preliminary evidence suggests that the lateral PFC does contribute to a later (600–1200 ms), frontally distributed effect recorded during the retrieval of contextual, or source, information about studied items (Swick et al., 1999). In this experiment, subjects listened to lists of words spoken by a male or female voice; each word was presented twice during the study phase to improve encoding. At test, subjects made old/new decisions, and for words judged old, a subsequent male/female voice decision was required. In agreement with their ERP deficit, source accuracy was impaired in the patients with frontal lesions. Previous studies have generally indicated that such patients show relatively intact recognition memory, but are impaired in free recall, contextual memory for details, and the application of strategies to assist memory processing (Shimamura, 1995). Future patient studies will examine the effects of frontal lesions on source memory ERPs more closely.

A final issue is that the neural sources participating in explicit and implicit forms of memory retrieval appear to make differing contributions to ERP old/new effects

(Rugg et al., 1991; Paller & Kutas, 1992; Paller, Kutas, & McIsaac, 1995). In a companion study to the continuous recognition experiment described above, the old/new effect was assessed in the same group of frontal patients using an incidental repetition paradigm (Swick, 1998). Words and nonwords were repeated after one of three delays, and stimuli were categorized in a lexical decision task. In controls, repeated words elicited more positive-going potentials than new words, beginning at 300 ms and lasting until 500 to 700 ms. This ERP repetition effect was reduced, but not eliminated, by PFC lesions (Swick, 1998). However, the behavioral manifestation of priming (RT facilitation) was intact in the patients, suggesting that PFC may modulate the neural generators in posterior cortical regions that are critical for priming, akin to the biased competition model (e.g., Desimone & Duncan, 1995). A more dramatic reduction was obtained in the encoding phase of the source memory experiment, in which the ERP repetition effect was completely abolished by left lateral PFC lesions (Larsen & Swick, 2000).

Error-Related Negativity (ERN)

The ERN, or Ne, was discovered independently by labs in the United States (Gehring et al., 1990) and Germany (Falkenstein et al., 1990). The ERN peaks at about 60 to 80 ms after incorrect responses and is largest at the frontocentral midline electrodes (FCz, Cz). The onset of the ERN can actually be seen in conjunction with EMG activity in the incorrect digit or limb. Several lines of evidence indicate that the ERN is elicited when a comparison between representations of the appropriate (correct) response and the actual response produces a mismatch (Coles et al., 2001). An alternate view holds that the ERN is not the result of a comparator process, but rather the manifestation of conflict between competing responses that can also occur on correct trials (Carter et al., 1998). Determining which of these two models better captures the data, as well as the brain regions involved in performance monitoring, have been of great interest.

Patients with lateral PFC lesions did not show differential electrophysiological activity on error trials and correct trials (Gehring & Knight, 2000). ERN amplitude was the same as controls, but the negativity on correct trials was enhanced. The effects of frontal lesions on compensatory behavior were mixed: the patients showed normal post-error slowing, but a reduction in error correction rates. Gehring and Knight (2000) concluded that the PFC interacts with the anterior cingulate cortex (ACC) to carry out performance monitoring functions. However, it is still an assumption that the ERN is generated in the ACC, because direct confirmation of this idea was not provided by this experiment.

An event-related fMRI study demonstrated that dorsal ACC showed increases in activity during error trials as well as correct trials with higher levels of conflict (Carter et al., 1998). As a result, the conflict monitoring hypothesis maintains that errors and conflicts are processed by the same region of the ACC (Carter et al., 1998). We tested this hypothesis in a unique patient, R.N., with a unilateral lesion restricted to the left

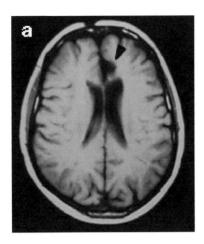
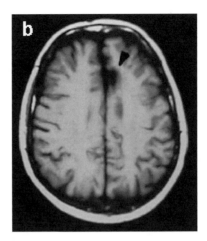

Figure 13.4

MRI scans showing R.N.'s lesion. (*a*, *b*) Horizontal sections illustrating the lesion in the left ACC (indicated by black arrowheads). (Adapted from figure 2 of Swick & Turken, 2002.)

rostral-dorsal ACC (figure 13.4). We used a Stroop-like task to examine if the conflict-related ERP on incongruent trials would be diminished in R.N., as the conflict monitoring hypothesis predicted (Carter et al., 1998). If not, this would suggest that ACC activations in the Stroop and other conflict tasks do not reflect activity that is strictly time-locked to conflict detection processes (Swick & Turken, 2002). Second, we also asked whether the ERN is intact in R.N.

In fact, the ERN was clearly reduced in R.N. (figure 13.5), accompanied by lower error correction rates (Swick & Turken, 2002). Conversely, the stimulus-locked component on correct conflict trials, the N450, was enhanced, and behavioral performance was impaired. Our interpretation was that intact regions of R.N.'s brain, such as lateral PFC, were still able to detect response conflict, but damage to the dorsal ACC impaired his ability to inhibit responses, perhaps due to disconnection from cingulate and supplementary motor areas. The results implicated the ACC in error monitoring, and suggested a dissociation between error and conflict detection processes.

Approach 2—Syndrome-Based

Three neurological syndromes that have experienced a growth in the application of ERP methodology to assess the nature of the impairment are (1) traumatic brain injury (Dupuis et al., 2000; Kaipio et al., 2000; Potter et al., 2001, 2002; Segalowitz, 2001; Polo et al., 2002), (2) hemispatial neglect and extinction of left-sided stimuli in patients with right hemisphere damage (Verleger et al., 1996; Deouell, Bentin, & Soroker, 2000;

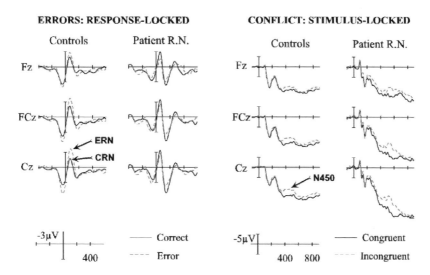

Figure 13.5

Dissociation of error-related and conflict-related ERPs in R.N. (*a*) The error-related negativity (ERN) and the correct-related negativity (CRN) in the response-locked waves at the frontocentral midline sites (Fz, FCz, Cz). Response onset occurs at the vertical bar (time = 0 ms), tic marks are 200 ms, and negative is plotted upward. (*b*) ERPs related to conflict (the N450 component) in the stimulus-locked waves at frontocentral midline sites. Stimulus onset occurs at the vertical bar (time = 0 ms). (Adapted from figure 3 of Swick & Turken, 2002.)

Deouell, Hamalainen, & Bentin, 2000; Vuilleumier et al., 2001; Eimer et al., 2002), and (3) aphasia (Hagoort & Kutas, 1995; Friederici, Hahne, & von Cramon, 1998; Friederici, von Cramon, & Kotz, 1999). The current review will focus on patients with aphasia, a disturbance in language production or comprehension that can follow damage to the left hemisphere.

Language is not just sandwiched
between Broca's and Wernicke's.
Heard, spoken or seen
meaning emerges from activities
in multiple sites
each scheming by all rights
at much the same time
to yield both the literal
and the metaphorical,
the banal
and the sublime.

—Marta Kutas (1998)

Aphasia

Assessment of residual language capacities in individuals with aphasia has proven to be one of the most fruitful areas of research using the syndrome-based approach. A major question about how language is affected by a left hemisphere lesion in aphasic individuals is whether lexical-semantic representations themselves are lost or if processing impairments lead to problems in accessing and integrating these representations. ERPs are particularly well suited to address this issue. For example, Hagoort and co-workers (1996) utilized a semantic priming paradigm to examine the effects of semantic relatedness on the N400 component. Elderly controls, aphasic patients, and nonaphasic patients with right hemisphere lesions passively listened to pairs of spoken words while ERPs were recorded. The stimulus pairs were associatively related ("bread-butter"), semantically related ("church-villa"), or unrelated ("table-book"). The semantic pairs are more distantly related than the associative pairs, and it is thought that the right hemisphere might contribute to the processing of such relations. Older control subjects showed the classic priming effect: in comparison to unrelated target words, the N400 to targets associatively or semantically related to the primes were reduced in amplitude. The results in aphasic patients with minor comprehension deficits were similar to those in controls. In aphasics with severe comprehension deficits, however, N400 priming effects were diminished for both associative and semantic word pairs. Right hemisphere lesioned patients generated a normal N400 effect for associatively related targets, but a mild reduction for the semantic relations.

A critical demonstration in this experiment was that the degree of language impairment was related to the size of the N400 deficit, and this finding cut across the diagnostic category of Broca's and Wernike's aphasia (Hagoort, Brown, & Swaab, 1996). Consequently, aphasic patients with severe comprehension deficits exhibited problems in integrating word meanings into a context. Another important observation was that the right hemisphere patients showed a small but selective deficit for the more distantly related word pairs, which agrees with its postulated involvement in coarse semantic coding (Beeman et al., 1994). Overall, this experiment illustrates the value of ERPs in groups of patients who might not be able to perform an explicit task.

Thus, another clear advantage of ERP recordings in people with aphasia is the ability to obtain direct brain measures of lexical-semantic processing during naturalistic language comprehension without the need for responses in a metalinguistic task such as lexical decision. Another experiment examined the ability of Broca's aphasics to access the meaning of ambiguous words in a sentence context (Swaab, Brown, & Hagoort, 1998). Comprehension deficits in such cases can result from difficulties with retrieving the less common usage of words with multiple meanings (e.g., "bank"), or from a delay in selecting the appropriate meaning in a given context. Spoken sentences were presented in one of three context conditions, followed by a target word either 100 ms or 1250 ms later (short and long ISIs, interstimulus intervals). In the unrelated condition, the final word of the sentence was unambiguous and unrelated to the target ("The boy petted the dog on the head"—RIVER). In the concordant condition, the ambiguous word was related to the correct meaning of the target ("The man planted a tree on the bank"—RIVER). In the discordant condition, the sentence context biased the alternate meaning of ambiguous word, which was unrelated to the target ("The man made a phone call to the bank"—RIVER). The size of the N400 effect was used as a measure of whether the subjects were able to select the contextually appropriate meaning of the ambiguous word. The N400 of older controls was similar in size to both the unrelated and discordant conditions, at both short and long ISIs, suggesting that selection of the correct meaning occurred within 100 ms after the sentence. The pattern of results in Broca's aphasics resembled those of controls at the long ISI. However, the patients were unable to select the contextually appropriate meaning of the ambiguous word at the short ISI, because N400 was significantly smaller in the discordant condition than in the unrelated condition. These results indicate that Broca's aphasics show a delay in integrating semantic information under conditions of lexical uncertainty.

The clinical utility of ERPs as assessment tools in aphasia is becoming more widely recognized, particularly for patients who cannot be evaluated with standard neuropsychological measures (Connolly et al., 2000). Connolly and his colleagues have adapted a version of the Peabody Picture Vocabulary Test-Revised (PPVT-R), a standardized measure of receptive vocabulary and language comprehension (Dunn & Dunn, 1981), for use with ERP recordings in aphasic patients (Connolly, Byrne, & Dywan, 1995; Marchand, D'Arcy, & Connolly, 2002; D'Arcy et al., 2003). In the traditional version of this test, the subjects are required to decide whether or not a spoken word matches a picture. In the computerized PPVT-R, behavioral responses were not required (D'Arcy et al., 2003). A picture was presented for 1700 ms, followed by a spoken word that is congruent or incongruent with the picture. For subjects with intact comprehension, ERPs time-locked to the onset of the spoken word should reveal an N400 for semantic incongruities. In the aphasic individuals, a statistically significant correlation between a derived measure of the N400 difference wave and the neuropsychological test score in the traditional PPVT-R was found (Marchand, D'Arcy, & Connolly, 2002; D'Arcy et al., 2003). Although the authors were conservative about the need for replication across different tasks and larger populations, they remain optimistic about the value of this methodology in patient populations.

Another research group (Cohen et al., 2001) tested aphasic patients and controls using a feature comparison task similar to the token test under four S1–S2 conditions: word-word, word-picture, picture-word, picture-picture. They assessed the slow wave (SW) and contingent negative variation (CNV) following S1 presentation. The authors noted that three alternative interpretations must be taken into account if the aphasics showed greater ERP amplitudes over the right hemisphere: (1) the patients might transform verbal information into pictorial representations, (2) the residual language capacities of the right hemisphere could compensate somewhat for language impairment due to left hemisphere damage, or (3) the patients require greater effort to perform the task, which could produce an enhancement over the right hemisphere. However, this result was not obtained for the SW. Unexpectedly, the patients (particularly the nonfluent aphasics, who presumably have large left frontal lesions) showed greater SW amplitudes than controls over the left hemisphere (Cohen et al., 2001). The anterior asymmetry for the SW was larger in aphasics than controls, but the converse was true for the CNV (i.e., the left > right asymmetry was larger in controls, with aphasics sometimes showing the reverse asymmetry). The CNV finding is consistent with prior studies demonstrating an ipsilesional reduction of CNV amplitude in patients with lateral PFC lesions (Rosahl & Knight, 1995; Zappoli et al., 2002). However, the SW result in the aphasics is difficult to reconcile with loss of tissue in left PFC, a region likely to be involved in retaining verbal information over a short delay, if the SW is related to this process. In the absence of detailed lesion information, this example points out the difficulties of drawing conclusions about the neural sources of a given component.

Conclusion

Application of the lesion technique has been a productive area of ERP research. Given the pervasiveness of neuroimaging studies of cognition, it is crucial to determine the conditions in which a given brain region is *essential* for cognitive performance. Likewise, it is important to utilize methods with a temporal resolution superior to that of hemodynamic measures in order to track the patterns of brain activity as they unfold in time. In the future, the combination of anatomically precise, voxel-based lesion-symptom mapping (Bates et al., 2003) with ERPs will allow more accurate localization of neural generators. Furthermore, joint fMRI and ERP studies in the same groups of patients can reveal the mechanisms of recovery of function after brain damage.

Acknowledgments

This work was supported by Grant DC03424 from the National Institute on Deafness and Other Communication Disorders and 98-47 CNS-QUA.05 from the James S. McDonnell Foundation. I also acknowledge the support of Robert T. Knight (NS21135 and NS17778 from NINDS) and the assistance of my colleagues and lab members over the years. Finally, I thank the patients for their enthusiastic participation.

References

Alain, C., Woods, D. L., & Knight, R. T. (1998). A distributed cortical network for auditory sensory memory in humans. *Brain Research, 812,* 23–37.

Alho, K., Woods, D. L., Algazi, A., Knight, R. T., & Naatanen, R. (1994). Lesions of frontal cortex diminish the auditory mismatch negativity. *Electroencephalography and Clinical Neurophysiology, 91*, 353–362.

Barceló, F., Suwazono, S., & Knight, R. T. (2000). Prefrontal modulation of visual processing in humans. *Nature Neuroscience, 3*, 399–403.

Bates, E., Wilson, S. M., Saygin, A. P., Dick, F., Sereno, M. I., Knight, R. T., & Dronkers, N. F. (2003). Voxel-based lesion-symptom mapping. *Nature Neuroscience, 6*, 448–450.

Beeman, M., Friedman, R. B., Grafman, J., Perez, E., Diamond, S., & Lindsay, M. B. (1994). Summation priming and coarse semantic coding in the right hemisphere. *Journal of Cognitive Neuroscience, 6*, 26–45.

Berg, P., & Scherg, M. (1994). A multiple source approach to the correction of eye artifacts. *Electroencephalography and Clinical Neurophysiology, 90*, 229–241.

Besson, M., Kutas, M., & Van Petten, C. (1992). An event-related potential (ERP) analysis of semantic congruity and repetition effects in sentences. *Journal of Cognitive Neuroscience, 4*, 132–149.

Bouillard, J. B. (1825). Recherches cliniques propres a demontrer que la perte de la parole correspond a la lesion des lobules anterieurs du cerveau. *Archives Generales de Medicine, 8*, 24–45.

Broca, P. (1861). Nouvelle observation d'aphemie produite par une lesion de la troisieme circonvolution frontale. *Bulletins de la Societe d'anatomie (Paris), 2e serie, 6*, 398–407.

Buckner, R. (2000). Neuroimaging of memory. In M. S. Gazzaniga (Ed.), *The new cognitive neurosciences*, 2nd Edition (pp. 817–828). Cambridge, MA: MIT Press.

Carter, C. S., Braver, T. S., Barch, D. M., Botvinick, M. M., Noll, D., & Cohen, J. D. (1998). Anterior cingulate cortex, error detection, and the online monitoring of performance. *Science, 280*, 747–749.

Cohen, R., Dobel, C., Berg, P., Köbbel, P., Schönle, P. W., & Rockstroh, B. (2001). Event-related potential correlates of verbal and pictorial feature comparison in aphasics and controls. *Neuropsychologia, 39*, 489–501.

Coles, M. G. H., Scheffers, M. K., & Holroyd, C. B. (2001). Why is there an ERN/Ne on correct trials? Response representations, stimulus-related components, and the theory of error-processing. *Biological Psychology, 56*, 173–189.

Connolly, J. F., Byrne, J. M., & Dywan, C. A. (1995). Event-related brain potentials reflect the receptive vocabulary of individuals as measured by the Peabody Picture Vocabulary Test-Revised: A study of cross-modal and cross-form priming. *Journal of Clinical and Experimental Neuropsychology, 17*, 548–565.

Connolly, J. F., D'Arcy, R. C., Lynn Newman, R., & Kemps, R. (2000). The application of cognitive event-related brain potentials (ERPs) in language-impaired individuals: Review and case studies. *International Journal of Psychophysiology, 38*, 55–70.

Conturo, T. E., Lori, N. F., Cull, T. S., Akbudak, E., Snyder, A. Z., Shimony, J. S., McKinstry, R. C., Burton, H., & Raichle, M. E. (1999). Tracking neuronal fiber pathways in the living human brain. *Proceedings of the National Academy of Sciences, 96*, 10422–10427.

Dale, A. M. (1994). *Source localization and spatial discriminant analysis of event-related potentials: Linear approaches*. Ph.D. Dissertation, University of California, San Diego.

Damasio, H., & Frank, R. (1992). Three-dimensional in vivo mapping of brain lesions in humans. *Archives of Neurology, 49*, 137–143.

D'Arcy, R. C. N., Marchand, Y., Eskes, G. A., Harrison, E. R., Phillips, S. J., Major, A., & Connolly, J. F. (2003). Electrophysiological assessment of language function following stroke. *Clinical Neurophysiology, 114*, 662–672.

Dejerine, J. (1892). Contribution a l'etude anatomopathologique et clinique des differentes varietes de cecite verbale. *Comptes Rendus Hebdomadaires des Seances et Memoires de la Societe de Biologie, 4*, 61–90.

Deouell, L. Y., Bentin, S., & Soroker, N. (2000). Electrophysiological evidence for an early (pre-attentive) information processing deficit in patients with right hemisphere damage and unilateral neglect. *Brain, 123*, 353–365.

Deouell, L. Y., Hamalainen, H., & Bentin, S. (2000). Unilateral neglect after right-hemisphere damage: Contributions from event-related potentials. *Audiology and Neurotology, 5*, 225–234.

Desimone, R., & Duncan, J. (1995). Neural mechanisms of selective visual attention. *Annual Review of Neuroscience, 18*, 193–222.

Donchin, E., & Coles, M. G. H. (1988). Is the P300 component a manifestation of context updating? *Behavioral Brain Sciences, 11*, 357–374.

Dunn, L. M., & Dunn, L. M. (1981). *Peabody Picture Vocabulary Test-revised*. Minnesota: American Guidance Service.

Dupuis, F., Johnston, K. M., Lavoie, M., Lepore, F., & Lassonde, M. (2000). Concussions in athletes produce brain dysfunction as revealed by event-related potentials. *Neuroreport, 11*, 4087–4092.

Düzel, E., Yonelinas, A. P., Mangun, G. R., Heinze, H.-J., & Tulving, E. (1997). Event-related brain potential correlates of two states of conscious awareness in memory. *Proceedings of the National Academy of Sciences, 94*, 5973–5978.

Eimer, M., Maravita, A., Van Velzen, J., Musain, M., & Driver, J. (2002). The electrophysiology of tactile extinction: ERP correlates of unconscious somatosensory processing. *Neuropsychologia, 40*, 2438–2447.

Falkenstein, M., Hoormann, J., Christ, S., and Hohnsbein, J. (2000). ERP components on reaction errors and their functional significance: A tutorial. *Biological Psychology, 51*, 87–107.

Falkenstein, M., Hohnsbein, J., Hoorman, J., & Blanke, L. (1990). Effects of errors in choice reaction tasks on the ERP under focused and divided attention. In C. H. M. Brunia, A. W. K. Gaillard, & A. Kok (Eds.), *Psychophysiological brain research* (pp. 192–195). Tilburg: Tilburg University Press.

Fernandez, G., Effern, A., Grunwald, T., Pezer, N., Lehnertz, K., Dumpelmann, M., Van Roost, D., & Elger, C. E. (1999). Real-time tracking of memory formation in the human rhinal cortex and hippocampus. *Science, 285*, 1582–1585.

Frank, R. J., Damasio, H., & Grabowski, T. J. (1997). Brainvox: An interactive, multimodal visualization and analysis system for neuroanatomical imaging. *Neuroimage, 5*, 13–30.

Friederici, A. D., Hahne, A., & von Cramon, D. Y. (1998). First-pass versus second-pass parsing processes in a Wernicke's and a Broca's aphasic: Electrophysiological evidence for a double dissociation. *Brain and Language, 62*, 311–341.

Friederici, A. D., von Cramon, D. Y., & Kotz, S. A. (1999). Language related brain potentials in patients with cortical and subcortical left hemisphere lesions. *Brain, 122*, 1033–1047.

Friedman, D. (1990). ERPs during continuous recognition memory for words. *Biological Psychology, 30*, 61–87.

Friedman, D., & Johnson, R. Jr. (2000). Event-related potential (ERP) studies of memory encoding and retrieval: A selective review. *Microscopy Research and Technique, 51*, 6–28.

Gehring, W. J., Coles, M. G. H., Meyer, D. E., & Donchin, E. (1990). The error-related negativity: An event-related brain potential accompanying errors. *Psychophysiology, 27*, S34.

Gehring, W. J., Goss, B., Coles, M. G. H., Meyer, D. E., & Donchin, E. (1993). A neural system for error detection and compensation. *Psychological Science, 4*, 385–390.

Gehring, W. J., & Knight, R. T. (2000). Prefrontal-cingulate interactions in action monitoring. *Nature Neuroscience, 3*, 516–520.

Gratton, G., Coles, M. G. H., & Donchin, E. (1983). A new method for off-line removal of ocular artifact. *Electroencephalography and Clinical Neurophysiology, 75*, 468–484.

Hagoort, P., Brown, C. M., & Swaab, T. Y. (1996). Lexical-semantic event-related potential effects in patients with left hemisphere lesions and aphasia, and patients with right hemisphere lesions without aphasia. *Brain, 119*, 627–649.

Hagoort, P., & Kutas, M. (1995). Electrophysiological insights into language deficits. In F. Paller & J. Grafman (Eds.), *Handbook of neuropsychology, Vol. 10* (pp. 105–134). Amsterdam: Elsevier Science B.V.

Halgren, E., Baudena, P., Clarke, J. M., Heit, G., Marinkovic, K., Devaux, B., Vignal, J.-P., & Biraben, A. (1995). Intracerebral potentials to rare target and distractor stimuli. II. Medial, lateral and posterior temporal lobe. *Electroencephography and Clinical Neurophysiology, 94*, 229–250.

Halgren, E., Squires, N. K., Wilson, C. L., Rohrbaugh, J. W., Babb, T. L., & Crandall, P. H. (1980). Endogenous potentials generated in human hippocampal formation and amygdala by infrequent events. *Science, 210*, 803–805.

Harlow, J. M. (1868). Recovery from the passage of an iron bar through the head. *Publications of the Massachusetts Medical Society, 2*, 327–346.

Johnson, R., Jr. (1988). Scalp-recorded P300 activity in patients following unilateral temporal lobectomy. *Brain, 111*, 1517–1529.

Johnson, R., Jr. (1995). On the neural generators of the P300: Evidence from temporal lobectomy patients. In G. Karmos, M. Molner, V. Csepe, & I. Czigler (Eds.), *Perspectives of Event-Related Potential Research* (EEG Suppl. 44: 110–129). Amsterdam: Elsevier.

Kaipio, M. L., Cheour, M., Ceponien, R., Ohman, J., Alku, P., & Naatanen, R. (2000). Increased distractibility in closed head injury as revealed by event-related potentials. *Neuroreport, 11*, 1463–1468.

Karayanidis, F., Andrews, S., Ward, P. B., & McConaghy, N. (1991). Effects of inter-item lag on word repetition: An event-related potential study. *Psychophysiology, 28*, 307–318.

Knight, R. T. (1984). Decreased response to novel stimuli after prefrontal lesions in man. *Electroencephalography and Clinical Neurophysiology, 59*, 9–20.

Knight, R. T. (1996). Effects of hippocampal lesions on the human P300. *Nature, 383*, 256–259.

Knight, R. T., & Scabini, D. (1998). Anatomic bases of event related potentials and their relationship to novelty detection in humans. *Journal of Clinical Neurophysiology, 15*, 3–13.

Knight, R. T., Scabini, D., Woods, D. L., & Clayworth, C. C. (1989). Contributions of temporal-parietal junction to the human auditory P3. *Brain Research, 502*, 109–116.

Kutas, M. (1998). Current thinking on language structures. *Cahiers de Psychologic Cognitive, 17*, 951–969.

Kutas, M., & Dale, A. (1997). Electrical and magnetic readings of mental functions. In: M. D. Rugg (Ed.), *Cognitive neuroscience* (pp. 197–242). Cambridge, MA: MIT Press.

Kutas, M., & Hillyard, S. A. (1980). Reading senseless sentences: Brain potentials reflect semantic incongruity. *Science, 207*, 203–205.

Kutas, M., & Van Petten, C. (1994). Psycholinguistics electrified: Event-related brain potential investigations. In M. Gernsbacher (Ed.), *Handbook of psycholinguistics* (pp. 83–143). New York: Academic Press.

Larsen, J., & Swick, D. (2000). Left frontal lesions eliminate the ERP repetition effect during repeated encoding of item and source information. *Society for Neuroscience Abstracts, 26*, 973.

Marchand, Y., D'Arcy, R. C., & Connolly, J. F. (2002). Linking neurophysiological and neuropsychological measures for aphasia assessment. *Clinical Neurophysiology, 113*, 1715–1722.

McCarthy, G., Wood, C. C., Williamson, P. D., & Spencer, D. D. (1989). Task-dependent field potentials in human hippocampal formation. *Journal of Neuroscience, 9*, 4253–4268.

Miller, E. K., & Cohen, J. D. (2001). An integrative theory of prefrontal cortex function. *Annual Review of Neuroscience, 24*, 167–202.

Näätänen, R. (1990). The role of attention in auditory information processing as revealed by event-related potentials and other brain measures of cognitive function. *Behavioral and Brain Sciences, 13*, 201–288.

Onofrj, M., Fulgente, T., Nobilio, D., Malatesta, G., Bazzano, S., Colamartino, P., & Gambi, D. (1992). P3 recordings in patients with bilateral temporal lobe lesions. *Neurology, 42*, 1762–1767.

Paller, K. A., & Kutas, M. (1992). Brain potentials during memory retrieval provide neurophysiological support for the distinction between conscious recollection and priming. *Journal of Cognitive Neuroscience, 4*, 375–391.

Paller, K. A., Kutas, M., & Mayes, A. R. (1987). Neural correlates of encoding in an incidental learning paradigm. *Electroencephography and Clinical Neurophysiology, 67*, 360–371.

Paller, K. A., Kutas, M., & McIsaac, H. K. (1995). Monitoring conscious recollection via the electrical activity of the brain. *Psychological Science, 6*, 107–111.

Pineda, J. A., Foote, S. L., & Neville, H. J. (1989). Effects of locus coeruleus lesions on auditory, long-latency, event-related potentials in monkey. *Journal of Neuroscience, 9*, 81–93.

Polich, J., & Squire, L. R. (1993). P300 from amnesic patients with bilateral hippocampal lesions. *Electroencephalography and Clinical Neurophysiology, 86*, 408–417.

Polo, M. D., Newton, P., Rogers, D., Escera, C., & Butler, S. (2002). ERPs and behavioural indices of long-term preattentive and attentive deficits after closed head injury. *Neuropsychologia, 40*, 2350–2359.

Potter, D. D., Jory, S. H., Bassett, M. R., Barrett, K., & Mychalkiw, W. (2002). Effect of mild head injury on event-related potential correlates of Stroop task performance. *Journal of the International Neuropsychological Society, 8*, 828–837.

Potter, D. D., Bassett, M. R., Jory, S. H., & Barrett, K. (2001). Changes in event-related potentials in a three-stimulus auditory oddball task after mild head injury. *Neuropsychologia, 39*, 1464–1472.

Reed, J. M., & Squire, L. R. (1997). Impaired recognition memory in patients with lesions limited to the hippocampal formation. *Behavioral Neuroscience, 111*, 667–675.

Rempel-Clower, N. L., Zola, S. M., Squire, L. R., & Amaral, D. G. (1996). Three cases of enduring memory impairment after bilateral damage limited to the hippocampal formation. *Journal of Neuroscience, 16*, 5233–5255.

Rosahl, S. K., & Knight, R. T. (1995). Role of prefrontal cortex in generation of the contingent negative variation. *Cerebral Cortex, 5*, 123–134.

Rugg, M. D., & Allan, K. (2000). Memory retrieval: An electrophysiological perspective. In M. S. Gazzaniga (Ed.), *The new cognitive neurosciences*, 2nd Edition (pp. 805–816). Cambridge, MA: MIT Press.

Rugg, M. D., Otten, L. J., & Henson, R. N. A. (2002). The neural basis of episodic memory: Evidence from functional neuroimaging. *Philosophical Transactions of the Royal Society of London, B, 357*, 1097–1110.

Rugg, M. D., Roberts, R. C., Potter, D. D., Pickles, C. D., & Nagy, M. E. (1991). Event-related potentials related to recognition memory: Effects of unilateral temporal lobectomy and temporal lobe epilepsy. *Brain, 114*, 2313–2332.

Sauvé, M. J., Walker, J. A., Massa, S. M., Winkle, R. A., & Scheinman, M. M. (1996). Patterns of cognitive recovery in sudden cardiac arrest survivors: The pilot study. *Heart and Lung, 25*, 172–181.

Segalowitz, S. J., Bernstein, D. M., & Lawson, S. (2001). P300 event-related potential decrements in well-functioning university students with mild head injury. *Brain and Cognition, 45*, 342–356.

Shimamura, A. P. (1995). Memory and the frontal lobe. In M. S. Gazzaniga (Ed.), *The cognitive neurosciences* (pp. 803–813). Cambridge, MA: MIT Press.

Smith, M. E. (1993). Neurophysiological manifestations of recollective experience during recognition memory judgments. *Journal of Cognitive Neuroscience, 5*, 1–13.

Smith, M. E., & Halgren, E. (1989). Dissociation of recognition memory components following temporal lobe lesions. *Journal of Experimental Psychology: Learning, Memory, and Cognition, 15*, 50–60.

Soltani, M., & Knight, R. T. (2000). Neural origins of the P300. *Critical Reviews in Neurobiology, 14*, 199–224.

Squires, N. K., Squires, K. C., & Hillyard, S. A. (1975). Two varieties of long-latency positive waves evoked by unpredictable auditory stimuli in man. *Electroencephalography and Clinical Neurophysiology, 38*, 387–401.

Stapleton, J. M., Halgren, E., & Moreno, K. A. (1987). Endogenous potentials after anterior temporal lobectomy. *Neuropsychology, 25*, 549–557.

Swaab, T. Y., Brown, C., & Hagoort, P. (1998). Understanding ambiguous words in sentence contexts: Electrophysiological evidence for delayed contextual selection in Broca's aphasia. *Neuropsychologia, 36*, 737–761.

Swick, D. (1998). Effects of prefrontal lesions on lexical processing and repetition priming: An ERP study. *Cognitive Brain Research, 7*, 143–157.

Swick, D., & Knight, R. T. (1998). Cortical lesions and attention. In R. Parasuraman (Ed.), *The attentive brain* (pp. 143–162). Cambridge, MA: MIT Press.

Swick, D., & Knight, R. T. (1999). Contributions of prefrontal cortex to recognition memory: Electrophysiological and behavioral evidence. *Neuropsychology, 13*, 155–170.

Swick, D., Kutas, M., & Neville, H. (1994). Localizing the neural generators of event-related brain potentials. In A. Kertesz (Ed.), *Localization and neuroimaging in neuropsychology* (pp. 73–121). San Diego: Academic Press.

Swick, D., Senkfor, A., Machado, L., & Van Petten, C. (1999). Frontal patients show impairments in behavioral and ERP measures of source memory. *Society for Neuroscience Abstracts, 25,* 649.

Swick, D., & Turken, A. U. (2002). Dissociation between conflict detection and error monitoring in the human anterior cingulate cortex. *Proceedings of the National Academy of Sciences, 99,* 16354–16359.

Tulving, E. (1985). Memory and consciousness. *Canadian Psychologist, 25,* 1–12.

Van Petten, C., Kutas, M., Kluender, R., Mitchiner, M., & McIsaac, H. (1991). Fractionating the word repetition effect with event-related potentials. *Journal of Cognitive Neuroscience, 3,* 131–150.

Vaughan, H. G. (1987). Topographic analysis of brain electrical activity. In R. J. Ellingson, N. M. F. Murray, & A. M. Halliday (Eds.), *The London symposia* (EEG Suppl. *39,* 137–142). Amsterdam: Elsevier.

Verleger, R. (1988). Event-related potentials and cognition: A critique of the context updating hypothesis and an alternative interpretation of P3. *Behavioral Brain Sciences, 11,* 343–427.

Verleger, R., Heide, W., Butt, C., Wascher, E., & Kompf, D. (1996). On-line brain potential correlates of right parietal patients' attentional deficit. *Electroencephalography and Clinical Neurophysiology, 99,* 444–457.

Vuilleumier, P., Hazeltine, E., Sagiv, N., Poldrack, R. A., Swick, D., Rafal, R. D., & Gabrieli, J. D. E. (2001). Neural fate of seen and unseen faces in visuospatial neglect: A combined event-related fMRI and ERP study. *Proceedings of the National Academy of Sciences, 98,* 3495–3500.

Yamaguchi, S., & Knight, R. T. (1991). Anterior and posterior association cortex contributions to the somatosensory P300. *Journal of Neuroscience, 11,* 2039–2054.

Zappoli, R., Zappoli, F., Picchiecchio, A., Chiaramonti, R., Arneodo, M. G., Zappoli Thyrion, G. D., & Zerauschek, V. (2002). Frontal and parieto-temporal cortical ablations and diaschisis-like effects on auditory neurocognitive potentials evocable from apparently intact ipsilateral association areas in humans: Five case reports. *International Journal of Psychophysiology, 44,* 117–142.

Zola-Morgan, S., Squire, L. R., & Amaral, D. G. (1986). Human amnesia and the medial temporal region: Enduring memory impairment following a bilateral lesion limited to field CA1 of the hippocampus. *Journal of Neuroscience, 6,* 2950–2967.

14 ERPs and Intracranial Recordings

Maryam Soltani, Erik Edwards, Robert T. Knight, and Mitchel S. Berger

The use of electrophysiology-based measures of brain activity dates back to the nineteenth century. In 1848, Du Bois-Raymond first demonstrated action potentials in nerves, and less than 30 years later, British psychologist Richard Caton described the electrical activity of the brain. In 1929, Hans Berger published the first report of the electroencephalogram (EEG) in humans, which in turn led to the first use of intra-operative EEG by Foerster and Alternberger in 1935. Beginning in the late 1930s, Wilder Penfield and Herbert Jasper further refined the technique of intraoperative EEG, demonstrating that it can be used to localize seizure activity during epilepsy surgery (Penfield & Jasper, 1954; see also Walker, Marshall, & Beresford, 1947).

In relation to questions of cortical function, tremendous advances in understanding were made by combining electrocorticographic (ECoG) recordings with electrical stimulation mapping (ESM)—the application of a brief electrical pulse to the cortex. For example, Penfield and Boldrey (1937) applied ESM to the motor cortex of awake human patients undergoing epilepsy surgeries. These studies produced a classic map for motor output referred to as the "motor homunculus," a map indicating which regions of motor cortex control which motor effectors. Over 25 years later, Penfield and Roberts (1959) introduced language mapping as a technique to spare critical language areas during surgical resection of cortical tissue. Specifically, they reported that the stimulation of language cortex could produce aphasic-like errors, information that could guide the extent of the surgical resection (Ojemann & Whitaker, 1978). Finally, in the 1970s, Ojemann and colleagues used ESM to map various cognitive functions (e.g., language and memory) in awake patients undergoing epileptic foci and tumor resections (Rao et al., 1995). Today, the technique is employed clinically to guide tissue resections and used experimentally to understand the neural mechanisms underlying cognitive function.

Methods of Intracranial Recording

Stereoelectroencephalography

Stereoelectroencephalography concerns recording electrical activity from electrodes inserted beneath the cortical surface. The stereotactic method was first used to investigate functioning of the thalamus and hypothalamus in patients with petit mal epilepsy (Spiegel & Wycis, 1950, 1951). Since its advent, stereoelectroencephalographic—or depth—recordings have been done with linear, multicontact arrays, and continue to be used for the localization of epileptic seizure activity. The electrodes are monitored within the subject for days to weeks, during which time researchers can do additional cognitive experiments. In terms of the electrode metals used, it is important to note that many metals when left in the brain for periods greater than a day can cause inflammatory reactions. For instance, cobalt, copper, nickel, and vanadium cause toxic reactions (Wieser, 1999); platinum, silver, chlorided silver, and tungsten can all cause reactions when left in for a period of weeks to months (Fischer, Sayre, & Bickford, 1957; Robinson & Johnson, 1961; Cooper & Crow, 1966; Cooper, Osselton, & Shaw, 1980). The thin wire used to make contemporary intracerebral electrodes is generally encapsulated with Teflon or some other type of nontoxic enamel (Cooper, Osselton, & Shaw, 1980).

In relation to ERPs, Halgren and colleagues have successfully used stereoelectro-encephalography to better localize the origins of various scalp recorded evoked potentials (Halgren et al., 1980; Halgren et al., 1995). For example, they have demonstrated that the scalp recorded P300 is a product of multiple cortical generators (Baudena et al., 1995; Clarke, Halgren, & Chauvel, 1999a, 1999b; Halgren et al., 1995a, 1995b; Halgren, Marinkovi, & Chauvel, 1998). They propose that the brain has developed a strategy in which it recruits all potentially useful regions in order to complete a task, even though the probability that each region will contribute to the immediate task is low. In turn, this widespread activation of multiple parallel-processing systems is assumed to facilitate interactions with the natural environment, where it is beneficial to rapidly identify and evaluate an event so that an adaptive response can be made (Halgren, Marinkovi, & Chauvel, 1998). Importantly, these studies demonstrate how intracranial recordings can contribute to both psychological and neuroscientific theory.

Critically, stereoelectroencephalographic methods continue to evolve. Halgren and colleagues have recently developed a thumbtacklike multielectrode with intercontact distances of 75–200 μm (Ulbert et al., 2001). This has allowed for the exploration of laminar patterns of cortical activity, including the firings of single units. Similarly, intracranial single-unit recordings in the medial temporal lobe and basal ganglia have provided important insights into memory and visual perception (Ojemann & Schoenfield-McNeill, 1999; Kreiman, Koch, & Fried, 2000), as well as motor control (Brown et al., 2002). Researchers have also applied stereoelectro-encephalographic methods to questions of functional connectivity. For instance, depth electrode recordings have revealed β-band oscillatory synchrony between extrastriate regions during short-term memory maintenance (Tallon-Baudry, Bertrand, & Fischer, 2001).

Electrocorticography

Electrocorticography (ECoG) concerns the recording of electrical potentials directly from the cortical surface.[1] In this domain, there are two main methods for ECoG recordings (Reid, 1989): (1) individual movable electrodes (IMEs), and (2) arrays of electrodes embedded in a flexible silastic sheet. The following sections detail the particulars of each electrode type and its uses.

Individual Moveable Electrodes   Individual Moveable Electrodes are typically ball-shaped electrodes made of silver, platinum, or carbon, and are attached to an apparatus affixed to the skull (figure 14.1, plate 8). An important use of these recordings is to monitor cortical after-discharges during electrical stimulation mapping (ESM). Ojemann and colleagues have conducted a limited number of studies using these intraoperative recordings for the investigation of language related potentials (Fried,

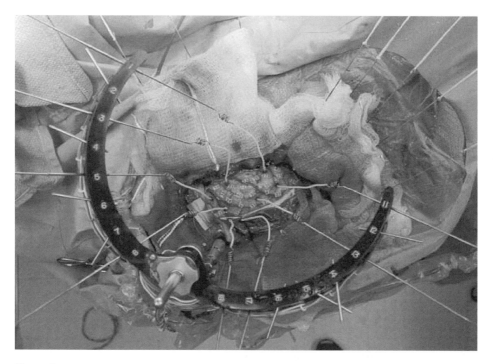

Figure 14.1
The picture depicts a typical electrode mounting apparatus, the horseshoe-shaped cortical crown. The carbon ball electrodes can be seen at the end of the white wires connected to the crown. The numbers tag the locations of cortical stimulation during language or motor mapping. (See plate 8 for color version.)

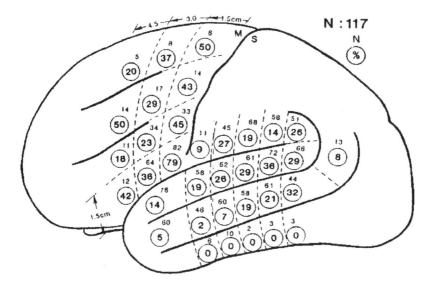

Figure 14.2
Essential language sites in 117 patients. The number within the circle is the percentage of patients
with an essential language site in that region. The number above the circle gives the number of
patients for whom that region was tested. (Courtesy of the *Journal of Neurosurgery*, in Ojemann
et al., 1989.)

Ojemann, & Fetz, 1981; Ojemann, Fried, & Lettich, 1989). Most notably, they mapped
essential language sites in 117 patients and demonstrated that, although there is some
concentration around traditional Broca's and Wernicke's areas, there is remarkable
intersubject variability in the number and location of essential language sites (Ojemann, Fried, & Lettich, 1989) (figure 14.2).

Silastic Sheets   The great majority of published ECoG studies of cognitive phenomena
employ silastic sheets, which are subdural arrays of electrodes imbedded in a flexible,
transparent sheet (figure 14.3). When laid on the surface of the patient's brain, the
sheet takes up the convexity of the cortex. Almost invariably, these electrodes are made
of platinum-iridium or stainless steel, have a diameter of ~3 mm, and have an inter-
electrode spacing of about 1 cm.

The most frequently studied region of the brain using silastic sheets has been the
sensorimotor system, where several centers have studied evoked potentials and spectral
activity (Baumgartner et al., 1991, 1992; Crone et al., 1998a, 1998b). An interesting
application of this research is the development of a direct brain interface for neuro-
prosthetic motor control in paralyzed individuals (Levine et al., 2000). Outside of the
sensorimotor cortex, a small number of studies have used subdural ECoG arrays to

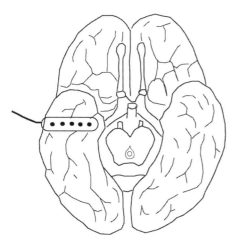

Figure 14.3
The figure illustrates electrodes embedded in a silastic strip. The silastic strip can be seen resting beneath the dura on the right temporal lobe. (Adapted from Reid, 1989.)

study visual processing (Arroyo et al., 1997), auditory processing (Crone et al., 2001a), or language (Nobre, Allison, & McCarthy, 1994; Nobre & McCarthy, 1995; McCarthy et al., 1995; Hart et al., 1998; Crone et al., 2001b).

Methodology

Recording
Often taking place in the operating room environment, ECoG recordings face a number of challenges: (1) electromagnetic interference from operating room equipment, (2) a nonsilent reference electrode, (3) recording of far field potentials, and (4) the influence of anesthetic agents, which can alter the EEG recordings. Consequently, anyone undertaking ECoG recordings should consider these issues carefully when designing, analyzing, and interpreting experiments.

Electromagnetic Interference The operating room is a haven of electromagnetic interference due to the fluorescent lighting and the abundance of electric and magnetic equipment (e.g., heart monitors, computers, MRI scanners). Three techniques that can facilitate the acquisition of relatively noise free data are low impedance electrodes, a differential amplifier with good common mode rejection (at least 100dB), and proper grounding and shielding of equipment and cables.

For an amplifier to perform maximally, electrode impedances should be kept at a value less than the amplifier's input impedance by a factor of 100 (Picton et al., 2000).

Impedance and noise are directly related. That is, the higher the electrode impedance the more likely that electromagnetic fields will contaminate the recordings (Picton et al., 2000). Furthermore, impedances should be kept constant across electrodes. Unequal electrode impedances will reduce the ability of the differential amplifier to reject common mode signals (Legatt, 1995; Picton et al., 2000). It is also important to use electrodes that are composed of the same material; using dissimilar metals can result in DC offsets between recording channels.

A differential amplifier with an excellent common mode rejection feature (e.g., a typical system on the market has a rejection ratio of 106dB, or a 200,000:1 reduction, in 60-Hz noise) is beneficial because it allows for the elimination of signals occurring in phase at each of the electrodes. Specifically, each active electrode will pick up signals that are both in and out of phase with respect to the reference electrode. However, based on the properties of a differential amplifier, whatever is in phase with the reference electrode—that is, the common signal—will be subtracted out. Furthermore, common mode rejection eliminates the data distorting that can occur with 60-Hz notch filters, which produce a damped oscillatory response when presented with a transient input (Cooper, Osselton, & Shaw, 1980).

Proper grounding and shielding techniques can also help reduce unwanted noise. One very basic step is to limit the length of all cables used and shield them thoroughly. Note that in order to activate a shield, it needs to be grounded. If the operating room has a designated ground, connect the shield wire to that terminal. If not, attach the shield wire to the amplifier chassis. As well, keep the amplifier and any head box cables as far away as possible from any AC cords or other electronic devices.

Nonsilent Reference Electrode   In a monopolar electrode arrangement or referential montage, voltage is recorded from an epicortical electrode (i.e., the active electrode) relative to an electrode placed approximately several centimeters away (i.e., the reference electrode). The reference electrode might be placed on the pia mater, on the dura mater, on the scalp, or on some other skin surface, such as the nose or neck. In any case, the reference is considered to be a neutral reference (i.e., a "silent reference" or "inactive reference"), such that any activity recorded on that channel can be ascribed to activity occurring at the site of the active electrode.

In reality, however, the ideal of a truly neutral reference is never accomplished in real recordings, due to contributions from electrically nearest neural or muscle activity. Reference electrodes on the pia mater, dura mater, or scalp will ultimately introduce neural activity into the channel, and reference electrodes on the scalp, nose, neck, or needle electrodes inserted into muscle will reflect muscle activity. Furthermore, with epicortical or epidural reference electrodes it is important to have them placed as far away from blood vessels as possible, which can also introduce unwanted artifacts into the EEG. As with scalp recordings, reference electrodes on the scalp or nose will also include ocular artifact from the corneoretinal dipole.

One method to determine the most silent reference is to record from numerous electrodes, create ERPs by averaging across trials, visually inspect the waveforms for the most silent electrode, and then re-reference off-line to that electrode. A predicted model of the original reference can also be created in order to obtain a better understanding of the signal. However, this method does not eliminate the problems inherent to a nonsilent reference, due to the fact that with differential amplifiers the original recording will always include an influence from the original reference electrode. As a consequence, its effects are not completely eliminated. But it does allow for some reduction in reference artifact contamination.

Crone et al. (2001a) argue for the use of a common average reference in analyzing ECoG data. The technique involves taking the average potential from all nonartifactual channels and then subtracting the result from the potential in each channel. This method allows for a reference independent calculation. The aforementioned calculation, however, does not allow for an evaluation of the original reference. To evaluate the activity at the original reference site, divide the sum of all channels by the number of all channels plus one (Dien, 1998). Nonetheless, it is important to note that with limited epicortical electrode coverage, one cannot assume that the common average reference can approximate an inactive reference. The technique is based on scalp EEG, which generally involves denser coverage, and satisfies the assumption that the signals—obtained from multiple scalp locations—relative to the average reference will approximate the true voltage over the head, namely average to zero (Bertrand, Perrin, & Pernier, 1985; Dien, 1998). Specifically, because the brain does not create nor destroy charge, its current sources (regions with net current outflow into the extracellular space) and sinks (regions with net current inflow into the neuron) should be equivalent. Hence, the potentials observed at the surface of the cortex or scalp (i.e., a spherical volume conductor) should average to zero (Bertrand, Perrin, & Pernier, 1985). As such the common average reference should act as a supplement to the common reference analysis. For a more detailed discussion of the common average reference, see Dien 1998.

Far- versus Local-Field Potentials   Relative to scalp-recorded ERPs, the advantage of ECoG recordings is their greater spatial localization of signal sources, which stems from recording local-field potentials on the cortical surface that are unrecordable on the scalp surface. On the other hand, far-field potentials—which comprise all cortical activity recorded on the scalp surface—arise from distant voltage sources, such as the corneoretinal dipole, subcortical dipoles, or distant cortical dipoles. Because the potential of a single dipole falls off in strength with the square of the distance from the

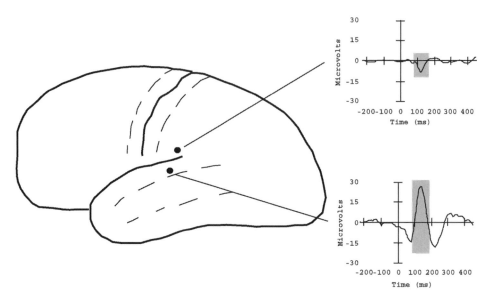

Figure 14.4
Illustration of far-field effects. The waveform depicts a typical response to a deviant auditory tone.
The generator is thought to be buried within the Sylvian fissure. Note the polarity reversal across
the fissure (see gray boxes).

dipole, the contribution of far-field potentials to ECoG recordings are considered to
be weak compared to the local-field potentials arising directly beneath or in the near
vicinity of the recording electrode. Also, unlike surface-recorded ERPs, the reference
electrode is often in relative proximity to the recording electrode, so it would tend to
cancel out far-field effects.

Nonetheless, far-field potentials often appear in ECoG recordings. Recordings in
animals from the crown of a gyrus can show far-field effects from the parts of the gyrus
buried within the sulcus (e.g., Pellegrini et al., 1987). Our own data from peri-Sylvian
areas of humans show auditory potentials originating from the superior temporal plane
buried within the Sylvian fissure (figure 14.4) (Soltani et al., 2003).

Effects of Anesthetic Agents   Anesthetic agents exert their effects by altering cerebral
metabolism, which in turn can affect the EEG by either exciting or depressing it (Sloan,
1998) (table 14.1). As a further complication, each anesthetic agent alters the evoked
response differently. Hence, general knowledge of commonly used anesthetics and
their effects on intraoperative electroencephalography is beneficial. As a rule of thumb,
halogenated inhalational agents decrease the amplitude and prolong the latency of
evoked potentials (EPs); *nitrous oxide* prolongs the latency and decreases the amplitude

Table 14.1

Effects of anesthetic agents on cortical EEG and evoked potentials (EPs)

Agents	EEG Effects	EP Effects
Halogenated Inhalational (e.g., desflurane, enflurane, halothane, isoflurane)	Varies based on agent used (see Sloan, 1998)	Decrease amplitude Increase latency
Nitrous Oxide	If used alone produces high frequency activity (>30 Hz) frontally	Decreases amplitude Increases latency
Barbiturates	Increase beta activity	Decrease amplitude Increase latency
Ketamine	Produces high amplitude theta activity and increase beta activity	Increases amplitude
Benzodiazepines	Low doses: Produces frontal beta activity with a decrease in alpha activity	Decrease amplitude No effect on latency
Etomidate		Increases amplitude
Propofol	Dose-dependent depression	Decreases amplitude, with rapid recovery upon termination
Muscle Relaxants	No effect	No effect

Data gathered from Sloan (1998).

of cortical EPs; *barbiturates* increase beta frequency activity in the EEG, decrease the amplitude and increase the latency of EPs; *ketamine* either does not effect EPs or it increases their amplitude; *benzodiazipines* increase beta activity, decrease EP amplitude, and have no effect on latency; *etomidate* causes an increase in both amplitude and latency of EPs; *propofol* decreases the amplitude of EPs but has a rapid recovery after termination; *narcotics* reduce EP amplitude; and *neuromuscular blockers* (muscle relaxants) demonstrate no significant effect on EPs (Sloan, 1998). For a more detailed review of the effects of anesthetic agents, see Sloan 1998.

Data Analysis

The analysis of ECoG data has many parallels to the analysis of scalp-recorded EEG. However, important differences exist as well, including both issues of method and interpretation. In the following sections we consider the particulars of artifact rejection, signal averaging, and time frequency analysis as they pertain to ECoG data.

Artifact Rejection Like deriving scalp-recorded ERPs, eliminating of artifact from the EEG data set is critical for intracortical ERPs. Generally there are four sources of artifact:

(1) EEG equipment (not discussed here; for a review, see Cooper, Osselton, & Shaw, 1980), (2) electromagnetic noise in the recording environment, (3) noisy electrodes and leads, and (4) noncerebral physiologic potentials. The rejection of such artifacts can best be accomplished with computer algorithms in conjunction with the visual inspection and the manual rejection of contaminated trials.

External electrical interference can be a serious contaminant of intraoperative data. The sources of the problem stem from electrostatic, electromagnetic, and radio-frequency pulses that can be traced to the abundance of electronic equipment in the operating room. We discussed solutions for reducing the electrical interference above. Nonetheless, the most effective way to remove the remaining electrical noise (e.g., 60-Hz line noise) involves conducting off-line low- and high-pass filters aimed at removing the contaminant frequency (see also Picton, Lins, & Scherg, 1995).

Artifacts from electrodes and leads generally result from poor contact between the electrode and the patient's cortex. The most obvious solution is to request that the electrode be reapplied to the brain. If, however, this is not possible, the electrode can be dropped either on- or off-line. Because the currents needed to measure electrode impedances are very low, researchers can use these measures to identify bad electrode contacts prior to recording. Furthermore, the contact between the electrode and the cortex may at times be disrupted by the surgical team and thereby cause the EEG amplifier to saturate. In recordings involving stimulation mapping, the current applied to the cortex can cause nearby electrode channels to saturate. Saturation can be prevented on-line with a gate that pauses the recording, or off-line with computer algorithms designed to remove those trials that are affected by and/or recovering from saturation. The most basic algorithm involves comparing each segment of the EEG time series with a maximum voltage threshold, and discarding that segment of the data when this threshold is exceeded (see chapter 6 of this volume).

The most common artifacts in EEG recordings are those that arise from the patient. Fortunately, unlike with scalp recordings, in the intraoperative setting eye movement, blink, and muscle potentials do not affect the EEG (an exception to this rule would result from an ill-placed reference electrode). This, however, does not mean that intraoperative data is free from physiologic artifact. For instance, the ECoG does contain a pulse artifact. When the brain is exposed, clear pulsations are visible with each heartbeat; this can cause a pulse artifact in the ECoG and is especially problematic if it arises in the reference electrode. Specifically, the electrodes rest on the surface of the brain and thereby move relative to the cortex. As with surface EEG recordings, creating a stable metal/liquid interface can minimize this artifact. One method for creating a stable interface, as Cooper, Osselton, and Shaw (1980) suggest, is "by using cotton wicks, soaked in saline solution, which rest on the brain surface and connect to wires supported by a clamp affixed to the skull." A second method requires interfacing the EKG machine with the ECoG acquisition machine, and directly recording the patient's heartbeat, so that the pulse artifact can be estimated and removed off-line. Finally a third involves filtering the data off-line with a high-pass filter set high enough to remove the patient's heart rate (~2 Hz, depending on heart rate and filter roll-off), but not so high that it removes potentially interesting slow waves (probably no higher than ~4 Hz).

Anesthetics can also introduce artifacts into the data, and can be difficult to interpret and reject. As table 14.1 details, a general understanding of the various anesthetics and their effects can facilitate the process. The best rejection method in this situation involves visually inspecting the data and manually removing those trials that demonstrate abnormal (or anesthetically induced) patterns of activity. Depending on the frequency of the artifact, high-pass filtering may also help.

Signal Averaging   The most basic method for analyzing ECoG data is to derive ERPs, which are simply the time-locked averages across many trials. The time-locking is typically done to a stimulus, such as an auditory tone, and the resulting ERP contains a series of positive and negative voltage fluctuations from the pre-stimulus baseline, termed components. Note, however, that the ERPs recorded from the cortical surface are much greater in amplitude than those recorded from the surface of the scalp. Indeed, single-trial event-related responses can sometimes be seen in ECoG data. However, in our own experience, the signal-to-noise for cortically recorded ERPs is still low enough that several tens of trials are needed to obtain a stable waveform in the ERP (figure 14.5).

Scalp-recorded ERPs provide a noninvasive measure of the temporal course of various cognitive processes, but they do lack in spatial resolution. That is, relative to the latest brain imaging techniques such as fMRI, ERPs do not provide adequate information regarding the neural generators of a particular brain potential. Nonetheless, high-density recording arrays in conjunction with sophisticated data analysis techniques have enabled researchers to extract some information regarding the location of various neural generators. For instance, researchers have employed dipole source localization techniques, wherein they seed dipoles, located in a region thought to be involved in the generation of a particular ERP component, into a source modeling algorithm. The algorithm, in turn, provides information regarding the scalp distribution of the seeded dipoles. If the distribution significantly resembles (or explains) that of the component in question, then one can conclude that the chosen region is a potential generator of that ERP component. This is also known as the forward solution. Note there is also an inverse problem, which states that scalp distribution cannot effectively be used to localize (or determine) neural generators, because there are an infinite number of solutions (or dipole positions) that can potentially sum to give rise to each scalp-recorded distribution (for a review of these issues, see chapter 7 of this volume).

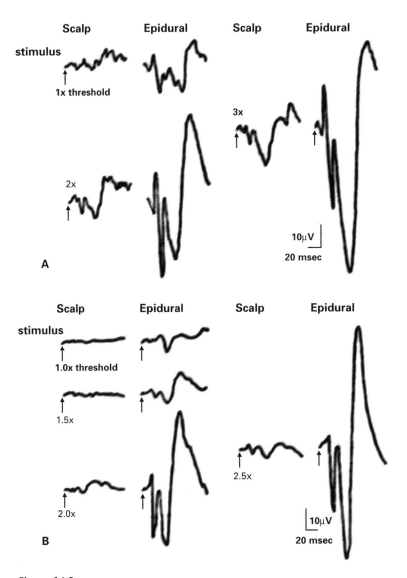

Figure 14.5

Averaged somatosensory-evoked responses in two patients under local anesthesia. A monopolar scalp needle and an epidural stainless steel ball electrode were placed over the hand area of the somatosensory cortex. The nasion served as the reference. The patient was fully awake, having received no prior medication except for local anesthesia at pressure points for the head holder and at the site of the scalp incision over the premotor area. The contralateral median nerve was stimulated at the wrist at a frequency of 4 cy/s with monopolar cathodal squarewave pulses of 0.2 msec duration at stimulus threshold and various increments as shown. The analysis time of 200 averaged response was 125 ms. The stimulus was applied at the arrow. The time base and microvolt calibration are as indicated. Negativity is upward. The records of two different subjects (*A* and *B*) are shown to illustrate some of the variability of the responses. (Courtesy of *Science*, in Domino et al., 1964.)

Like scalp EEG, intracranial EEG has very high temporal resolution, but unlike scalp EEG, it also has very high spatial resolution. The spatial resolution of intracranially recorded ERPs is effectively limited by electrode size and spacing, and as such the technique can identify local ERP generators (Halgren, Marinkovic, & Chauvel, 1998). In this method, if a locally recorded ERP component is much larger in amplitude than in neighboring structures, and it changes in polarity over short distances, then one can conclude that the structure in question is a generator of the observed ERP component (see figure 14.4).

Finally, in interpreting the waveforms one should consider the stimuli used to elicit the ERP and the properties of the scalp-recorded ERP (i.e., amplitude, latency, and spatial distribution) in order to obtain a clear understanding of what the intracranially recorded ERP represents. As a general rule of thumb, earlier components are most commonly associated with sensory events and the later with more cognitive events. The amplitude generally provides information regarding the extent of the neural activation, the latency the onset of the activation, and the scalp distribution the underlying activity or pattern of brain activation (Friedman, Cycowicz, & Gaeta, 2001).

Time-Frequency Analysis   Time-frequency analysis allows for the investigation of the event-related spectral perturbations of the brain (e.g., gamma activity or 40 Hz). For instance, animal electrophysiological studies have demonstrated that synchronized brain activity in the gamma frequency range may be the correlate to feature binding (Gray et al., 1989). In line with the animal findings, induced gamma activity may correlate with feature binding in humans (Müller et al., 1996). Researchers can also use event-related coherence measures to investigate functional connectivity between various brain regions. For example, by examining how the gamma activity observed in two different brain structures "correlate" with one another.

The same time-frequency methods used in scalp EEG, mainly moving-window fast Fourier transforms (FFTs) and wavelet-based methods (see chapter 11 in this volume), are used for intracranial data. Once again by bypassing the low-pass filter characteristics of the skull, intracranial recordings allow for the examination of high frequencies. Using subdural electrodes, Crone et al. (2001a) reported high-frequency gamma activity (~80–100 Hz) in the auditory cortex during a phoneme discrimination task. In a simple intraoperative mismatch negativity (MMN) task, we also acquired high-frequency gamma activity (70–170 Hz) to deviant tones, but when we conducted the same task using scalp recorded EEG we did not observe the high-frequency activity (70–170 Hz). Finally, intracranial recordings have also provided information on high-frequency "ripples" (100–500 Hz) in hippocampal and epileptic human cortex (Staba et al., 2002a, 2002b), and have shown that successful memory performance is accompanied by rhinal-hippocampal gamma band coupling (Fell et al., 2001). Hence, those undertaking time-frequency analyses should examine the higher frequencies as well.

Unless 60 Hz is a major recording issue, the amplifier low-pass filter (LPF) should be set higher for ECoG than what is typical of scalp recordings.

Applications

Intracranially recorded EEG can be applied to many of the same questions of cortical function addressed with scalp-recorded EEG, albeit with a higher degree of certainty regarding the loci of EEG signal sources. However, there are also questions that may be tractable only with intracranial recordings. Here we consider two questions uniquely addressed via intracranial methodology.

The Effect of the Skull on EEG

In relation to scalp-recorded EEG, the skull is thought to act as a low-pass filter. Toward validating this assumption, Pfurtscheller and Cooper (1975) investigated the low-pass properties of the skull by recording simultaneous ECoG and EEG in a single patient. Specifically, they directly applied sinusoidal voltages of varying frequencies through two IMEs, and measured the responses at the remaining IMEs and on the surface of the scalp. Applying this method, they found that the low-pass characteristics of the skull (as measured by scalp EEG) are due to a decrease in signal coherence across space as signal frequency increases. Thus, as signal frequency increases, there is a reduction in the degree to which signal phases align and thus the signals at higher frequencies tend to cancel out. In short, amplitude in the scalp EEG is a function of amplitude plus coherence in the ECoG, and at the scalp surface both amplitude and coherence decrease with frequency. In further comparing scalp EEG to cortical ECoG, considerable differences in signal spectra can be observed in ECoG electrodes spaced just millimeters apart, which is not generally the case for scalp-recorded EEG (Cooper et al., 1965).

The Size of Functional Units in Cortex

A second question relevant to intracranial recordings concerns elucidating the size of functional units in cortex. The question is particularly amenable to the analysis of synchrony in EEG frequency bands. The local domain of EEG synchrony, at least for gamma rhythms, is about 1 cm^2 (Menon et al., 1996, discussed further below). In conjunction from converging evidence from other domains, this suggests that the size of specialized cortical "modules" is on the order of a square centimeter or so. The techniques used to discover the locations and overall functions of these modules might be termed "macroscopic." A technique that looks at spatiotemporal patterns of activity within a module in order to determine how its primary computational units (cortical columns of the order of 1 mm in diameter) interact might be termed "mesoscopic."

Clearly, the uses of ECoG are essentially macroscopic, because the diameter and spacing of the electrodes are such that 1 cm^2 regions of cortex are sampled, and many tens of cortical columns are sampled beneath each electrode. However, Walter Freeman and Helmuth Petsche pioneered electrocorticography with grids of more closely spaced electrodes in animals in the 1970s. Both have argued convincingly for mesoscopic imaging (Petsche, Pockberger, & Rappelsberger, 1982, 1984; Freeman, 2000). For example, Petsche studied penicillin-induced seizure activity in rabbits using a 4×4 grid of electrodes with 0.3 mm diameter and spacings of 1 or 2 mm (Petsche, 1978; Petsche, Pockberger, & Rappelsberger, 1982). He modeled synchronization as arising from interactions of many elementary generators, each producing a unique signal. These generators are about 1 mm in diameter and probably correspond to cortical columns.

In humans, Freeman and colleagues have also examined synchrony of gamma activity and the spatial resolution of its underlying generators. Menon et al. (1996) used a standard silastic sheet with 1 cm spacing between electrodes to look for domains of spatially correlated gamma activity, as had been previously identified in animals. They reported negative results, suggesting that domains of locally correlated gamma activity existed on spatial scales smaller than 2 cm^2. They concluded that a denser array of electrodes, with spacings no greater than 0.5 mm, would be needed to study patches of local correlation. In a second study (Freeman et al., 2000), a new array was created that had closer spacings between electrodes. The new array had 0.1 mm diameter stainless steel electrodes embedded in a linear arrangement at an interelectrode spacing of 0.5 mm. The results of the study were consistent with a 1 cm^2 size for the domains of local gamma synchrony, but the linear array left other analyses wanting. They concluded that the optimal array would have "an electrode interval of 1.25 mm and an 8×8 spatial window of at least 10 mm." In sum, mesoscopic imaging in humans awaits such an electrode array.

Conclusion

Even though intracranial EEG provides excellent temporal and spatial resolution, it is still not without problems. For example, the technique does not employ healthy, normal working brains. As well, intracranial investigations are limited to recording from restricted brain regions. That is, the method provides information relating to a limited number of brain regions that have not necessarily been identified through experimental requirements. Fortunately, however, imaging techniques, such as functional magnetic resonance imaging (fMRI), provide excellent spatial resolution. As such, neuroimaging techniques can complement the intracranial findings by allowing for noninvasive investigations of the entire healthy human brain. Indeed, lesion and imaging studies have revealed a mosaic of interacting cortical modules that specialize in different functions. The technique thus offers the unique opportunity to look at the patterns of activity within these modules to better understand how they perform their specialized task. Proper analysis of the high-density data should also allow for clarification of issues relating to far-field effects and activity at the reference electrode.

Another lucrative possibility is to perform functional connectivity analyses on preoperative fMRI data sets, and then position two high-density electrode arrays over potentially interacting regions. The technique may allow for the observation of interareal synchronization between regions identified as functionally connected in fMRI (Bressler, 1995; von Stein, Chiang, & König, 2000). ESM mapping could also be used to identify regions that interact during a certain task or function. The spatial resolution of a high-density electrode array will also allow for testing broader hypothesis of neural transient interactions and interareal mutual information, of which interareal synchronization is but a subset (Friston, 1995, 1997). Such studies will undoubtedly lead to new insights concerning neocortical dynamics and information processing.

Note

1. Although these electrodes technically rest on top of the pia mater and some arachnoid, in the literature they are typically referred to as "epicortical."

References

Arroyo, S., Lesser, R. P., Poon, W. T., Webber, W. R., & Gordon, B. (1997). Neuronal generators of visual evoked potentials in humans: Visual processing in the human cortex. *Epilepsia, 38,* 600–610.

Baudena, P., Halgren, E., Heit, G., & Clarke, J. M. (1995). Intracerebral potentials to rare target and distractor auditory and visual stimuli: III. Frontal Cortex. *Electroencephalography and Clinical Neurophysiology, 94,* 251–264.

Baumgartner, C., Barth, D. S., Levesque, M. F., & Sutherling, W. W. (1991). Functional anatomy of human hand sensorimotor cortex from spatiotemporal analysis of electrocorticography. *Electroencephalography and Clinical Neurophysiology, 78,* 56–65.

Baumgartner, C., Barth, D. S., Levesque, M. F., & Sutherling, W. W. (1992). Human hand and lip snsorimotor cortex as studied on electrocorticography. *Electroencephalography and Clinical Neurophysiology, 84,* 115–126.

Bell, A. J., & Sejnowski, T. J. (1995). An information-maximization approach to blind separation and blind deconvolution. *Neural Computation, 7,* 1129–1159.

Berger, H. (1929). Uber das electrenkephalogramm des menschen. *Archives of Psychiatry, 87,* 527–570.

Bertrand, O., Perrin, F., & Pernier, J. (1985). A theoretical justification of the average reference in topographic evoked potential studies. *Electroencephalography and Clinical Neurophysiology, 62,* 462–464.

Bressler, S. L. (1995). Large-scale cortical networks and cognition. *Brain Research (Brain Research Reviews), 20*, 288–304.

Brown, P., Williams, D., Aziz, T., Mazzone, P., Oliviero, A., Insola, A., Tonali, P., & Di Lazzaro, V. (2002). Pallidal activity recorded in patients with implanted electrodes predictively correlates with eventual performance in a timing task. *Neuroscience Letters, 330*, 188–192.

Clarke, J. M., Halgren, E., & Chauvel, P. (1999a). Intracranial ERPs in humans during lateralized visual oddball task: I. Occipital and peri-Rolandic recordings. *Electroencephalography and Clinical Neurophysiology, 110*, 1210–1225.

Clarke, J. M., Halgren, E., & Chauvel, P. (1999b). Intracranial ERPs in humans during a lateralized visual oddball task: II. Temporal, parietal, and frontal recordings. *Electroencephalography and Clinical Neurophysiology, 110*, 1226–1244.

Cooper, R., & Crow, H. J. (1966). Toxic effects of intra-cerebral electrodes. *Medical and Biological Engineering, 4*, 575–581.

Cooper, R., Osselton, J. W., & Shaw, J. C. (1980). *EEG technology*. London: Butterworths and Co.

Cooper, R., Winter, A. L., Crow, H. J., & Walter, W. G. (1965). Comparison of subcortical, cortical, and scalp activity using chronically indwelling electrodes in man. *Electroencephalography and Clinical Neurophysiology, 18*, 217–228.

Crone, N. E., Miglioretti, D. L., Gordon, B., Sieracki, J. M., Wilson, M. T., Uematsu, S., & Lesser, R. P. (1998a). Functional mapping of human sensorimotor cortex with electrocorticographic spectral analysis: I. Alpha and beta event-related desynchronization. *Brain, 121*, 2271–2299.

Crone, N. E., Miglioretti, D. L., Gordon, B., & Lesser, R. P. (1998b). Functional mapping of human snsorimotor cortex with electrocorticographic spectral analysis: II. Event-related synchronization in the gamma band. *Brain, 121*, 2301–2315.

Crone, N. E., Boatman, D., Gordon, B., & Hao, L. (2001a). Induced electrocorticographic gamma activity during auditory perception. *Clinical Neurophysiology, 112*, 565–582.

Crone, N. E., Hao, L., Hart, J., Boatman, D., Lesser, R. P., Irizarry, R., & Gordon, B. (2001b). Electrocorticographic gamma activity during word production in spoken and sign language. *Neurology, 57*, 2045–2053.

Dien, J. (1998). Issues in the application of the average reference: Review, critiques, and recommendations. *Behavior Research Methods, Instruments and Computers, 35*, 745–754.

Domino, E. F., Matsuoka, S., Waltz, J., & Cooper, I. (1964). Simultaneous recordings of scalp and epidural somatosensory-evoked responses in man. *Science, 145*, 1199–1200.

Fell, J., Klaver, P., Lehnertz, K., Grunwald, T., Schaller, C., Elger, C. E., & Fernandez, G. (2001). Human memory information is accompanied by rhinal-hippocampal coupling and decoupling. *Nature Neuroscience, 4*, 1259–1264.

Fischer, G., Sayr, G. P., & Bickford, R. G. (1957). Histologic changes in the cat's brain after introduction of metallic and plastic coated wire used in EEG. *Proceedings of Staff Meeting the Mayo Clinic, 32*, 14.

Freeman, W. J. (2000). Mesoscopic neurodynamics: From neuron to brain. *Journal de Physiologie, 94*, 303–322.

Freeman, W. J., Rogers, L. J., Holmes, M. D., & Sibergeld, D. L. (2000). Spatial spectral analysis of human electrocorticograms including the alpha and gamma bands. *Journal of Neuroscience Methods, 95*, 111–121.

Fried, I., Ojemann, G. A., & Fetz, E. E. (1981). Language-related potentials specific to human language cortex. *Science, 212*, 353–356.

Friedman, D., Cycowicz, Y. M., & Gaeta, H. (2001). The novelty P3: An event-related brain potential (ERP) sign of the brain's evaluation of novelty. *Neuroscience and Biobehavioral Reviews, 25*, 355–373.

Friston, K. J. (1995). Neuronal transients. *Proceedings of the Royal Society of London. Series B: Biological Sciences, 261*, 401–405.

Friston, K. J. (1997). Another neural code? *Neuroimage, 5*, 213–220.

Gray, C. M., Konig, P., Engel, A. K., & Singer, W. (1989). Oscillatory response in the cat visual cortex exhibit intercolumnar synchronization which reflects global stimulus properties. *Nature, 338*, 334–337.

Halgren, E., Baudena, P., Clarke, J. M., Heit, G., Liegeois, C., Chauvel, P., & Musolino, A. (1995a). Intracerebral potentials to rare target and distractor auditory and visual stimuli: I. Superior temporal plane and parietal lobe. *Electroencephalography and Clinical Neurophysiology, 94*, 191–220.

Halgren, E., Baudena, P., Clarke, J. M., Heit, G., Marinkovic, K., Devaux, B., Vignal, J., & Birabin, A. (1995b). Intracerebral potentials to rare target and distractor stimuli: II. Medial, lateral, and posterior temporal lobe. *Electroencephalography and Clinical Neurophysiology, 94*, 229–250.

Halgren, E., Marinkovi, K., & Chauvel, C. (1998). Generators of the late cognitive potentials in auditory and visual oddball tasks. *Electroencephalography and Clinical Neurophysiology, 106*, 1152–1337.

Halgren, E., Squires, N. K., Wilson, C. L., Rohrbaugh, J. W., Babb, T. L., & Crandell, P. H. (1980). Endogenous potentials generated in the human hippocampus formation and amygdala by infrequent events. *Science, 210*, 803–805.

Hart, J., Crone, N. E., Lesser, R. P., Sieracki, J., Miglioretti, D. L., Hall, C., Sherman, D., & Gordon, B. (1998). Temporal dynamics of verbal object comprehension. *Proceedings of the National Academy of Sciences of the United States of America, 26*, 6498–6503.

Johnson, M. D., & Ojemann, G. A. (2000). The role of the human thalamus in language and memory: Evidence from electrophysiological studies. *Brain and Cognition, 42*, 218–230.

Kreiman, G., Koch, C., & Fried, I. (2000). Imagery neurons in the human brain. *Nature, 16*, 357–361.

Legatt, A. D. (1995). Impairment of common mode rejection by mismatched electrode impedances: Quantitative analysis. *American Journal of EEG Technology, 35*, 296–302.

Levine, S. P., Huggins, J. E., BeMent, S. L., Kushwaha, R. K., Schuh, L. A., Rohde, M. M., Passaro, E. A., Ross, D. A., Elisevich, K. V., & Smith, B. J. (2000). A direct brain interface based on event-related potentials. *IEEE Transactions in Rehabilitative Engineering, 8*, 180–185.

McCarthy, G., Nobre, A. C., Bentin, S., & Spencer, D. D. (1995). Language-related field potentials in the anterior-medial temporal lobe: I. Intracranial distribution and neural generators. *Journal of Neuroscience, 15*, 1080–1090.

Menon, V., Freeman, W. J., Cutillo, B. A., Desmond, J. E., Ward, M. F., Bressler, S. L., Laxer, K. D., Barbaro, N., & Gevins, A. S. (1996). Spatio-temporal correlations in human gamma band electro-corticograms. *Electroencephalography and Clinical Neurophysiology, 98*, 89–102.

Muller, M. M., Bosch, J., Elbert, T., Kreiter, A., Sosa, M. V., Sosa, P. V., & Rockstroh, B. (1996). Visually induced gamma-based responses in human electroencephalographic activity—a link to animal studies. *Experimental Brain Research, 112*, 96-1-2.

Nobre, A. C., Allison, T., & McCarthy, G. (1994). Word recognition in the human inferior temporal lobe. *Nature, 372*, 260–263.

Nobre, A. C., & McCarthy, G. (1995). Language-related field potentials in the anterior-medial temporal lobe: II. Effects of word type on semantic priming. *Journal of Neuroscience, 15*, 1090–1098.

Ojemann, G. A., & Whitaker, H. A. (1978). Language localization and variability. *Brain and Language, 6*, 239–260.

Ojemann, G. A., Fried, I., & Lettich, E. (1989). Electrocorticographic (ECoG) correlates of language: I. Desynchronization in temporal language cortex during object naming. *Electroencephalography and Clinical Neurophysiology, 73*, 453–463.

Ojemann, G. A., Ojemann, J., Lettich, E., & Berger, M. (1989). Cortical language localization in left dominant hemisphere: An electrical stimulation mapping investigation in 117 patients. *Journal of Neurosurgery, 71*, 316–326.

Ojemann, G. A., & Schoenfield-McNeill, J. (1999). Activity of neurons in human temporal cortex during identification and memory for names and words. *Journal of Neuroscience, 19*, 5674–5682.

Pellegrini, A., Curro-Dossi, R., Ermani, M., Zanotto, L., & Testa, G. (1987). On the intracortical activity during recruiting responses: An analysis of laminar profiles before and after topical application of GABA to cortex. *Experimental Brain Research, 66*, 409–420.

Penfield, W., & Boldrey, E. (1937). Somatic motor and sensory representation in the cerebral cortex of man as studied by electrical stimulation. *Brain, 60*, 389–443.

Penfield, W., & Jasper, H. (1954). *Epilepsy and the functional anatomy of the human brain.* Boston: Little, Brown and Co.

Penfield, W., & Roberts, L. (1959). *Speech and brain-mechanisms.* Princeton NJ: Princeton University Press.

Petsche, H. (1978). EEG synchronization in seizures: Facts and models. *Electroencephalography and Clinical Neurophysiology (Supplement), 34,* 299–308.

Petsche, H., Pockberger, H., & Rappelsberger, P. (1982). The micro-EEG: Methods and application to the analysis of the antiepileptic action of benzodiazepines. In Herrman (Ed.), *EEG and drug research* (pp. 159–182). New York: Gustav Fischer.

Petsche, H., Pockberger, H., & Rappelsberger, P. (1984). On the search for the sources of the electroencephalogram. *Neuroscience, 11,* 1–27.

Pfurtscheller, G., & Cooper, R. (1975). Frequency dependence on the transmission of the EEG from cortex to scalp. *Electroencephalography and Clinical Neurophysiology, 38,* 93–96.

Picton, T. W., Bentin, S., Berg, P., Donchin, E., Hillyard, S. A., Johnson, R., Miller, G. A., Ritter, W., Ruchkin, D. S., Rugg, M. D., & Taylor, M. J. (2000). Guidelines for using human event-related potentials to study cognition: Recording standards and publication criteria. *Psychophysiology, 37,* 127–152.

Picton, T. W., Lins, O. G., & Scherg, M. (1995). The recording and analysis of event-related potentials. In F. Boller & J. Grafman (Eds.), *Handbook of Neuropsychology* (pp. 3–73). New York: Elsevier Science.

Rao, S. M., Binder, J. R., Hammeke, T. A., Bandettini, P. A., Bobholz Frost, Myklebust, B. M., Jacobson, J. S., & Hyde, J. S. (1995). Somatotopic mapping of the human primary motor cortex with functional magnetic resonance imaging. *Neurology, 45,* 919–924.

Reid, S. A. (1989). Toward the ideal electrocorticography array. *Neurosurgery, 25,* 135–137.

Robinson, F. R., & Johnson, H. T. (1961). Histopathological studies of tissue reactions to various metals implanted in cat brains. In *ASD technical reports* (pp. 61–397). Ohio: Wright-Patterson Air Force Base.

Sloan, T. B. (1998). Anesthetic effects on electrophysiological recordings. *Journal of Clinical Neurophysiology, 15,* 217–226.

Soltani, M., Erik, E., Deouell, L., Knight, R. T., & Berger, M. S. (2003). Comparison of mismatch and pure sensory responses from epicortical recordings in awake patients. *Third International Workshop on Mismatch Negativity and Auditory Functions and Dysfunctions.*

Spiegel, W. A., & Wycis, H. T. (1950). Thalamic recordings in man, with special reference to seizure discharges. *Electroencephalography and Clinical Neurophysiology, 2,* 23–29.

Spiegel, W. A., & Wycis, H. T. (1951). Diencephalic mechanisms in petit mal epilepsy. *Electroencephalography and Clinical Neurophysiology, 3,* 473–475.

Staba, R. J., Wilson, C. L., Fried, I., & Engel, J. (2002a). Single neuron burst firing in the human hippocampus during sleep. *Hippocampus, 12*, 724–734.

Staba, R. J., Wilson, C. L., Bragin, A., Fried, I., & Engel, J. (2002b). Quantitative analysis of high-frequency oscillations (80–500 Hz) recorded in human epileptic hippocampus and entorhinal cortex. *Journal of Neurophysiology, 88*, 1743–1752.

Tallon-Baudry, C., Bertrand, O., & Fischer, C. (2001). Oscillatory synchrony between human extrastriate areas during visual short-term memory maintenance. *Journal of Neuroscience, 21*, RC177.

Ulbert, I., Halgren, E., Heit, G., & Karmos, G. (2001). Multiple microelectrode-recording system for human intracortical applications. *Journal of Neuroscience Methods, 106*, 69–79.

von Stein, A., Chiang, C., & König, P. (2000). Top-down processing mediated by interareal synchronization. *Proceedings of the National Academy of Sciences of the United States of America, 97*, 14748–14753.

Walker, A. E., Marshall, C., & Beresford, E. M. (1947). Electrocorticographic characteristics of the cerebrum in posttraumatic epilepsy. *Research in Nervous and Mental Disorders, 26*, 502–515.

Wieser, H. G. (1999). Stereoelectroencephalography and Foramen Ovale electrode recording. In E. Niedermeyer & F. L. Da Silva (Eds.), *Electroencephalography: Basic principles, clinical application, and related fields* (pp. 725–739). Baltimore, MD: Lippincott Williams and Wilkins.

Whitaker, H. A., & Ojemann, G. A. (1995). From Bartholow to Penfield: The historical development of electrical stimulation of the human brain from 1874 to 1928. *Brain and Language, 51*, 60–62.

15 Combining Electrophysiology with Structural and Functional Neuroimaging: ERPs, PET, MRI, and fMRI

Joseph B. Hopfinger, Wayne Khoe, and Allen Song

Event-related potentials (ERPs) are a vital tool for investigating the temporal dynamics of human cognition. The ability to identify the precise location of the underlying neural generators, however, is limited. In this chapter, we describe improved localization via realistic head models derived from structural magnetic resonance imaging (MRI). We then describe the advantages in spatial and temporal resolution that can be gained through combining ERPs with hemodynamic neuroimaging methods. Finally, we describe recent advances in MRI techniques that may further improve the integration of these methods.

Combining ERPs with Structural MRIs

Modeling Scalp-Recorded ERPs

Event-related brain potentials (ERPs) provide an excellent temporal resolution measure of neural processing, and thereby add significantly to theories of mental functioning. In addition to providing precise information regarding *when* mental events occurr, ERPs can also provide information regarding *where* in the brain such processing occurrs. However, the ability to precisely identify where these activities occur is limited, due to the distance between the neural generator and scalp recorded responses, and the assumptions one must make when modeling the transduction of the electrical signal through the intervening materials.

If the precise location and orientation of an active neuronal population is known, a unique pattern of activity on the outer surface of the human scalp can be calculated (known as the "forward solution"). The forward solution consists of calculating the voltage distribution at the scalp from known current sources within the brain. However, the situation faced with ERP data is the opposite—attempting to determine the neural generator of the activity recorded at the scalp. As described previously (e.g., chapter 7 of this volume), there is no unique solution to account for a specific pattern of activity recorded on the scalp, because any given pattern of activity on the scalp can be modeled by numerous different combinations and configurations of intracranial neural generators. Therefore, the localization of the neural generator of a scalp-recorded potential is inherently an ill-posed problem (known as the "inverse problem"). Despite the fact that there is no unique solution, it is still possible to achieve meaningful results. Relevant prior knowledge, such as the structure of the underlying anatomy, can further constrain the realm of possible solutions.

To solve for the inverse solution, an iterative error minimization algorithm is applied, measuring the differences between the fields calculated from the forward solution and the fields actually measured on the scalp with electrodes. Often, a simplifying assumption is made, so that a population of active neurons is approximated by a single source—an "equivalent current dipole" (ECD). To calculate a dipole solution, a model of volume conduction must be specified. The calculation typically includes solving for dipole parameters such as location within the head, orientation, and strength of activity. Through each iteration, the dipole parameters are adjusted to minimize the difference between the fields measured at the scalp and the forward solution (calculated from the hypothesized dipoles). A least-squares estimation is used to evaluate the goodness-of-fit between the scalp-recorded data and forward solutions. The accuracy of the inverse solution (measured as residual error variance) is dependent upon the precision of the volume conduction model chosen. In particular, small errors in modeling the forward solution (i.e., scalp distribution of the current) will translate into large errors of source parameter (e.g., dipole) estimation. Two major factors that contribute to the difficulty of solving for dipole sources are the low conductivity of the skull and the relatively high conductivity of the scalp. The skull and scalp conductivity determine the distribution and strength of the voltages measured at the scalp. Thus, it is important to choose an appropriate volume conduction model to describe and estimate the scalp current distribution when calculating the forward solution. Approaches used to model the head as a volume conductor include spherical and realistic head models. In both models, the brain, skull, and scalp tissue are segmented into various layers. Each layer is assigned a conductivity index, the amount of charge that passes through the layer. Depending on the model specified, the layers may be represented by concentric spherical shells or anatomically realistic layers or compartments. Assumptions of conductivities and shape of each layer play a significant role in the accuracy of the forward solution. Below we describe a few of these models in more detail.

Spherical Shell Models

The simplest volume conduction model is the spherical head model. Early efforts at modeling ERP components utilized a spherical head model to calculate the intracranial generators that best accounted for the data recorded on the scalp. These early efforts sometimes modeled the entire head and all internal material as a single homogeneous sphere, or "shell." Previous limits in computing power somewhat necessitated this simplifying assumption that the head could be modeled this way. However, there were serious limitations to this approach. Two of the most obvious limitations concern the

facts that the brain and head are not perfect spheres, and that there are multiple surfaces between the neural generators and the recording electrode. Furthermore, these
different surfaces have different electrical conductivities. The computational advantage
of this formulation is that it provides an analytic solution, a unique solution, to the
forward problem. However, this simple model may produce large estimation errors, especially because it does not take into account the low conductivity of the skull (Ary
et al., 1981).

Therefore, more recent source modeling attempts have used three-sphere models,
which model the brain, skull, and scalp as concentric spheres. The "brain" in these
three-sphere models refers to everything contained within the cortical sheet—all the
cortical gray and white matter, in addition to the cerebral spinal fluid. The "skull" layer
refers to skeletal structure surrounding the brain. The "scalp" layer refers to the layer
of scalp tissue surrounding the skull. Each layer is assigned an isotropic conductivity
index (i.e., each layer is assumed to have homogenous conductivity throughout).
However, in reality, conductivities may not be entirely homogenous within a layer.
Future models may thus incorporate further fractionating of each layer. Even if the
model does not incorporate these differences in conductivities, distinguishing the
"brain" from the "skull" and "scalp" has led to more accurate models. Researchers
generally assume that the skull, in particular, has a significantly different conductivity
than the brain and scalp, and therefore, some mathematical models using three concentric shells have assumed relative conductivities of 1 for the brain and scalp and
.0125 for the skull. Although this makes a simplification by assuming homogeneous
conductivities within each layer, the three-sphere model does significantly improve the
localization of the spherical head models over the single shell models (Ary et al., 1981).

MRI-Derived Realistic Head Models

The spherical shell model is a rough approximation of both the geometrical and electrical properties of the head. In particular, the conductivity of the skull contains
local variations that cannot be modeled in a spherical head model. The limitation of
assuming isotropic conductivities becomes more apparent for sources located deeper
within the brain. For example, Menninghaus and colleagues (1994) found dipole localization errors increased from 3 mm to 8 mm when the distance between the dipole
and inner surface of the skull increased from 1 cm to 3 cm. In addition, the spherical
approximation of each layer is insufficient for modeling regions where the tissue
boundaries deviate significantly from sphericity. Deviations from sphericity can produce significant changes in the scalp voltage topography produced by sources near the
nonsphericities, thus affecting the accuracy of the forward solution (e.g., Cuffin, 1990).
Hamalainen and Sarvas (1989) demonstrated dipoles located in frontal and temporal
regions were poorly localized due to the poor fit between the spherical representation
and the aforementioned cortical areas. In frontal regions, the upper portion of the
skull is roughly spherical, whereas the bottom is flat. In temporal regions, the sphere

provides a poor fit with the flat portion of the region. Although spherical head models are computationally advantageous in providing a relatively quick analytic solution to the forward problem, the approximation of compartment shape and assignment of homogeneous conductivities to each layer can lead to errors in localization on the order of centimeters.

In contrast to spherical models of the head, realistic head models rely on three-dimensional surfaces that are typically constructed using anatomical and geometrical details extracted from MRI images. Specifically, these models extract the boundaries between different tissues and different features of the head, based on the signal intensity differences in anatomical MRI images. Compartments are constructed to represent the brain, skull, and scalp. Some recent models may include a fourth layer, the cerebral spinal fluid, between the brain and skull. Figure 15.1 illustrates these compartments as derived from a typical T1-weighted MRI anatomical set of images. The electrical potential produced by a dipole source is then computed by solving a system of integral equations governing the potential at these different layers. Extracting realistic compartments improves the forward solution, because the calculated scalp voltage topography takes into account the unique anatomy of the layers. Realistic head models can improve the dipole locations by up to approximately 2 cm due to the extraction of boundary surfaces from the MRI (Roth et al., 1993; Yvert et al., 1997).

Models employing these methods include the boundary element model (BEM) (Fuchs et al., 1998; Hamalaninen & Sarvas, 1989; Meijs et al., 1989) and finite element model (FEM) (Awada et al., 1997; Le & Gevins, 1993). In both models, the conducting volumes are parceled into a specific number of elements. In the BEM, the outer boundary of each compartment is defined and approximated by a mesh of (usually triangular) elements on the surface of the compartment; each compartment is assigned an isotropic conductivity. In other words, homogeneous conductivities are assigned to each layer, dividing the head into separate regions of constant conductivities. Given that within each boundary there are different types of material, however, the assumption of isotropic conductivities within each compartment is not ideal. For example, the skull consists of different bone types that may have considerably different conductivities. Unlike the surface triangulation of the different compartments in the BEM, FEM typically applies regularly shaped tetrahedral elements to approximate the volume of each compartment. More importantly, each volume element can be assigned an individual, anisotropic conductivity. Assigning individual conductivities to each element can improve the dipole solution by up to 5 mm. However, the gains in accuracy using a FEM can be smaller than the errors that could occur by assigning erroneous conductivities. In other words, obtaining accurate conductivity values for each region is more important than just modeling the volumes (Awada et al., 1998). Furthermore, the computational power needed to carry out the complex calculation used in the forward solution for the FEM is quite large relative to the computational load needed to calculate the forward solution in the BEM.

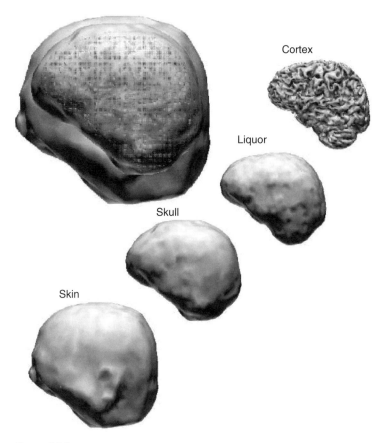

Figure 15.1
An anatomical T-1 weighted MRI image was acquired with a standard gradient echo sequence with isotropic 1 mm voxels. The image was then segmented (using CURRY 4.0 from Neuroscan, Inc.) into the compartments shown here: cortex, liquor (e.g., cerebrospinal fluid), skull, and skin compartments.

Distributed Source Models

In contrast to modeling the electrical activity recorded at the scalp with a small number of "equivalent current dipoles" (ECD), one may instead model the EEG signal as a weighted estimate of the activity over the entire cortical surface using a continuous estimation approach (Dale & Halgren, 2001; Dale & Sereno, 1993). Specifically, after segmenting the head into various compartments and layers, the cortical surface is flattened and divided into a large number of small patches (i.e., ~10,000 in Dale and Sereno's 1993 paper). An ECD is positioned in *each* patch perpendicular to the cortical surface. A continuous estimation approach then results in weighted estimates of activation being assigned to each ECD, thus approximating the patterns of neuronal sources over the cortical surface that may give rise to the distribution of synaptic currents observed on the scalp. The continuous estimation approach emphasizes the smoothness of the solution. In other words, the solution must take into account that neighboring neurons are most likely to activate simultaneously and synchronously. Similar to the cortical surface reconstruction approach proposed by Dale and Sereno (1993) is a method termed low-resolution brain electromagnetic tomography (LORETA) (Pascual-Marqui, Roth, & Lehmann, 1994; Pascual-Marqui et al., 2002). LORETA is similar to other distributed source models in that the brain is divided into discrete elements. However, unlike other approaches, LORETA emphasizes a 3D solution to the inverse problem. In LORETA, the brain is represented as a dense 3D grid with an ECD located at each grid point, and the orientation of each ECD is allowed to rotate during the continuous estimation algorithm. The spatially continuous nature of the solution from distributed source models thus allow solutions from individual subjects to be combined into an average, after aligning the MRI images into a common reference space (Dale et al., 2000; Fischl et al., 1999).

Co-Registration between ERP and MRI Data

When using a realistic head model, issues of integrating data from different imaging modalities into a common coordinate system become critical. In particular, spatially aligning electrode locations to the 3D anatomical MRI datasets must be performed prior to solving for the inverse solution. The position of each recording electrode must be determined in exact reference to the realistic head model. Researchers have proposed several co-registration techniques to address the problem of co-registration between the two imaging modalities, including landmark and surface coordinate based registration techniques (see Maintz & Viergever, 1998 for review).

Landmark based registration methods are the most common and simple of the co-registration methods available. Image registration proceeds by placing the electrode locations into a common reference frame relative to the locations of standard anatomical landmarks (i.e., the nasion and the left and right pre-auricular points). Experimenters have employed electromagnetic or acoustic digitization systems to measure the locations of the electrodes in three-dimensional space. To co-register MRI images to the electrode location, one can attach MR-visible oil-filled capsules (e.g., vitamin E capsules) to anatomical landmarks during the MRI scan. Although experienced researchers may identify the anatomical landmarks directly from high-resolution anatomical MRI scans, oil capsules allow the landmarks to be seen easier in the MRI images. To co-register the electrode locations and the MRI data, the landmarks specified in the MRI and digitization sessions are transformed into the same space. To ensure that the landmarks specified in the digitization procedure and MRI scan are at the same locations, one must be careful when specifying the landmarks because they are typically done in separate sessions. If the landmark locations vary across the two sessions, this will translate to errors in co-registration that can lead to errors in source localization. One method to ensure that the same landmarks are being specified in both procedures is to use ear molds custom fit to the subject's head (e.g., Woldorff et al., 2002). During the MRI scan, researchers can push MR-visible oil-filled capsules down into the ear molds to help identify the landmarks. Subjects can wear the same ear molds during the electrode digitization procedure to ensure measurement of the same landmark locations.

Other co-registration techniques include surface based techniques. The surface registration method is based on a contour fit algorithm that matches digitized scalp surface points or electrode locations with the segmented skin surface from the MRI image (Huppertz et al., 1998; Pelizzari et al., 1989; Willemesen et al., 1998). These methods are also known as "hat-on-the-head" methods. For example, the electrode locations or the scalp surface points are transformed into a "hat," whereas the scalp surface extracted from the MRI is the "head." To achieve the best fit between hat and head, researchers use an algorithm that minimizes the distance between the segmented surface and the contour points on the surface.

Combining ERPs with Hemodynamic Neuroimaging

Introduction: Hemodynamic Neuroimaging Methods

Positron Emission Tomography Hemodynamic neuroimaging methods measure properties of blood flow that correlate strongly with neural activity. Positron emission tomography (PET) refers to a method of neuroimaging where trace amounts of a radioactive material are injected into the blood stream. Highly sensitive coincidence detectors are then able to localize where the radioactive material is, by detecting the gamma rays produced when positrons from the radioactive material are annihilated upon combination with free electrons. Researchers can use different types of radioactive material to investigate a wide range of functions (e.g., radioactive fluoride ^{18}F to investigate glucose metabolism; [^{11}C]CFT to investigate dopamine reuptake). For studies of human cognition, however, the most common method is to use water tagged with an oxygen isotope (^{15}O). By radioactively tagging oxygen molecules, experimenters can inject water into the blood stream (via a saline intravenous drip), and compare the regional cerebral blood flow across different experimental conditions. Although the exact mechanisms are still not completely understood, there is a high correlation between neural activity and increased blood flow. Therefore, PET can provide a high spatial resolution view into the areas of the brain activated by a given cognitive process.

Functional Magnetic Resonance Imaging Functional magnetic resonance imaging (fMRI) initially also used contrast agents injected into a patients' blood stream to localize relative increases and decreases in blood flow. However, over a decade ago,

Ogawa and colleagues (1990) showed that intrinsic properties of the blood could be used to obtain measures of blood flow without the need for injected contrast agents. With this advancement, fMRI quickly became one of the preferred methods for investigating the neural mechanisms of human cognition. Indeed, the excellent spatial resolution of fMRI allows precise localization of brain regions corresponding to cognitive functions. However, as noted above, the exact mechanism whereby neural activity leads to an increase in blood flow is still unknown, and fMRI measures something even more removed from the actual neural activity: the relative concentration of oxygenated to deoxygenated hemoglobin. Again, although there is a very consistent correlation between increased neural activity, increased blood flow, and increased fMRI signal (due to an increased ratio of oxygenated to deoxygenated hemoglobin), it can be useful to keep in mind that hemodynamic neuroimaging methods are not directly measuring neural activity.

Limitations of Hemodynamic Neuroimaging   Although both PET and fMRI provide excellent spatial resolution, their temporal resolution is insufficient to identify the neural dynamics underlying cognitive processes. PET scanning typically averages over a 30- to 60-s interval to provide the necessary power to detect differences in activity across conditions. The temporal resolution of PET is constrained by the half-life of the radioactive isotope being utilized. For ^{15}O studies, this translates to at least 10 min between different experimental conditions. Although researchers can combine clever experimental designs with this method to investigate different brain states, it is too poor of a temporal resolution to accurately identify neural dynamics between multiple active brain regions. FMRI studies can collect whole-brain data once every second. Although this is an improvement over PET scanning, the major limiting factor is still the sluggishness of the hemodynamic response, which does not peak until 6–8 s after the initial activity. This does not provide the necessary resolution to determine the order of neural activity or the interactions of brain regions involved in mental processing. Therefore, although hemodynamic neuroimaging methods provide a significant advance in research possibilities, methods that directly measure neural activity remain necessary tools in cognitive neuroscience. As the following sections describe, combining ERPs with PET or fMRI data can provide the spatiotemporal resolution that neither alone can provide.

General Framework for Integrating ERPs and Neuroimaging

Experimental Design   Here we describe the experimental design controls that permit a stronger integration of ERP and hemodynamic neuroimaging. Previously, we described a "frames of reference" logic for combining different methodologies (Mangun, Hopfinger, & Heinze, 1998). According to this approach, there are four main reference frames that one should ideally address in any study that combines multiple methodologies. The first is that an identical *experimental* frame of reference should be established by utilizing identical experimental conditions in each session. Although the most powerful experimental design for one recording methodology may be different than the most powerful design in a second methodology, it is important that the experimental design remain the same across both sessions. By ensuring that factors such as timing parameters, task instructions, response requirements, and expectations of the participants are the same in each session, one can have greater confidence that the mental processing should be the same in each case. In addition, this allows the comparisons of interest to be calculated from the identical conditions in each session. This is another important factor in establishing a relation between the data from the different sessions. (In this section, we are referring to the more common case where the ERP and neuroimaging sessions are performed separately; however, later we describe in more detail the advantages and disadvantages of simultaneously recording ERPs directly during the fMRI session).

A second reference frame is the *sensory* reference frame. This refers to having identical stimuli in all recording sessions, in order to prevent any differences from arising due to different stimulus parameters. Although most ERP sessions utilize a computer monitor to present stimuli, this may not be a possible method of presentation in neuroimaging sessions. In a previous combined ERP/PET experiment (Mangun et al., 1997), we were able to use identical monitors in both sessions; however, the strong magnetic fields of MRI scanners preclude using a typical computer monitor during fMRI experiments. Instead, one must use specialized projection systems or goggle systems. One method to ensure the best control of the sensory frame of reference would be to use the identical goggle system (or projection system) during ERP sessions as those used in the MRI scanner. As a practical matter, however, the equipment designed for the MRI environment is typically significantly more expensive than standard equipment used in ERP studies, and therefore it may not be an option to simply purchase MRI-compatible equipment for an ERP lab. Therefore, in order to ensure a similar sensory frame of reference, investigators should take care to calibrate and carefully measure the equipment in both environments. (Note that even when using the identical presentation systems in each recording session, there may still be differences inside and outside of the MRI scanner due to the strong magnetic fields). Although an identical sensory reference frame would always be the ideal situation, the control of this sensory reference frame is an especially large concern for experimenters investigating sensory systems; it may not be as critical when investigating higher order aspects of cognition that are less sensitive to simple physical differences in the stimuli. Though the above discussion dealt with visual displays, one faces similar problems when presenting stimuli in other sensory modalities as well.

A third reference frame requires that the same subject(s) be used in all sessions. We refer to this as the *biological* reference frame. In order to integrate the multiple methodologies more completely, a common "spatial" reference frame is desirable. This final *spatial* frame of reference requires putting the data into a common space to establish a more firm relationship between the ERP effects and the hemodynamic neuroimaging activations. In order to do this, we must utilize all available information about the possible spatial localization of the ERP effects. This can be done using dipole modeling, as described earlier in this chapter. As we noted earlier, however, the inverse solution from scalp-recorded electrical data has no unique solution, and thus, it may appear paradoxical now to consider using it to aid in answering the question of how neuroimaging and ERP effects relate. However, although modeling ERP data alone cannot give one unique solution, the addition of neuroimaging activations can provide additional constraints on the modeling, resulting in functionally and anatomically plausible solutions.

Theoretical Relation Between ERP and Hemodynamic Neuroimaging Measures   In attempting to relate ERP and PET/fMRI results, it is helpful to consider the nature of the mapping between electromagnetic recordings and measures of regional cerebral blood flow (rCBF). Much previous research has provided evidence that ERP responses reflect the electrical current generated directly by postsynaptic activity in neurons (see Nunez, 1981). ERPs time-locked to a stimulus measure a transient-evoked response that is composed of one of two types of neural activity: exogenous (stimulus driven) and endogenous (non-stimulus driven, but observed time-locked to a stimulus or behavioral response) responses. ERPs may also reveal changes in cortical excitability, as indexed by slow shifts in scalp voltage such as the contingent negative variation (CNV). Whereas ERPs directly measure neuronal activity, PET and fMRI methods view this activity indirectly by measuring the blood flow changes that are coupled to neuronal activity. It remains unknown whether the fMRI and PET effects primarily reflect transient stimulus-evoked activity, changes in cortical excitability that is not stimulus evoked, or both. Although ERP and hemodynamic neuroimaging measures are reflections of different physiological signals, they may nonetheless arise as the result of identical information processing activities occurring in the neuronal population. However, one must consider various possible mappings between the ERP and PET effects.

   The possible mapping of ERPs to PET/fMRI include: (1) the ERP and hemodynamic measures may be reflections of identical neuronal activity—for example, both may result from either (a) stimulus-evoked activity, or (b) cortical excitability that is not stimulus-evoked per se; (2) the ERP and rCBF measures may be reflecting different aspects of neuronal activity, but in the same neurons and as the result of the same mental state—for example, the sensory-evoked ERPs could be transient-evoked activities, whereas the rCBF changes could be more closely associated with changes in excitability and background firing rates, but in the same neuronal population; (3) the ERP and rCBF measures may be reflections of a similar mental state, but in entirely separate neuronal populations, because each is either reflecting different types of neuronal activity or similar types of activity segregated in different brain areas. In principle, another possibility exists, that they have no relationship whatsoever. However, if the experiment has been designed under the constraints of the "frames of reference" approach discussed earlier, this latter possibility is unlikely because the ERP and PET/fMRI effects are by definition related via the experimental circumstances under which they were revealed—same stimuli, same tasks, same experimental comparisons, same subjects. Of the foregoing possibilities, all are probably going to be true to varying extents depending upon the process and brain system under investigation. They key question is, How correlated are the two measures in any given brain region or for any given behavioral or cognitive task? It is probably best not to assume perfect correspondence, but rather carefully to build an experimental framework in which the effects are both related to a specific mental operation (as defined by the study, and specific comparisons), and then to ask via modeling and experimentation just how the measures might be related for each brain activity and cognitive process under investigation.

Importantly, there is no a priori reason to assume that every effect observed in one modality should necessarily have a correlate in recordings done using another method, due to the unique sensitivities of each recording modality. Thus, the idea that the problem is merely how to match rCBF activations to electromagnetic effects is incorrect. One must formulate experimental designs with the specific goal of integrating these distinct measures, execute analyses in such a way as to make the results comparable, and utilize procedures that allow the combination of the results to more rigorously test hypotheses of the spatiotemporal dynamics of mental processes.

In the following two sections we describe two methods to assist in the matching between these measures. One is the use of electrical modeling. Combining methodologies provides a means for constraining the inverse problem using information from functional neuroimaging as an extension of prior attempts to constrain such exercises using only anatomical information (e.g., Dale & Sereno, 1993). Another method is the analysis of covariation between effects from different recording modalities across multiple tasks, which can add to the benefit of combining these approaches. Indeed, in many cases the most powerful approach for relating electromagnetic to blood flow measures may be to demonstrate that they covary over a wide range of manipulations.

Identifying Covariations between ERP and Neuroimaging Results

When an experiment is designed to allow examination of interactions or parametric effects, one can look for covariations in these effects. For example, previously we reported data from a study of visual selective attention, wherein we investigated the localization of an early visual-evoked ERP component, the P1, in a study that combined PET and ERPs (Mangun et al., 1997). Participants ($N = 11$) were required to maintain fixation upon a centrally located cross, while pairs of symbols flashed bilaterally (50-ms duration, 250–550-ms stimulus onset asynchrony) to the right and left upper visual fields. In separate blocks, participants were instructed either to attend to the pair of symbols on the left, attend to the pair on the right, or simply passively to view the stimuli. There were also three types of instructions. Participants were instructed on some blocks to press a button whenever the two symbols matched (a difficult discrimination), on other blocks to press a button whenever a small dot appeared somewhere within the area where the symbols were flashing (a simple detection task), or to simply passively view the stimuli in yet other blocks. Participants completed PET and ERP sessions on separate days. MRI scans were also obtained from each participant.

If the same neural and computational processes generate both the ERP and PET/fMRI effects, then the effects recorded through each methodology should covary with one another as a function of stimulus and task demands. The comparisons of interest here were the main effects of (1) attending to the right versus left visual field, (2) the hard versus easy task conditions, and (3) the interaction of attention-direction and task-condition. In the ERP data, a significant main effect of attention was obtained for the P1 component in both tasks (figure 15.2, top). This result was expected as numerous previous studies have shown that voluntary selective attention can modulate the neural processing that generates the P1. In addition, however, we found a significant interaction between attention and task. This resulted from the more difficult form discrimination task inducing larger attention effects in P1 amplitude than did the detection task (figure 15.2, bottom). In the PET data, we found a significant main effect of attention (attend left versus attend right) in two different visual processing regions of the brain: the posterior fusiform gyrus and the middle occipital gyrus, both contralateral to the attended hemifield (figure 15.3, top). Given two alternative generators of the P1 component, we then investigated the interaction of task and attention to determine if either or both of these regions would show the same interaction with task that we observed on the P1 attention effect. An analysis of the interaction of attention by task revealed that only the fusiform gyrus activation was significantly modulated in a similar manner to the P1 attention effect; the middle occipital did not show evidence of an interaction with task difficulty (figure 15.3, bottom). This covariation between the P1 effect and the fusiform gyrus PET effect provided further evidence that the stage of visual processing indexed by the P1 component (that begins around 80 ms latency) occurs in extrastriate cortex in the posterior fusiform gyrus. This method of utilizing different task parameters to analyze covariations between attention effects observed in different recording modalities can serve as a strong test of hypothesized relationships, especially when the measures have been recorded from the same group of human subjects.

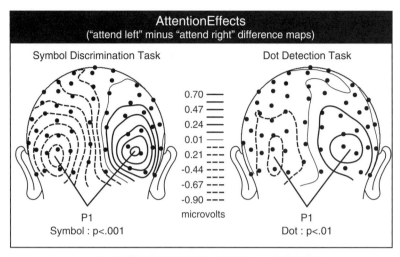

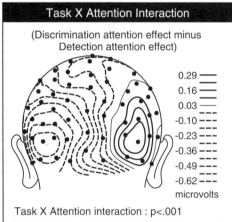

Figure 15.2

(*Top*) Topographic voltage maps of P1 attention effect, for attend right minus attend left differences. Both the symbol discrimination task (left column) and dot detection task (right column) resulted in significant effects over lateral occipital scalp sites during the 110–140 ms time range, corresponding to the peak of the P1 component. (*Bottom*) Topographic voltage map of the difference between symbol-discrimination and dot-detection attention effects in the 110–140 ms time range. This difference shows a significant task by attention interaction, which is localized at a similar scalp region as the P1 component. (Reprinted from Mangun, Hopfinger, & Heinze, 1998, with permission from Psychonomic Society.)

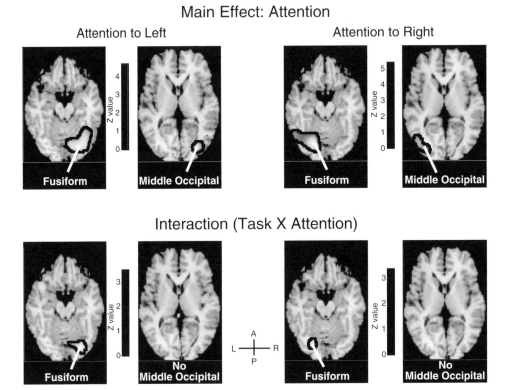

Figure 15.3

(*Top*) Main effects for the symbol (form) discrimination task, showing effects of attending left (left two images) and attending right (right two images), superimposed upon MRI images. Shown are horizontal brain sections low in the brain and slightly more dorsal. Attention produced activation in the fusiform gyrus (seen in the lower slices) and middle occipital gyrus (seen in the more dorsal slices) in the hemisphere contralateral to the attended location. (*Bottom*) Interactions of attention and task showing significant effects in the fusiform gyrus contralateral to the attended hemifield. Thus, the fusiform gyrus effect was modulated by task in the same manner as the P1 attention effect in the ERP data. (Adapted from Mangun, Hopfinger, & Heinze, 1998, with permission from Psychonomic Society.)

Comparing across multiple conditions increases the ability to investigate these types of interactions. Of course, a strong constraint here is that as the number of experimental conditions increases, the smaller the number of trials within each condition. Given a limited amount of time within a PET or fMRI scanner, or limits in the number of ERP sessions that an individual can participate, it may not be tenable to include more than one condition if one is looking at small effects. If experimental effects are large enough to allow the use of more conditions, parametric type analyses allow even greater potential for analyzing covariations between the results from different methodologies.

For example, in the above description, we directly contrasted attend left versus attend right conditions to examine the effects of selective attention on visual processing. However, there are numerous attention related processes engaged within a task that do not depend upon the precise locus of spatial attention, but rather are engaged regardless of where attention is directed. Therefore, in other analyses, we have investigated the brain regions involved in non-directionally sensitive aspects of attention. Recent studies of attentional "load" (Lavie & Tsal, 1994) have shown that the allocation of attentional resources is not an all-or-none phenomenon, but rather depends on factors such as perceptual and task difficulty. Therefore, recently we reported the results of a "parametric" style analysis across the three task types of this same study to investigate regions of the brain in which activity changed systematically with increasing task difficulty, or recruitment of attentional resources (Hopfinger et al., 2001). For the purposes of this analysis, we interpreted the passive viewing condition as being the least attention demanding "task," the detection of simple luminance targets as the next most attention demanding, and the symbol discrimination task as having the highest attentional load.

In our analysis, we found that multiple brain regions that had not shown selective attention effects (differences in attend left versus attend right) were revealed as being involved in the more general, non-directionally sensitive aspects of attentional engagement. This analysis revealed activity that our previous analysis of selective attention effects had not, such as in the right pulvinar and bilateral parietal regions. These regions of cortex have previously been implicated in attention, and here we showed that they are engaged to a greater extent as the task difficulty increases, possibly involved in the recruitment or allocation of attentional resources. We found a particularly strong modulation across tasks in a region of the supplementary motor area, extending into the mid-cingulate gyrus (figure 15.4, left). This area is very similar to the area activated by the target stimuli in recent event-related fMRI experiments (e.g., Hopfinger et al., 2000; Woldorff et al., 2001). Although recent event-related fMRI studies were able to attribute this activity to target processing (as opposed to cue invoked preparatory processing), they could not precisely specify when the activity was occurring. Therefore, from the fMRI data alone, it's difficult to infer the stage of

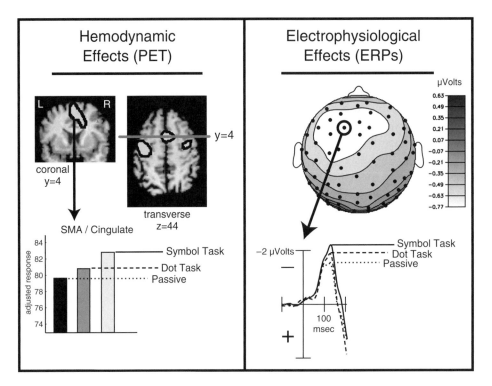

Figure 15.4

Parametric analyses of PET effects and corresponding ERP effects with increasing levels of task difficulty. The coronal section at left is taken at the anterior-posterior level indicated in the horizontal section displayed to the right. At the bottom left, the pattern of activation for the SMA/ cingulate activation (stereotactic coordinates 0, 4, 44; $Z = 5.10$) is shown graphically (the y-axis "adjusted response" refers to blood flow measurements after all scans were scaled to have a mean whole brain level of 50 ml/min/dl, and after removal of confounding factors). At bottom right, the ERP waveform from a single frontocentral electrode site is displayed for the three levels of the task. An increase in the anterior N1 ERP component (peaking at about 140 ms) can be seen with increasing task difficulty. The scalp distribution of this effect is shown at top right, by plotting the difference map for the symbol task minus the passive viewing condition. (Adapted from Mangun, Hopfinger, & Jha, 2000 with permission from Lippincott, Williams, & Wilkins, 2000.)

processing at which this area of the brain is involved in target processing. However, even though PET alone has a much poorer temporal resolution than fMRI alone, our combined PET/ERP study provided superior temporal information. Specifically, we were able to examine the ERP data for activity that varied with task difficulty, in addition to testing for parametric modulations in the PET data. A negative polarity peak, occurring at approximately 100 ms latency after target onset and recorded at scalp locations overlying the SMA/cingulate region, was found to show a parametric increase with increasing attentional load (figure 15.4, right). Although we have not conducted electrical modeling of the intracranial currents associated with this ERP activity, the scalp distribution of this ERP effect is consistent with a generator in midline anterior regions of the brain. This covariation between the PET and ERP effects, combined with the spatial position of these effects, suggests that this region of cortex may be active approximately 100 ms following the presentation of the target. Researchers can use this information to constrain the interpretation of the operation(s) being performed by this region, for example by excluding the possibility that it is only involved in a final response generation after perceptual analyses have been thoroughly completed.

Neuroimaging-Constrained ERP Modeling

As mentioned previously, a great strength of combined ERP/neuroimgaing studies is that the neuroimaging results may provide important constraints for modeling ERP data. In our study described above, the effects of selective attention were increased blood flow in two separate loci within visual cortex (fusiform gyrus and middle occipital gyrus). In the previous section, we described how researchers can use covariations across experimental manipulations to infer the correspondence between attention effects seen in neuroimaging results and attention effects on specific components of the ERP waveform. Here, we describe how we used the brain loci identified by PET to constrain our inverse dipole modeling of that ERP data (cf. Heinze et al., 1994; Martinez et al., 1999).

For the present data, we used a boundary element approach in a realistic head model (Hopfinger et al., 2001). We derived the details of the brain, skull, and scalp anatomy from anatomical MR images of the participants. The ERP data were coregistered with the MR-derived realistic head model by fitting the 3D electrode array (digitized from each participant's head during recording) to the MR image surface using a minimization algorithm and fiducial landmarks. With two candidate regions (fusiform and middle occipital gyrus) in each hemisphere defined by our PET activations, it was possible to seed dipoles to either the fusiform gyrus or middle occipital gyrus and then to test which of these produced the best model of the recorded ERP data at a specific time.

We found that when dipoles were placed in the fusiform gyrus, the model provided a better explanation (i.e., lower residual variance) for the recorded data in the time range

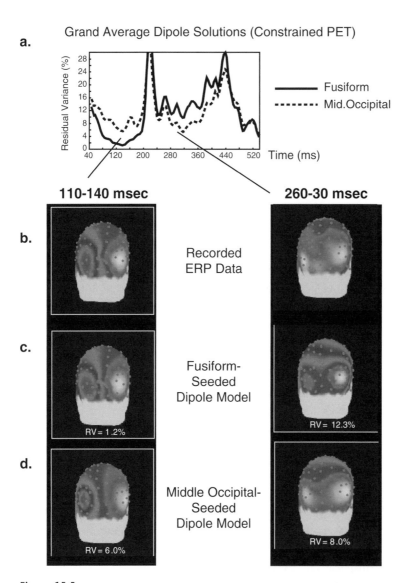

Figure 15.5
(*a*) Graph depicting the percentage of scalp voltage variance not accounted for ("residual variance") when measuring the goodness of fit between dipole models and the observed ERP scalp distribution for the attend left minus attend-right difference waveform (note that a lower value on the residual variance graph represents a better goodness of fit). Dipole models were constrained by the PET activations (left and right fusiform gyri, and left and right middle occipital gyri) elicited by the attend left versus attend right comparison. The fusiform gyrus model (solid line in the graph) produced a better fit than the middle occipital model (1.2 percent versus 6.0 percent, re-

from 110 to 140 ms than did placement of the dipoles in the more lateral PET activations in the middle occipital gyrus (figure 15.5, top graph and left column; see plate 9). This time range conforms closely to the P1 ERP attention effect, and provides more evidence that the fusiform attention effect is occurring at this time, as proposed previously (Heinze et al., 1994; Mangun et al., 1997). Interestingly, we observed the inverse pattern for an ERP component in a later time range. Specifically, in the 260–300 ms latency range, the middle occipital gyrus dipoles produced a better model solution than did those in the fusiform gyrus (figure 15.5, top graph and right column). These findings support our prior conclusion that activity in the region of the fusiform is related to attentional modulations of early sensory processing, and extends this result by showing that activations in more lateral regions of visual cortex are related to attentional modulations at longer latencies, in line with the organization of the ventral visual processing stream (e.g., Tootell et al., 1998). These results provide an illustration of the ability of a combined approach to elucidate the temporal sequence of even closely spaced brain activity.

Simultaneous versus Parallel EEG and fMRI Sessions

Although more standard EEG equipment could be used in most PET machines, only recently have advances in EEG amplifier technology made it possible to acquire EEG inside the MRI scanner. This raises the issue of whether it still makes sense to acquire EEG and neuroimaging in separate sessions, or whether it would always be preferable to collect the EEG and neuroimaging data simultaneously. According to the logic laid out above, simultaneous recording would be preferable in the sense of having the mental mechanisms be identical. However, there are numerous issues to consider.

One of the most severe limiting factors may be the interactions between MR imaging pulses (electromagnetic and magnetic) and EEG signal reception. Such interactions are generally mutual, in that MR would affect EEG and vice versa. The interference of

Figure 15.5 (continued)

spectively) in the latency range of 110–140 ms, corresponding to the P1 ERP attention effect. In contrast, at a latency range of 260–300 ms, the middle occipital gyrus model (thick dashed line) produced a better fit than did the fusiform model (8.0 percent versus 12.3 percent). (*b–d*) Recorded topographic maps of attention effects (*b*) corresponding to the attend left minus attend-right difference waveform, and model data topographic maps (*c* and *d*) for dipoles placed at the location of the PET defined fusiform gyrus attention effects (*c*) or the location of the PET defined middle occipital gyrus attention effects (*d*). The maps are for the time period of the P1 component (110–140 ms) in the left column, and for a later sustained positivity (260–300 ms) in the right column. The difference between the recorded and model data, expressed as percent residual variance (RV), is shown below each model head. The view of the heads is from the rear (left on left). The locations of electrodes are indicated by gray disks. (Reprinted from Hopfinger et al., 2001, with permission from Elsevier Science.) (See plate 9 for color version.)

the EEG recording system to MR signal can be minimized by properly isolating and shielding the power sources of the EEG system such that it does not alter the uniformity of the electromagnetic and magnetic fields used for MR imaging. On the other hand, it is a significant challenge to minimize the impact of the electromagnetic and switching magnetic fields on the EEG signal. One effective method may be the spike-triggered EEG recording technique (Lemieux et al., 2001) that ensures EEG acquisition only occurs during the "quiet" period of MRI, that is, the period when no MR imaging pulses are broadcast.

Another issue may be the increased cost of the system for MR compatibility. Because special EEG leads and special amplifiers must be used to allow EEG recording in the MRI environment, the cost of these systems can be significantly greater than the cost of a typical EEG set-up. A related issue is then the portability of the unit. Specifically, due to the time required to set up the systems in an imaging environment, it would likely require a dedicated system to remain at the imaging center. Although this does not suggest that it is preferable to do the recordings separately, it is a factor that one may need to consider.

There is also a limit to the density of the electrode montage that can be used. Specifically, the MRI compatible systems generally contain a reduced number of electrode recoding sites compared to standard systems. Previous research has shown that the ability to localize EEG sources is significantly impaired as one reduces the number of electrode locations. Therefore, although one may gain the knowledge that the mental states were exactly the same during the EEG and neuroimaging collection, localization of the EEG sources could be compromised by having too few channels. In this sense, it may actually be preferable to perform a separate recording session outside of the magnet with a higher density array of electrode locations.

Finally, the number of trials required to obtain sufficient signal to noise ratios for EEG signal may exceed the time limit allowed for a typical fMRI session. Although some ERP components are large enough to obtain a high signal-to-noise ratio with relatively few trials, many ERPs require a large number of trials, even in a shielded room. It may be very difficult to obtain clean measures of these ERP components in the electrically noisy environment of an MRI scanner; at the very least it is likely to require a large number of trials. However, it may not be possible to obtain the necessary signal-to-noise in a single MRI session, although the fMRI signal may be sufficiently strong from a single session. Considering the high cost and uncomfortable environment of MRI scanning, it is likely that participants would provide higher quality EEG data outside the MRI environment for a number of experiments. Due to the fact that inverse-dipole source-modeling is very sensitive to noise, obtaining data with a high signal-to-noise ratio is critical in these endeavors. Therefore, it may be preferable to record the sessions separately so that one can provide the best possibility for success, in terms of being able to accurately model the ERP data.

Therefore, whether it is preferable to obtain EEG and neuroimaging methods in separate or simultaneous sessions must be decided on a case-by-case basis, with a strong consideration of the effects of interest in the study. For example, one specific case in which it would be preferable to obtain data simultaneously is the study of human learning mechanisms. If one hypothesizes that learning is happening throughout the task, it may not make sense to record a second session, if the learning of interest has already occurred. It may also be preferable to attempt simultaneous acquisition in situations where both blood oxygenation level dependent (BOLD) and EEG signals are likely to be very strong and do not require too large a number of trials. However, there still remain many instances where it is likely preferable to obtain data in separate sessions, and to use high-density EEG recordings to enhance the ability to localize the generators of more subtle scalp-recorded events.

Recent Advancements in MRI: Implications for Enhancing Multimethodology Integration

As mentioned above, the blood oxygenation level dependant (BOLD) signal detected in most fMRI studies does not reflect neural activity directly, but rather measures a change of the deoxygenated blood. Although this signal correlates very strongly with neural activity, experimenters must keep in mind that it is not a direct measure of neural activity. This is especially apparent in the fact that the BOLD signal can be highly sensitive to draining veins. Because of this, the activity detected by BOLD methods often extends beyond the region of actual neural activity, and may include spurious "activations" as well (e.g., veins, motion artifacts). Below we describe a few techniques that hold promise for more precisely identifying the actual regions of active tissue. We also discuss recent MRI methods that may allow for the measurement of electrical conductivities of different volumes within the head. Combined with advances in modeling techniques that utilize MRI images to create realistic head models, these methods could provide even greater localization of the neural sources of EEG and MEG data.

Improving the Localization of Neural Activity Using Hemodynamic Contrast Mechanism

Although the first fMRI experiment was conducted in 1991, it is still unclear what MR imaging method is the "best" for mapping brain function. The reasons are many, including: the complex hemodynamics of the human vascular system in the event of neuronal activities influences the spatial accuracy of the co-localization of the BOLD signal; the multidimensional parameter space of fMRI contrast manipulation changes the amplitude and spatial extent of the functional signal; the lack of a clear gold standard in the human functional imaging literature to determine what signal is the most accurate in spatial and temporal co-localization with the neuronal activities. Despite this difficulty in choosing the most accurate imaging technique, the workhorse method has been the gradient-recalled echo-planar imaging (EPI) method because of its sensitivity to the inhomogeneity underlying the BOLD signal and its high temporal resolution. This technique is appealing in practice as it produces the largest signal changes with neuronal activation. However, it has been reported and is now gaining wide acceptance that the bulk of the signal observed by the gradient-recalled EPI method is from the large veins and their surroundings (Boxerman et al., 1995; Lai et al., 1993; Song et al., 1995, 1996). Signal arising from these sites may be distant from the true neuronal activities.

Optimal Scanning Sequences   Refined methods that minimize these distant activations are desireable. For example, researchers have reported that diffusion weighting can selectively eliminate contaminating signals from the large veins (Boxerman et al., 1995; Popp et al., 1998; Song et al., 1996). These techniques are critical in achieving more accurate co-localization, but they often result in a much smaller functional signal at the typical magnet strength used in most cognitive neuroimaging studies (1.5 tesla). Some have proposed alternative methods using T2 contrast (e.g., spin-echo EPI) to reduce extra-vascular contribution from large vessels (Baker, 1993; Bandettini, 1994), but these also result in reduced overall activation. Moreover, such signals still contain intravascular contribution from the large veins, which could still be distant. A parallel use of diffusion weighting is still necessary, which further diminishes the functional signal. As a result, although diffusion weighting and/or spin echo EPI seem to have some advantages over the more typical EPI method, these techniques are less often used for most functional experiments on 1.5 T scanners.

An implication for combining ERP and fMRI data is that using the more typical gradient-recalled EPI sequences may produce sites of "activation" that are not true sources of neural activity. Because these "false activations" can sometimes appear larger than real activations, one may mistakenly use the false activations as "seeded-dipoles" in source modeling the ERP data. On the other hand, using alternative fMRI sequences and parameters (e.g., spin-echo EPI) may better protect against false activity sources, but has the limitation of decreased signal. This could prove even worse for some instances of source modeling efforts, as the reduced magnitude fMRI signal may not allow detection of the true activity underlying some ERPs. One must remain aware of the limitations of the fMRI sequences being used when attempting to work with these data in source modeling efforts.

The Initial "Dip"   Recent optical spectroscopy and fMRI data (Malonek & Grinvald, 1996, 1997; Vanzetta & Grinvald, 1999; Hu, Le, & Ugurbil, 1997; Kim, Duong, & Kim, 2000) suggest that the spatial specificity of BOLD could be further and more dramatically improved if a—hypothesized—initial *decrease* of MR signals can be utilized for functional imaging formation. Some suggest that the event immediately following focal neuronal activity is an increase in local oxygen consumption, consequent to the increased neuronal firing rate of active neurons. The resultant increase of deoxy-hemoglobin content would be detected as a transient decrease in MR signal using appropriate (i.e., T2 or T2* weighted) imaging sequences. As fresh blood enters the capillaries in response to the increased metabolism, the oxygenation level will reverse such that the MR signal will experience an eventual increase—giving rise to the conventional BOLD signal. Grinvald and co-authors (Malonek et al., 1997; Malonek & Grinvald, 1996) hypothesized a fundamentally distinct functional specificity for these two events: The initial deoxygenation, as a consequence of an increase in oxidative metabolism, should be co-registered with the site of electrical activity up to the level of individual cortical columns. The delayed oxygenation of the cortical tissue on the other hand, is far less specific due to the spread of hemodynamic activity beyond the site of original neural activity. Both the existence of "biphasic" BOLD response *per se*, and the suggested differences in functional specificity has been the subject of heated controversies in recent years (Buxton, 2001). Although the initial deoxygenation signal in fMRI (termed "initial dip") has been reported in awake behaving humans (Hu, Le, & Ugurbil, 1997) and anesthetized monkeys (Logothetis et al., 1999), most studies in rodents failed to detect any significant initial decrease in BOLD signal following sensory stimulation (Lindauer et al., 2001; Marota et al., 1999; Silva & Kim, 2000), although some did (Mayhew et al., 2001). The question of whether the use of initial dip would indeed improve the spatial specificity of BOLD has been far more difficult to address experimentally, largely because of its low contrast-to-noise ratio (CNR) and coarse spatial resolution. As such, only the results from ultra-high magnetic field can reliably demonstrate this initial decrease of MR signal, as Kim, Duong, and Kim (2000) show.

The impact of this for combined ERP/fMRI studies is still unclear. The ability to localize neural activity at a cortical column resolution is unlikely to make a significant difference in modeling ERPs due to the blurring effect that the brain, skull, and scalp have on the electrical activity. However, the ability of this method to better localize activity, in terms of not highlighting "activations" from draining veins, could be a great benefit. The better localization of actual neural activity should improve the ability to correctly model scalp recorded activity. However, the decrease in signal strength of the initial dip (as compared to the subsequent BOLD increase in signal) may hinder modeling attempts if neural generators cannot be identified from the background noise.

Recapture Signal from Areas with Susceptibility Artifacts   A limitation in using fMRI activations to constrain source-localization modeling is that there are regions of the brain that standard fMRI sequences do not cover well. Specifically, there is very significant signal loss in areas where there is a rapid change in tissue density (such as between tissue and air). This "susceptibility artifact" means, in effect, that fMRI is likely to miss any potential ERP generators in those regions. The orbitofrontal regions (near the nasal sinus cavities) and basal temporal regions (near the ear canals) are especially problematic regions. However, recent advances in acquisition sequences have been shown to be able to recover signal in these areas (Song, 2001; Glover & Law, 2001). These sequences allow recovery of signals in inhomogeneous regions without sacrificing temporal resolution—a common shortcoming in the earlier methods. These new improved methods would be critical in imaging activation and modeling ERP sources in the ventral brain regions.

Perfusion Imaging   On a different front, parallel development in perfusion imaging methodology has led to its extended usage in fMRI. By employing an arterial spin labeling (ASL) scheme, perfusion weighted images can be made sensitive to the blood flow changes from upstream arterial networks to the capillaries. Because of the exchange mechanism in the capillaries and the diminishing sensitivity in large veins due to T1 recovery, the optimized perfusion contrast is believed to have better spatial localization ability (Luh et al., 2000; Yang et al., 2000; Detre & Wang, 2002) compared to the BOLD imaging methods. This finding was also confirmed in animal experiments, which demonstrated the existence of the orientation columns in cat visual cortex (Duong et al., 2001). However, perfusion imaging does have limitations, most notably the necessity for the wait time for the labeled upstream blood to arrive at the imaging plane, the often undetermined mean transit time, and the inevitable T1 recovery, all of which lead to low temporal resolution and limited spatial coverage.

Dynamic Water Diffusion Imaging   Recent results using refined diffusion weighting methodology also showed promises in achieving improved spatial localization. Improved from early diffusion weighted acquisitions, such methods were further adapted for fMRI research, leading to several recent studies (Song & Popp, 1998; Darquie et al., 2001; Gangstead & Song, 2002; Song et al., 2002) that detected the dynamic changes of the apparent diffusion coefficient (ADC: a quantity that defines the diffusion mobility of the proton pools). Dynamic use of the mild diffusion weighting strategies is sensitive to the intravoxel incoherent motion (IVIM) (Le Bihan et al., 1986; Le Bihan & Turner, 1992), and differs from early studies that simply employed static weighting strategies to eliminate proton pools of large mobility. Indeed, it is not sensitive to the aforementioned extravascular component of large vessels as parenchyma tissue near a large vessel does not change mobility over time. Our initial results demonstrated that ADC contrast holds strong promise for better spatial localization, because it has intrinsic sensitivity to the blood flow changes that originate upstream, diminishing downstream (Gangstead & Song, 2002; Song et al., 2002). By setting appropriate and mild diffusion weighting range for IVIM weighting, ADC contrast can be made uniquely sensitive to the capillary networks. Furthermore, dynamic ADC contrast is advantageous compared to the traditional BOLD methods in that (1) it does not require an ultra-high field, as it is detecting the blood mobility changes, (2) it has higher contrast-to-noise ratio (CNR) and lower power consumption compared to the spin-echo BOLD methods that are believed to be another alternative for capillary localization, and (3) it has higher CNR compared to the initial-dip BOLD signal.

Dynamic ADC contrast is also advantageous compared to another popular fMRI method using CBF contrast in that (1) it does not require the long transit and exchange time between tagging and image acquisition, thus affording much higher temporal throughput, and (2) it intrinsically has much larger spatial coverage. Darquie and Le Bihan (2001) recently presented a close relative of this type of ADC contrast, using much stronger diffusion weighting factors such that the vascular signals were mostly eliminated. Instead of the usual increase of ADC values during brain activation, they found a synchronized decrease of ADC, which could be caused by neuronal activation-induced cell swelling. Though its signal changes are not as robust as those detected using smaller diffusion weighting, and its mechanism is still under investigation, it has opened a new avenue for alternative contrast that may ultimately lead to better spatial localization.

Advantages and Limitations of Higher Magnetic Field Strength The use of higher magnetic fields (e.g., 3T and 4T scanners) affords the possibility to improve the functional resolution in investigations of human brain function. There are many theoretical benefits of higher field studies; two of the most pronounced are (1) increased baseline signal that can be used to increase the spatial resolution while still maintaining sufficient signal-to-noise ratio (SNR), and (2) increased proportion of the parenchymal participation in functional signal. The physics of the first advantage is well known because the static magnetization increases linearly with field strength. The increase of the static MR signal can be used to improve the spatial resolution by reducing partial volume effects—by reducing the spatial averaging effect of the idling brain tissue, the functional activity may become larger and easier to identify. The second improvement is less well known but generally accepted by the fMRI community. As the field strength goes up, the field gradient around the capillaries becomes larger and extends further into the parenchyma, thus increasing the participation of the brain tissue in functional signal while reducing the contribution from the large veins. As a result, the weighting of the near capillary signal becomes more significant and thus the functional signal is better co-localized with neuronal activities. However, researchers have not quantitatively determined how much better the functional signal is at high field, nor have they identified the most suitable methods for achieving the greatest improvements.

Although the signals of interest are increased with higher field scanners, challenges also arise in achieving homogeneous electromagnetic and magnetic fields necessary for imaging. For example, it is harder to achieve uniform excitation at high fields. Consequently, the anatomical images may suffer from signal nonuniformity and spatial distortions, which will make co-registration to ERP results difficult. This poses problems for combined studies at two stages: (1) spatial distortions will impair the ability to build correct head models, and (2) the data between the two sessions may not align properly. Refined coil designs are thus needed (Vaughan et al., 1994; Wen, Chesnick, & Balaban, 1994; Wong, Tan, & Hyde, 1993). Another common but very serious limitation to high-field fMRI is the pronounced susceptibility artifact that causes signal loss and geometric distortions in brain regions that may be of considerable interest to the neuroscientist. If fMRI is unable to pick up activation in a given region of the cortex that contributes to a scalp recorded potential, the integration of ERP and fMRI datasets will be hampered. Specially designed local phase compensation during the spin excitation can be used to minimize signal losses at the cost of temporal resolution (Yang et al., 2000; Stenger, Boada, & Noll, 1999; Cho & Ro, 1992; Glover & Lai, 1998; Mao & Song, 1999), or more recently, without sacrificing temporal resolution (Glover & Law, 2001; Song, 2001). In addition, reliable linear and high order magnetic field shimming (Wen, 1994; Spielman, Adalsteinsson, & Lim, 1998; Jesmanowicz & Hyde, 1997) and explicit knowledge of the magnetic field can minimize image distortions (Weisskoff & Davis, 1992; Jezzard & Balaban, 1995).

Measuring Brain Conductivities

Although realistic head models can provide more accurate source localization, most models still rely on the oversimplifying assumptions that brain and scalp can be modeled with standard conductivity estimates. Further improvements in source analysis can be achieved if the actual conductivities of individual subjects are known. However, most researchers do not typically measure these conductivities. A relatively straightforward but non-MR imaging tool for direct imaging of brain conductivity is electrical impedance tomography (EIT), which measures the brain impedance distribution through electrical conduction, based on a wide range of impedances across all brain tissue types. To measure the impedance, a minute current must flow through the scalp, skull, and brain tissues, and the resulting voltages be measured. In practice the current is injected from surface electrodes, much like those used in the ERP measurements. To better resolve spatial information, experimenters may use a grid of electrodes across the scalp to allow multiple measurements. EIT is relatively new, and its clinical utilities are still under evaluation. However, the equipment necessary to do this is not standard on most ERP recording set ups, and furthermore, the added risk (although slight) and time required may inhibit investigators from doing this. An exciting possibility, however, would be to obtain conductivity estimates using MRI techniques, while the subject is participating in that portion of the experiment. Although it remains unknown how well this may work, evidence suggests that it may in fact be possible (George et al., 2002).

Using Diffusion Weighted Imaging to Define Connectivity   Recent advances in diffusion tensor imaging (Xue et al., 1999; Basser et al., 2000; Poupon et al., 2000) could depict nerve fiber structures and track neural pathways in vivo among functional regions. Such a process is made possible by characterizing the preferred direction of water diffusion patterns in the human brain, based on the known fact that water molecules would diffuse with more ease along the myelinated nerve fiber instead of across the fiber. Upon validation, such a method can reveal conduction pathways of the neuronal communication and would likely see increased usage in the integrated use of ERP and fMRI.

Measuring Magnetic Neural Activity Directly with MRI   It would be beneficial to combine the advantages of the ERP recording and the fMRI technique—more specifically, to use MRI to image the neuronal electrical activity directly. This possibility motivated investigations in trying to image electrical activities similar to those in biological systems.

In particular, a study by Joy, Scott, and Henkelman (1989) used spin-echo phase imaging to assess the field perturbation of electrical currents in phantom and in vivo. This study suggested that the physiological current in the biological systems may potentially be detected by acquiring phase maps during stimulation. However, because these techniques do not take advantage of the strong magnetic field and the available high-power gradient systems of the MRI scanner, it may thus be intrinsically limited by the small magnitude of induced field inhomogeneity.

A new method was proposed that can detect minute electrical activity in a strong magnetic field. It uses displacement encoding to detect small spatial displacement induced by Lorentz force on the conducting materials; hence the term Lorentz effect imaging (LEI) (Song & Takahashi, 2001). With increased sensitivity from improved hardware capabilities or signal averaging, one may use this technique to detect spatial displacements induced by small currents comparable to neuronal electrical current. The initial results using the LEI technique demonstrated a spatial accuracy on the order of 10 μm, which may provide insight in assessing the feasibility of using MRI to non-invasively detect the neuronal electrical activities.

Bodurka and Bandettini (2002) recently proposed an alternative method based on selective detection of rapidly changing magnetic fields and suppression of slowly changing fields. The technique is sensitive to phase changes that reflect transient and subtle changes in magnetic field in cortical tissue associated with electrical currents consequent to neuronal activity. The method was tested on a phantom that contains wires in which current can be modulated. The sensitivity and flexibility of the technique was demonstrated by modulation of the temporal position and duration of the stimuli-evoked transient magnetic field relative to the 180 RF pulse in the imaging sequence-requiring precise stimulus timing. Currently, this method can detect magnetic field changes as small as 2×10^{-10} T (200 pT) and lasting for 40 ms.

To reliably detect neuronal and physiological currents may be more difficult in vivo. However, researchers using state of the art hardware and software have demonstrated the technical capability and feasibility of the approach. We may see initial use of such technology in humans in the near future, indicating a true integration of ERP principles into modern MRI.

Conclusion

Combining multiple methodologies promises to greatly enhance the ability to specify the neural dynamics underlying mental processes. Combining ERP with MRI-derived anatomical models of the head allows for a significant increase in the ability to localize where in the brain the scalp activity originates. Combining ERPs with PET or fMRI data promises even greater gains in building models of mental processes that include both the precise localization and precise timing of neural activity. As described in this chapter, there are multiple issues that one should consider before attempting to combine methodologies. There may not be a single best solution, but rather one should consider on a case-by-case basis the best strategy for combining methodologies. Although each methodology has its own strengths, effectively integrating ERPs with MRI, fMRI, and PET can significantly enhance the understanding of neural processes underlying mental functions in a way that is more than simply the sum of the separate parts.

References

Ary, J. P., Klein, S. A., & Fender, D. H. (1981). Location of sources of evoked scalp potentials: Corrections for skull and scalp thicknesses. *IEEE Transactions on Biomedical Engineering, 28*, 447–452.

Awada, K. A., Jackson, D. R., Williams, J. T., Wilton, D. R., Baumann, S. B., & Papanicolaou, A. C. (1997). Computational aspects of finite element modeling in EEG source localization. *IEEE Transactions on Biomedical Engineering, 44*, 736–752.

Awada, K. A., Jackson, D. R., Baumann, S. B., Williams, J. T., Wilton, D. R., Fink, P. W., & Prasky, B. R. (1998). Effect of conductivity uncertainties and modeling errors on EEG source localization using a 2-D model. *IEEE Transactions on Biomedical Engineering, 45*, 1135–1145.

Baker, J. R., Hoppel, B. E., Stern, C. E., Kwong, K. K., Weisskoff, R. M., & Rosen, B. R. (1993). Dynamic functional imaging of the complete human cortex using gradient-echo and asymmetric spin-echo echo-planar magnetic resonance imaging. *Proceedings of International Society of Magnetic Resonance in Medicine*, p. 1400.

Bandettini, P. A., Wong, E. C., Jesmanowicz, A., Hinks, R. S., & Hyde, J. S. (1994). Spin-echo and gradient-echo EPI of human brain activation using BOLD contrast: A comparative study at 1.5 T. *NMR in Biomedicine, 7*, 12–20.

Basser, P. J., Pajevic, S., Pierpaoli, C., Duda, J., & Aldroubi, A. (2000). In vivo fiber tractography using DT-MRI data. *Magnetic Resonance in Medicine, 44*, 625–632.

Bodurka, J., & Bandettini, P. A. (2002). Toward direct mapping of neuronal activity: MRI detection of ultraweak, transient magnetic field changes. *Magnetic Resonance in Medicine, 47*, 1052–1058.

Boxerman, J. L., Bandettini, P. A., Kwong, K. K., Baker, J. R., Davis, T. L., Rosen, B. R., & Weisskoff, R. M. (1995). The intravascular contribution to fMRI signal change: Monte Carlo modeling and diffusion weighted studies in vivo. *Magnetic Resonance in Medicine, 34*, 4–10.

Buxton, R. B. (2001). The elusive initial dip. *Neuroimage, 13*, 953–958.

Cho, Z. H., & Ro, Y. M. (1992). Reduction of susceptibility artifact in gradient-echo imaging. *Magnetic Resonance in Medicine, 23*, 193–196.

Cuffin, B. N. (1990). Effects of head shape on EEG's and MEG's. *IEEE Transactions on Biomedical Engineering, 37*, 44–52.

Dale, A. M., & Halgren, E. (2001). Spatiotemporal mapping of brain activity by integration of multiple imaging modalities. *Current Opinion in Neurobiology, 11*, 202–208.

Dale, A. M., Liu, A. K., Fischl, B. R., Buckner, R. L., Belliveau, J. W., Lewine, J. D., & Halgren, E. (2000). Dynamic statistical parametric mapping: Combining fMRI and MEG for high-resolution imaging of cortical activity. *Neuron, 26*, 55–67.

Dale, A. M., & Sereno, M. I. (1993). Improved localization of cortical activity by combining EEG and MEG with MRI cortical surface reconstruction: A linear approach. *Journal of Cognitive Neuroscience, 5*, 162–176.

Darquie, A., Poline, J. B., Poupon, C., Saint-Jalmes, H., & Le Bihan, D. (2001). Transient decrease in water diffusion observed in human occipital cortex during visual stimulation. *Proceedings of the National Academy of Sciences, USA, 98*, 9391–9395.

Detre, J. A., & Wang, J. (2002). Technical aspects and utility of fMRI using BOLD and ASL. *Clinical Neurophysiology, 113*, 621–634.

Duong, T. Q., Kim, D. S., Ugurbil, K., & Kim, S. G. (2001). Localized cerebral blood flow response at submillimeter columnar resolution. *Proceedings of the National Academy of Sciences, USA, 98*, 10904–10909.

Fischl, B., Sereno, M. I., Tootell, R. B. H., & Dale, A. M. (1999). High-resolution inter-subject averaging and a coordinate system for the cortical surface. *Human Brain Mapping, 8*, 272–284.

Fuchs, M., Drenckhahn, R., Wischmann, H., & Wagner, M. (1998). An improved boundary element method for realistic volume-conductor modeling. *IEEE Transactions on Biomedical Engineering, 45*, 980–997.

Gangstead, S. L., & Song, A. W. (2002). On the timing characteristics of the apparent diffusion coefficient contrast in fMRI. *Magnetic Resonance in Medicine, 48*, 385–388.

George, J. S., Schmidt, D. M., Rector, D. M., & Wood, C. (2002). Dynamic functional neuroimaging integrating multiple modalities. In P. Jezzard, P. M. Matthews, & S. M. Smith (Eds.), *Functional MRI: An introduction to methods* (pp. 353–382). Oxford: Oxford University Press.

Glover, G., & Lai, S. (1998). Reduction of susceptibility effects in BOLD fMRI using tailored RF pulses. *Proceedings of International Society of Magnetic Resonance in Medicine*, p. 298.

Glover, G. H., & Law, C. S. (2001). Spiral in and out. Spiral-in/out BOLD fMRI for increased SNR and reduced susceptibility artifacts. *Magnetic resonance in medicine, 46*, 515–522.

Hamalainen, M. S., & Sarvas, J. (1989). Realistic conductivity geometry model of the human head for interpretation of neuromagnetic data. *IEEE Transactions on Biomedical Engineering, 36*, 165–171.

Harter, M. R., & Aine, C. J. (1984). Brain mechanisms of visual selective attention. In R. Parasuraman & D. R. Davies (Eds.), *Varieties of attention* (pp. 293–321). London: Academic Press.

Heinze, H. J., Mangun, G. R., Burchert, W., Hinrichs, H., Sholz, M., Munte, T. F., Gos, A., Scherg, M., Johannes, S., Hundeshagen, H., Gazzaniga, M. S., & Hillyard, S. A. (1994). Combined spatial and temporal imaging of brain activity during selective attention in humans. *Nature, 372*, 543–546.

Hopfinger, J. B., Buonocore, M. H., & Mangun, G. R. (2000). The neural mechanisms of top-down attentional control. *Nature Neuroscience, 3*, 284–291.

Hopfinger, J. B., Jha, A. P., Hopf, J. M., Girelli, M., & Mangun, G. R. (2000). Electrophysiological and neuroimaging studies of voluntary and reflexive attention. In J. Driver & S. Monsell (Eds.), *Attention & performance XVIII: The control over cognitive processes* (pp. 125–153). Oxford: Oxford University Press.

Hopfinger, J. B., Woldorff, M. G., Fletcher, E. M., & Mangun, G. R. (2001). Dissociating top-down attentional control from selective perception and action. *Neuropsychologia, 39*, 1277–1291.

Hu, X., Le, T. H., & Ugurbil, K. (1997). Evaluation of the early response in fMRI in individual subjects using short stimulus duration. *Magnetic Resonance in Medicine, 37*, 877–884.

Huppertz, H.-J., Otte, M., Kristeva-Feige, R., Grimm, C., Mergner, T., & Lücking, C. H. (1998). Estimation of the accuracy of automatic surface matching technique for registration of EEG and MRI data. *Electroencephalography and Clinical Neurophysiology, 106*, 409–415.

Jesmanowicz, A., & Hyde, J. S. (1997). Single-pass automatic 3D shimming. *Proceedings of International Society of Magnetic Resonance in Medicine*, p. 1983.

Jezzard, P., & Balaban, R. S. (1995). Correction for geometric distortions in echo-planar images from Bo field variations. *Magnetic Resonance in Medicine, 34*, 65–73.

Joy, M., Scott, G., & Henkelman, M. (1989). In vivo detection of applied electric currents by magnetic resonance imaging. *Magnetic Resonance Imaging, 7*, 89–94.

Kim, D. S., Duong, T. Q., & Kim, S. G. (2000). High-resolution mapping of iso-orientation columns by fMRI. *Nature Neuroscience, 3*, 164–169.

Lai, S., Hopkins, A. L., Haacke, E. M., Li, D., Wasserman, B. A., Buckley, P., Friedman, L., Meltzer, H., Hedera, P., & Friedland, R. (1993). Identification of vascular structures as a major source of signal contrast in high resolution 2D and 3D functional activation imaging of the motor cortex at 1.5 T: Preliminary results. *Magnetic Resonance in Medicine*, 387–392.

Lavie, N., & Tsal, Y. (1994). Perceptual load as a major determinant of the locus of selection in visual attention. *Perception & Psychophysics, 56*, 183–197.

Le, J., & Gevins, A. (1993). Method to reduce blur distortion from EEG's using a realistic head model. *IEEE Transactions on Biomedical Engineering, 40*, 517–528.

Le Bihan, D., Breton, E., Lallemand, D., Grenier, P., Cabanis, E., & Laval-Jeantet, M. (1986). MR imaging of intravoxel incoherent motions: Application to diffusion and perfusion in neurologic disorders. *Radiology, 161*, 401–407.

Le Bihan, D., & Turner, R. (1992). The capillary network: A link between IVIM and classical perfusion. *Magnetic Resonance in Medicine, 27*, 171–178.

Lemieux, L., Salek-Haddadi, A., Josephs, O., Allen, P., Toms, N., Scott, C., Krakow, K., Turner, R., & Fish, D. R. (2001). Event-related fMRI with simultaneous and continuous EEG: Description of the method and initial case report. *NeuroImage, 14*, 780–787.

Lindauer, U., Royl, G., Leithner, C., Kuhl, M., Gold, L., Gethmann, J., Kohl-Bareis, M., Villringer, A., & Dirnagl, U. (2001). No evidence for early decrease in blood oxygenation in rat whisker cortex in response to functional activation. *NeuroImage, 13*, 988–1001.

Logothetis, N. K., Guggenberger, H., Peled, S., & Pauls, J. (1999). Functional imaging of the monkey brain. *Nature Neuroscience, 2*, 555–562.

Luh, W. M., Wong, E. C., Bandettini, P. A., Ward, B. D., & Hyde, J. S. (2000). Comparison of simultaneously measured perfusion and BOLD signal increases during brain activation with T1-based tissue identification. *Magnetic Resonance in Medicine, 44*, 137–143.

Maintz, J. B. A., & Viergever, M. A. (1998). A survey of medical image registration. *Medical Image Analysis, 2*, 1–36.

Malonek, D., & Grinvald, A. (1996). Interactions between electrical activity and cortical microcirculation revealed by imaging spectroscopy: Implications for functional brain mapping. *Science, 272*, 551–554.

Malonek, D., & Grinvald, A. (1997). Vascular regulation at sub millimeter range. Sources of intrinsic signals for high resolution optical imaging. *Advances in Experimental Medical Biology, 413,* 215–220.

Mangun, G. R., Hopfinger, J. B., & Heinze, H.-J. (1998). Integrating electrophysiology and neuroimaging in the study of human cognition. *Behavior Research Methods, Instruments, & Computers, 30,* 118–130.

Mangun, G. R., Hopfinger, J. B., Kussmaul, C. L., Fletcher, E. M., & Heinze, H.-J. (1997). Covariations in ERP and PET measures of spatial selective attention in human extrastriate visual cortex. *Human Brain Mapping, 5,* 273–279.

Mangun, G. R., Hopfinger, J. B., & Jha, A. P. (2000). Integrating electrophysiology and neuroimaging in the study of human brain function. In P. Williamson, A. M. Siegel, D. W. Roberts, V. M. Thandi, & M. S. Gazzaniga (Eds.), *Neocortical epilepsies* (pp. 35–49). Philadelphia: Lippincott, Williams, & Wilkins.

Mao, J., & Song, A. W. (1999). Intravoxel rephasing of spins dephased by susceptibility effect for EPI sequences. *Proceedings of International Society of Magnetic Resonance in Medicine,* p. 1982.

Marota, J. J., Ayata, C., Moskowitz, M. A., Weisskoff, R. M., Rosen, B. R., & Mandeville, J. B. (1999). Investigation of the early response to rat forepaw stimulation. *Magnetic Resonance in Medicine, 41,* 247–252.

Martinez, A., Anllo-Vento, L., Sereno, M. I., Frank, L. R., Buxton, R. B., Dubowitz, D. J., Wong, E. C., Heinze, H. J., & Hillyard, S. A. (1999). Involvement of striate and extrastriate visual cortical areas in spatial selective attention. *Nature Neuroscience, 2,* 364–369.

Mayhew, J., Johnston, D., Martindale, J., Jones, M., Berwick, J., & Zheng, Y. (2001). Increased oxygen consumption following activation of brain: Theoretical footnotes using spectroscopic data from barrel cortex. *NeuroImage, 13,* 975–987.

Meijs, J. W. H., Weier, O. W., Peters, M. J., & Van Oosterom, A. (1989). On the numerical accuracy of the boundary element method. *IEEE Transactions on Biomedical Engineering, 36,* 1038–1049.

Menninghaus, E., Lutkenhoner, B., & Gonzalez, S. L. (1994). Localization of a dipolar source in a skull phantom: Realistic versus spherical head model. *IEEE Transactions on Biomedical Engineering, 41,* 986–989.

Motter, B. C. (1993). Focal attention produces spatially selective processing in visual cortical areas V1, V2, and V4 in the presence of competing stimuli. *Journal of Neurophysiology, 70,* 909–919.

Nunez, P. L. (1981). *Electrical fields of the brain: The neurophysics of EEG.* New York: Oxford University Press.

Ogawa, S., Lee, T. M., Kay, A. R., & Tank, D. W. (1990). Brain magnetic resonance imaging with contrast dependent on blood oxygenation. *Proceedings of the National Academy of Sciences USA, 87,* 9868–9872.

Pascual-Marqui, R. D., Esslen, M., Kochi, K., & Lehmann, D. (2002). Functional imaging with low resolution brain electromagnetic tomography (LORETA): A review. *Methods & Findings in Experimental & Clinical Pharmacology, 24*, 91–95.

Pascual-Marqui, R. D., Michel, C. M., & Lehmann, D. (1994). Low resolution electromagnetic tomography: A new method for localizing electrical activity in the brain. *International Journal of Psychophysiology, 18*, 49–65.

Pelizzari, C. A., Chen, G. T. Y., Spelbring, D. R., Weichselbaum, R. R., & Chen, C. T. (1989). Accurate three-dimensional registration of CT, PET, and/or MR images of the brain. *Journal of Computer Assisted Tomography, 13*, 20–26.

Popp, C. A., Song, A. W., Wong, E. C., & Hyde, J. S. (1998). T1 selective functional MRI with diffusion weighting. *NMR in Biomedicine, 11*, 405–413.

Poupon, C., Clark, C. A., Frouin, V., Regis, J., Bloch, I., Le Bihan, D., & Mangin, J. (2000). Regularization of diffusion-based direction maps for the tracking of brain white matter fascicles. *NeuroImage, 12*, 184–195.

Roth, B. J., Balish, M., Gorbach, A., & Sato, S. (1993). How well does the three-spheres model predict dipoles in a realistically-shaped head? *Electroencephalography and Clinical Neurophysiology, 87*, 175–184.

Silva, A. C., Lee, S. P., Iadecola, C., & Kim, S. G. (2000). Early temporal characteristics of cerebral blood flow and deoxyhemoglobin changes during somatosensory stimulation. *Journal of Cerebral Blood Flow and Metabolism, 20*, 201–206.

Song, A. W. (2001). Single-shot EPI with signal recovery from susceptibility-induced losses. *Magnetic Resonance in Medicine, 46*, 407–411.

Song, A. W., & Popp, C. A. (1998). fMRI using ADC contrast. *Proceedings of International Society of Magnetic Resonance in Medicine, 6*, 1438.

Song, A. W., Wong, E. C., Jesmanowicz, A., Tan, S. G., & Hyde, J. S. (1995). Diffusion weighted FMRI at 1.5 T and 3 T. *Proceedings of International Society of Magnetic Resonance in Medicine*, p. 457.

Song, A. W., Wong, E. C., Tan, S. G., & Hyde, J. S. (1996). Diffusion weighted fMRI at 1.5 T. *Magnetic Resonance in Medicine, 35*, 155–158.

Song, A. W., & Takahashi, A. M. (2001). Lorentz effect imaging. *Magnetic Resonance Imaging, 19*, 763–767.

Song, A. W., Woldorff, M., Gangstead, S. L., Mangun, G. R., & McCarthy, G. (2002). Enhanced spatial localization of neuronal activation using simultaneous apparent-diffusion-coefficient and blood-oxygenation functional MRI. *NeuroImage, 17*, 742–750.

Spielman, D. M., Adalsteinsson, E., & Lim, K. O. (1998). Quantitative assessment of improved homogeneity using higher-order shims for spectroscopic imaging of the brain. *Magnetic Resonance in Medicine, 40*, 376–382.

Stenger, V. A., Boada, F. E., & Noll, D. C. (1999). Gradient compensation method for the reduction of susceptibility artifacts for spiral fMRI data acquisition. *Proceedings of International Society of Resonance in Medicine*, p. 538.

Tootell, R. B., Hadjikhani, N., Hall, E. K., Marrett, S., Vanduffel, W., Vaughan, J. T., & Dale, A. M. (1998). The retinotopy of visual spatial attention. *Neuron, 21*, 1409–1422.

Van Voorhis, S., & Hillyard, S. A. (1977). Visual evoked potentials and selective attention to points in space. *Perception & Psychophysics, 22*, 54–62.

Vanzetta, I., & Grinvald, A. (1999). Increased cortical oxidative metabolism due to sensory stimulation: Implications for functional brain imaging. *Science, 286*, 1555–1558.

Vaughan, J. T., Hetherington, H. P., Oto, J. O., Pan, J. W., & Pohost, G. M. (1994). High frequency volume coils for clinical NMR imaging and spectroscopy. *Magnetic Resonance in Medicine, 32*, 206–218.

Weisskoff, R. W., & Davis, T. L. (1992). Correcting gross distortions on echo-planar images. *Proceeds of International Society of Magnetic Resonance in Medicine*, p. 4515.

Wen, H. (1994). *High field magnetic resonance imaging.* Unpublished PhD thesis, University of Maryland.

Wen, H., Chesnick, A. S., & Balaban, R. S. (1994). The design and test of a new volume coil for high field imaging. *Magnetic Resonance in Medicine, 32*, 492–498.

Willemsen, S., Fuchs, M., Wagner, M., & Wischmann, H. A., & Theissen, A. (1998). Automatic registration of MR-images with digitized head contours. *Brain Topography, 11*, 78.

Woldorff, M. G., Fichtenholtz, H. M., Song, A. W., & Mangun, G. R. (2001). Separation of cue and target related processing in a fast rate compound-event visual attention cueing paradigm. *Cognitive Neuroscience Society Meeting Abstracts.*

Woldorff, M. G., Liotti, M., Seabolt, M., Busse, L., Lancaster, J. L., & Fox, P. T. (2002). The temporal dynamics of the effects in occipital cortex of visual-spatial selective attention. *Cognitive Brain Research, 15*, 1–15.

Wong, E. C., Tan, G., & Hyde, J. S. (1993). A quadrature transmit-receive encapped birdcage coil for imaging of human head at 125 MHz. *Proceeds of International Society of Magnetic Resonance in Medicine*, p. 1344.

Xue, R., van Zijl, P. C., Crain, B. J., Solaiyappan, M., & Mori, S. (1999). In vivo three-dimensional reconstruction of rat brain axonal projections by diffusion tensor imaging. *Magnetic Resonance in Medicine, 42*, 1123–1127.

Yang, Q. X., Dardzinski, B. J., Li, S., Eslinger, P. J., & Smith, M. B. (1997). Multi-gradient echo with susceptibility compensation (MGESIC): Demonstration of fMRI in the olfactory cortex at 3T. *Magnetic Resonance in Medicine, 37*, 331–335.

Yang, Y., Engelien, W., Pan, H., Su, S., Silbersweig, D. A., & Stern, E. (2000). A CBF-based event-related brain activation paradigm: Characterization of impulse-response function and comparison to BOLD. *NeuroImage, 12*, 287–297.

Yvert, B., Bertrand, O., Thévenet, M., Echallier, J., & Pernier, J. (1997). A systematic evaluation of the spherical model accuracy in EEG dipole localization. *Electroencephalography and Clinical Neurophysiology, 102*, 452–459.

Contributors

Mitchel S. Berger
Department of Neurological Surgery
University of California, San Francisco
San Francisco, California

Niko A. Busch
Max Planck Institute of Cognitive
Neuroscience
Leipzig, Germany, and
Department of Biological Psychology
Otto von Guericke University
Magdeburg, Germany

Tracy DeBoer
Institute of Child Development and
Center for Neurobehavioral Development
University of Minnesota
Minneapolis, Minnesota

Joseph Dien
Department of Psychology
Tulane University
New Orleans, Louisiana

J. Christopher Edgar
Department of Psychology
University of Illinois
Champaign, Illinois

Erik Edwards
Department of Psychology and Helen
Wills Neuroscience Institute
University of California, Berkeley
Berkeley, California

Gwen A. Frishkoff
Department of Psychology
University of Oregon
Portland, Oregon

Maren Grigutsch
Max Planck Institute of Cognitive
Neuroscience
Leipzig, Germany

Todd C. Handy
Department of Psychology
University of British Columbia
Vancouver, BC, Canada

Christoph S. Herrmann
Max Planck Institute of Cognitive
Neuroscience
Leipzig, Germany, and
Department of Biological Psychology
Otto von Guericke University
Magdeburg, Germany

Joseph B. Hopfinger
Department of Psychology
University of North Carolina at Chapel
Hill
Chapel Hill, North Carolina

Wayne Khoe
Department of Neurosciences
University of California, San Diego
La Jolla, California

Robert T. Knight
Department of Psychology and Helen
Wills Neuroscience Institute
University of California, Berkeley
Berkeley, California

Steven J. Luck
Department of Psychology
University of Iowa
Iowa City, Iowa

Gregory A. Miller
Director, Biomedical Imaging Center
University of Illinois
Urbana, Illinois

Charles A. Nelson
Institute of Child Development, Center
for Neurobehavioral Development, and
Department of Pediatrics
University of Minnesota
Minneapolis, Minnesota

Leun J. Otten
Institute of Cognitive Neuroscience and
Department of Psychology
University College, London
London, United Kingdom

Michael D. Rugg
Center for the Neurobiology of Learning
and Memory
University of California, Irvine
Irvine, California

Alecia M. Santuzzi
Department of Psychology
Tulane University
New Orleans, Louisiana

Lisa S. Scott
Institute of Child Development and
Center for Neurobehavioral Development
University of Minnesota
Minneapolis, Minnesota

Scott D. Slotnick
Department of Psychology
Harvard University
Cambridge, Massachusetts

Maryam Soltani
Department of Psychology and Helen
Wills Neuroscience Institute
University of California, Berkeley
Berkeley, California

Allen Song
Departments of Radiology and
Biomedical Engineering
Duke University
Durham, North Carolina

Kevin M. Spencer
Psychiatry Department
Harvard Medical School/VA Boston
Healthcare System
Brockton, Massachusetts

Ramesh Srinivasan
Department of Cognitive Science
University of California, Irvine
Irvine, California

Jennifer L. Stewart
Department of Psychology
University of Illinois
Champaign, Illinois

Diane Swick
Department of Neurology
VA Northern California Health Care
System and University of California,
Davis
Davis, California

Durk Talsma
Center for Cognitive Neuroscience
Duke University
Durham, North Carolina

Marty G. Woldorff
Center for Cognitive Neuroscience
Duke University
Durham, North Carolina

Index